Nutrition and Diet Therapy

Dr. Sheel Sharma
Professor and Head
Department of Food Science and Nutrition
Banasthali University
P. O. Banasthali Vidyapith - 304022
Rajasthan

PEEPEE
PUBLISHERS AND DISTRIBUTORS (P) LTD.

Nutrition and Diet Therapy

Published by
Pawaninder P. Vij and Anupam Vij

Peepee Publishers and Distributors (P) Ltd.
Head Office: 160, Shakti Vihar, Pitam Pura
Delhi-110034 (India)

Correspondence Address: 7/31, First Floor, Ansari Road
Daryaganj, New Delhi-110002 (India)
Ph: 65195868, 23246245, 9811156083
e-mail: peepee160@yahoo.co.in
e-mail: peepee160@rediffmail.com
e-mail: peepee160@gmail.com
www.peepeepub.com

First Edition: **2014**

ISBN : 978-81-8445-145-0

Dedicated to the fond memory of my endearing father, Dr Shami Sharma,

a poet, littérateur, Vedic scholar and, above all,

a relentless worker with an indomitable spirit.

May the tribe of such people coming on this earth

increase by leaps and bounds

to make it a happier and habitable place.

FOREWORD

Professor Sheel Sharma is one such teacher of Biochemistry and Human Nutrition who ploughs back into academics what he learns from his experiences as a teacher and researcher and **Nutrition and Diet Therapy**, the book in the offing, is his another such attempt. Though the work appears to be an illustrious instance of Prof Sheel Sharma's resourcefulness, the real test of its true acclaim would lie in the receptivity and usage of his work by the academic fraternity; teachers and the students. Proof of the pudding, as some one has said wisely, always lies in the eating.

I am confident that the book would prove its worth among its prospective readers by becoming a treasure trove of information related to normal and therapeutic nutrition. I shall also hail Prof Sharma adding more titles to his name in future with each having a definite focus and philosophy. I cannot imagine a better way of beginning the academic session 2013-14 than reaffirming one's credentials as an author of substance. Kudos to Prof Sharma for never being on a sticky wicket as far as academics are concerned.

Dr. Gul Mathur
Professor, Foods and Nutrition
Dayalbagh Educational Institute
Dayalbagh, Agra

PREFACE

Pancake with cooked lentil (*dal roti* in Indian parlance, undoubtedly with an adequate admix of vegetables, fruits, milk and water) is what becomes instrumental in binding the body and breaths together to make human machine run efficiently day after day. Evidently, this every day fuelling or the process of supplying the living body with the substances needed for healthy physiological functioning is called Nutrition. Nutrition as a science, on the other hand, is–*a growing body of systematically arranged facts about the consumption and utilization of food by the people*. Being well past its infancy, in the ever changing childhood–adolescent period, this science is truly on the throes of 'coming of age'. The pace at which new information is emerging in Nutrition and calling for the reinterpretation of the older facts, and the rapidity with which new areas of application of this science are gaining ground, all point towards this being a truly dynamic science.

As a matter of fact, the nascent **'Nutrition and Diet Therapy'** seeks to make readers comprehend *Nutrition* as a process in the light of systematically arranged facts of *Nutrition* as a science. The very facts have been arranged into laws and principles over the years, collected and supported by research studies and controlled testing procedures called the 'Scientific Method'.

Of plan of the book, in keeping with its name, it has been divided into two parts, viz. **Nutrition and Diet Therapy**. The first part presents a brief overview of Nutrition along with the physiological, biochemical and regulatory mechanisms that operate in the internal environment or *milieu anterior* of human organism to maintain its consistency or *homeostasis* and the role of **Nutrition** in everyday life for various life stages and situations. The applied aspects such as 'Food toxicity perishability and preservation as well as 'Formulation of diets and planning of meals' have also been dealt with in this part. The second part or the **Diet Therapy** emphasizes the basics that come handy in the care of patients that suffer from diseases caused by nutritional impairments as well as of those suffering from *diseases that cause nutritional impairments*.

To ingrain impressions on the reader's mind in a subtle, nonchalant manner; certain learning aids, such as diagrams, figures and tables have also been added, interspersed with the text. Further, each chapter opens with a layout of the topic to aid both, systematic study and sporadic skimming, and closes with study questions, to help ready appraisal.

In a nutshell, the book endeavours to touch upon the important contours of this multifaceted science at the fundamental level to provide an understanding of the basic facts and principles of the science of *Nutrition* so as to make users broadly plan diets for individuals as well as communities, both in conditions of normal and ill health, and to explain how these facts and principles can be integrated with the physiologic and socio-economic factors and traditional practices in the selection and planning of meals.

It is my fond hope that **Nutrition and Diet Therapy** would do both, whet and satiate the cerebral appetite of a wide cross-section of readership in Nutrition making them move towards understanding the transformation of the molecules of food into the kind of molecules that make the body. May we all within the ambit of science of Nutrition contribute our humble pie to make people add not only years to the life but also life to the years. Om Sai Ram!

Prof Sheel Sharma
Professor and Head
Dept of Food Science and Nutrition
Banasthali University
P. O. Banasthali Vidyapith - 304022

ACKNOWLEDGEMENTS

Banasthali University, the institution where I work, a fountainhead of women education in the country, with its idyllic surroundings and sylvan serenity, created congenial conditions, conducive to the preparation of this manuscript, meriting a special first mention here. Likewise, the academic excellence and administrative acumen of Prof Aditya Shastri, Vice Chancellor, Banasthali University, cannot go without appreciative mentioning for being a source of academic exhortation.

I shall be amiss if I don't underscore the help and enthusiasm of my research group and family members in the pursuit of preparation of this manuscript. Quick acting quadruple of Ruchi, Nidhi, Archana and Preeti, the diligent doctorate pursuers, came forward in a big way with their contribution in manuscript preparation meriting a special mention here. *Nidhi Agarwal, a delineation of diligence that she is, came up with some sporadic formating, typing and proof reading, qualifying for a second time mention here.* Other colleagues who also double up as members of my research group—Ms Geeta Bisla, Dr Neelam Chaturvedi, Dr Ekta Singh and Ms Shubhra Saraswat have also been providing inputs from time to time.

My inane enthusiasm in putting more efforts and time on the manuscript to make it better reading was deftly thwarted by my wife Amita by handing me a quote from ***William Osler proclaiming—in seeking absolute truth, we aim at unattainable, and must be content with broken portions*** making me beat instant and hasty retreat towards publisher's den. Incidently, Amita teaches English literature which she never fails to try on her unsuspecting half for making her domination. Son Sharv and daughter Ashesha, though appreciative of my 'at desk dexterity', place a higher, premium on their mother's 'management skills'. Obviously, instant wit always impacts a fathom deeper or, at times, even rides roughshod over cool, slow spinning, intellect.

Professor Gul Mathur, an erudite university teacher of long standing in Foods and Nutrition has been considerate enough to go through the manuscript, give purposeful suggestions and write the Foreword. I really can't thank her enough for her mentorship and magnanimity. Prof Rajeshwar Sharma, my esteemed teacher, has been a guiding deity, always and ever and thus can never go without acknowledgement and expression of indebtedness.

I am grateful to the Peepee Publishers and Distributors (P) Ltd., Daryaganj, Delhi for their unfailing courtesy and undiluted patience, through out the writing and publishing of this book. The fact that the book has come into print in a remarkable short time, speaks highly about their commitment.

While making a reverential bow to the memory of *dada*, venerable late Prof Diwakar Shastri, former president and moving spirit behind Banasthali University, I cannot but remember the motivation provided by him for all the twenty-five years of my being as a member of *Banasthali Parivar*. The act, with all its material and sublime connotations, can only be felt and recapitulated and not described in words.

Prof Sheel Sharma
Professor and Head
Dept of Food Science and Nutrition
Banasthali University
P. O. Banasthali Vidyapith - 304022

CONTENTS

Nutrition

Diet Therapy

CHAPTER 1

Human Nutrition and Diet Therapy: An Overview

Chapter Outlines

- Eat to live dictum
- Food as fuel for human body
- Nutrition as a science
- Foods and nutrition in the social context
- Proximate principles of food analysis
- Applying facts of nutrition to nourishment and health
- Study questions

EAT TO LIVE DICTUM

An urge to eat almost anything one manages to get into one's mouth is the instinctive reaction to hunger as it is present at birth. It is only later experience of life that makes one distinguish food from inedible material. That is why in ancient times, even before the dawn of civilization, human beings believed in 'live to eat' or 'eat to live' notions, because probably, these were the first and fundamental lessons they could learn from the experience of existence and survival. It was Socrates, the great Greek philosopher of olden times, who put the matter in correct perspective by stating, "Other people live to eat while I eat to live". Obviously, he wanted every human being to eat only to live. As time passed, with the advent of civilization, more facts about food and eating came to the limelight. The man also acquired discretion and realized that one of the important determinants of quality life is the nature and content of food that he eats. Maharshi Charaka, the sage and physician of ancient times, emphatically observed—"The body is the outcome of food; the distinction between ease and disease arising, totally or partially, due to faulty food or diet"—thus laying down the bedrock of foods, nutrition and health relationship.

The term 'Food' is conventionally used while referring to the materials of solid or liquid nature which, when ingested, serve one or more functions of growth, maintenance and energy provision. Consuming foods appropriate in both content and kind promotes nutrition and health.

Nutrients are the components of food and drink that provide for growth, replacement and energy needs of the body. Not all components of food can qualify for this distinction, some of them, such as those providing flavour, colour or aroma; undoubtedly enhance our pleasure of eating food, yet they are not branded as nutrients. A nutrient, therefore, can be defined as the chemical substance or active principle present in food which acts as the nourishing material to ensure proper reproduction, growth and maintenance. Chemically, nutrients are the different classes of molecules, atoms or ions that are indispensable to the functioning of body. Components of food that do not serve any nourishing function are called non-nutrients. For example, the compound that gives garlic its pungent flavour, the pigments that give tomato its dark red colour. There are a large number of such compounds present in various types of foodstuffs. Many of them act as health promoters and others prove toxic. For instance, lycopene present in tomato is a beneficial substance but a goitrogen present in cabbage is harmful, though these substances are present in the foodstuffs in very small amounts.

Hence food is a complex mixture of nutrients and non-nutrients. Nutrients present in food have been classified into six groups—carbohydrate, protein, fat, water, vitamins and minerals. Whereas carbohydrate and fat primarily act as energy sources, proteins perform body building and maintenance functions. Together, these three are termed as macronutrients as they quantitatively comprise the bulk of our diet. Vitamins and minerals are present in the diet in much smaller amounts and thus they are called micronutrients. They are needed for the utilization of macronutrients as well as for some other essential functions of the body. Water is the solvent vehicle required for the processing and utilization of nutrients and thus acts not less than a nutrient. Human body is made up of nutrient materials arranged in different ways.

Apart from nourishment, people also turn to food for comfort and pleasure; even for seeking cure for some ailments. Thus food means many things to people, and many cultural and social traditions have been attached to the preparing, serving, eating and sharing of food. Due to the interplay of these factors, some people can be omnivores—who eat foods of all kinds; of both plant and animal origin including animal flesh, or they can be vegetarians—who exclude from their diet animal flesh and possibly eggs, milk and cheese. Vegetarians can be of three types:

i. *Lactovegetarians*: Vegetarians who use milk and milk products in their diets.

ii. *Lacto-ovo-vegetarians*: Vegetarians who use milk, milk products and also eggs in their diets.

iii. *Vegans*: Vegetarians who include no animal derived products, not even milk, cheese and other milk products.

In general, the daily food choices of people are based on the following factors:

i. *Personal preference*: People like to eat those foodstuffs the most which they like.

ii. *Habit*: Familiar foods are eaten more than those that are less familiar.

iii. *Tradition, values and beliefs*: Foodstuffs of our ethnic group and those compatible with our cultural traditions and religious beliefs are preferred the most.

iv. *Availability, convenience and economy*: Foods that are there to readily choose from, easy to prepare and within our means are eaten more than others.

v. *Social pressure:* Foods that are offered the most are eaten more frequently.

vi. *Positive associations:* Foods eaten by people we admire, or the ones that imply status are eaten preferentially.

vii. *Emotional needs:* Foods that we think can make us feel better, become our choicest ones.

viii. *Nutritive value:* As aware individuals, we tend to place preference on nourishing and health promoting foods.

FOOD AS FUEL FOR HUMAN BODY

To live, human body needs food as fuel for supplying energy for moving and doing work. The energy that fuels the body for doing work comes indirectly from the sun via plants. Plants trap and store energy of the sun in their tissues as they grow. Thus by eating plant based foodstuffs, such as—grains, vegetables and fruits—we obtain and utilize the energy of the sun, stored in various structural forms of foods by the plants. When animals eat plant based foodstuffs, they also obtain and utilize solar energy in the way similar to that in humans. When we eat animal based foodstuffs, such as—milk and meat—we obtain and utilize energy originally coming from the sun. As a matter of fact, energy from the sun is first stored in the plants that are consumed by animals and the same energy stored in plants is passed on to the animal tissues which eventually gets transferred to human beings through the consumption of milk and meat.

NUTRITION AS A SCIENCE

The study of how food nourishes the body is nutrition. It is a field of knowledge that consists of facts which scientists have obtained by systematically observing what people eat and noting how healthy they are. These facts have also been obtained and validated by experimentation to see the effects of various foods and diets on human health.

Because science is a step by step information gathering and testing process from finding after finding, the information thus collected is assembled to make the conceptual framework of a specific area of the scientific discipline of nutrition, such as—diet therapy or food analysis. To understand this, we take the analogy from the example of movie making. One single picture frame cannot make a movie. In fact, we need one picture frame moving after the other to make the characters of the movie move, dance and fight. Exactly in the same vein, we need a long trail of facts, one after the other, established through evidence, to create knowledge base and build up of a scientific discipline. Unlike other sciences, such as—physics and chemistry—nutrition is a young science as most of the facts have come up as a consequence of research conducted in the last century after 1900. However, this science of nutrition is an active growing and changing body of knowledge with new concepts and interpretations finding acceptance and recognition, some of them, at the expense of earlier ones. It is only when a research finding stands upto rigorous, repeated testing in several kinds of experiments performed and validated by different research groups, it is finally considered confirmed.

Frontiers of the science of nutrition, therefore, extend from food analysis, selection, preparation; to its digestion, absorption, assimilation, nutrient requirements of the body, their metabolic functions and health implications of under and over nourishment. Besides, nutrition also integrates itself with certain facets of health, biological, agriculture and social sciences and food processing, food technology and biotechnology. So it is but natural that this science incorporates those aspects of these disciplines which are relevant to its study (Table 1.1). Nutrition, therefore, has the distinction of transcending various scientific disciplines and hence is also termed as inter-disciplinary science in the true sense of the term.

Table 1.1: Relevance of 'Foods and Nutrition'

1. In food selection and preparation.
2. In understanding metabolic functions of nutrients.
3. In application of nutritional principles to health and disease.
4. In understanding sociological impact of nutrition in communities.
5. In assessing nutritional implications of food processing and food technology.
6. In integration of nutrition and agriculture.

FOODS AND NUTRITION IN THE SOCIAL CONTEXT

Indispensability of diet for sustaining life is a cardinal fact. Since the evolution of human race on mother earth and throughout its sailing on the high, often stormy, seas of life on the voyage of survival and development; food has been the focus of importance and attention. Communities or population groups in older times evolved their dietary preferences by the processes of 'trial and error' and 'natural selection'. However, the present era has witnessed a great change on earth involving degradation of environment, widening of social and economic gulfs, resulting in lopsidedness in food availability and ensuing nourishment levels between the rich and poor.

A marked effect of such rapidly changing values was that people became rebellious and less inclined in selecting foods on the basis of tradition and ethos. In turn, factors such as prosperity and availability of foods, dictated the food priorities and choices. Simultaneously, the biological and allied sciences, including foods and nutrition, have taken rapid strides in terms of rapid flow of information and knowledge, applications of which can enrich quality of human life on earth.

Of late, the science of foods and nutrition has been grappling with problems of finding the subtle relationships between different nutrient components of diet, health and disease. Simultaneously, it is also endeavouring hard to find scientific basis for food selection, cooking and preservation. With the coming of new information and expertise, efforts are being made to solve problems concerning food scarcity and undernutrition.

PROXIMATE PRINCIPLES OF FOOD ANALYSIS

Based upon the abundance of a certain type of nutrients in foods, they are grouped into energy rich (carbohydrate and fat rich), body building (protein rich) and protective (vitamin, mineral and protein rich) foods.

The total sum of different food combinations consumed over one single day by a person is referred to as his diet. A good diet supplies nutrients in requisite amounts, and comprise a variety of foods. 'Nutrition' as a scientific discipline dealing with foods and their nourishing abilities has come into being as a result of our realization that our well-being and quality of life are clearly influenced by the nature and amount of foods we eat. Though nutrition can be defined in an array of ways, the most exhaustive of these definitions interprets nutrition *as the science of foods, nutrients and other substances therein, their action, interaction and balance in relation to health and disease and the process by which the organism ingests, digests, absorbs, transports, utilizes and excretes food substances. In addition, nutrition also studies the social, economical, cultural and psychological implications of food and eating.*

Thus food gives the sustenance and we eat to keep our bodies effectively functioning getting the necessary inputs for growth and maintenance of tissue components of the body from the diet. However, nutrients present in foods have to undergo mechanical and biochemical processing, in order to render themselves available for the functioning of the body. Nutrition is the science which studies subtleties of these processes and interprets the relationship between intake of foods and functioning of human organism on a rational basis (Table 1.2).

APPLYING FACTS OF NUTRITION TO NOURISHMENT AND HEALTH

We eat food to satisfy hunger. We also enjoy tasty food and consider it to be an important part of social interaction

Table 1.2: Proximate principles of food analysis

Organic	Nitrogenous	Protein	Dispensable amino acids	Glutamic acid, aspartic acid alanine, serine, hydroxyproline
			Semidispensable amino acids	Arginine, glycine, histidine, cystine, tyrosine, proline
			Indispensable amino acids	Lysine, typtophan, phenylalanine, methionine, valine, threonine, leucine, isoleucine,
		Non-protein		Nucleic acids, amines, etc.
	Lipid	Neutral	Acylglyceroles	Triglycerides
			Steroles	Cholesterol, Vitamin D, etc.
			Terpenoids	Carotene, Vitamin A, xanthophylis, etc.
		Polar Phospholipids	Phosphoglycerides	Lecithins
			Sphingolipids	Sphingomyelins
	Nitrogen-free extract COH_2		Water-soluble vitamins	Thiamin, riboflavin, niacin, vitamin B_6 Pantothenic acid, biotin, folacin, vitamin B_{12}, ascorbic acid
			Monosaccharides	Simple pentose or hexose sugars
			Oligosaccharides	Compound sugars
			Polysaccharides ("soluble")	Starches
	Crude fiber		Polysaccharides ("insoluble")	Cellulose Hemicelluloses
Inorganic	Ash	Essential elements	Macro	Ca, Mg, Na, K, P, Cl, S
			Micro	Mn, Fe, Cu, I, Zn, Co, Mo, Se, Cr
		Potentially toxic elements		As, Cd, F, Pb, Hg, Si
		Non-essential elements		Al, Sb, Bi, B, Ge, Au, Pb, Hg, Rb, Ag.

and a means to satisfy our cultural, social, psychological and emotional patterns within the constraints of our setup or environment. We also need to eat right to lead healthy, happy and productive lives. Scientific evidence suggests that a lopsided or ill-balanced diet is a risk factor for the occurrence of major chronic diseases that become leading cause of adult death, namely—coronary heart disease, stroke, hypertension, diabetes mellitus and certain types of cancers. It has also been said that much of the consequences of present day living are 'afflictions of affluence' or 'diseases of prosperity' and understanding and application of nutrition can offer enormous scope in terms of preventive and remedial ways.

Nutritional principles can well be applied to therapeutic interventions for individuals down with illness. Diet therapy in the form of diets ranging from moderately modified in texture for being supportive and restorative to majorly altered to cure life threatening ailments by administration through external and parenteral routes, can make people combat, manage and overpower diseases.

This becomes possible by the combined efforts of nutritionists, food and biological scientists and physicians. An instance of the significance of diet therapy can be taken from the fact that despite tremendous technological and biomedical developments of the present era, the major means of survival and longevity for patients suffering from *inborn errors of metabolism* is prudently modified diet.

STUDY QUESTIONS

1. Explain the terms: Food, nutrient and diet.
2. Define 'Nutrition' and explain the relevance of 'Foods and Nutrition' as a scientific discipline.
3. Name various nutrients and explain their basic functions.
4. Write a critical note on 'Nutrition in the social context'.
5. Explain how does food act as a fuel for the body.

Nutrition

CHAPTER 2

Carbohydrates

Chapter Outlines

- Introduction
- Occurrence
- Classification
- Carbohydrates as sweeteners
- Carbohydrates as body nourishers
- Carbohydrate rich foods and glycemic response
- Role of dietary fiber as health promoter
- Artificial sweeteners or sugar substitutes
- Study questions

INTRODUCTION

In India, as we all know, diets are cereal based. Chapatti, rice or any other cereal food always find a place in the meal plan. Since carbohydrates are the major constituents of cereals, in India where diets are cereal based in general, around 65 to 75 percent of the total energy in the diet is contributed by carbohydrates.

Convenience in the cultivation of cereals, affordable prices and cultural acceptance make them the foodstuffs of choice.

OCCURRENCE

Carbohydrates are hydrates of carbon (CH_2O). The name was given by early researchers who found that heating carbohydrates (sugars) in dry test tubes resulted in the condensation of water droplets at the mouth of the tubes and a black residue (carbon) at the bottom. Subsequent chemical analyses conclusively proved the presence of carbon, hydrogen and oxygen in the ratio 1:2:1 in most of the carbohydrates. They are most abundant in plants contributing as much as 55 to 90 percent of their dry mass because plants synthesize carbohydrates from carbon dioxide and water in the presence of sunlight, the process being known as photosynthesis (Fig. 2.1). Being products

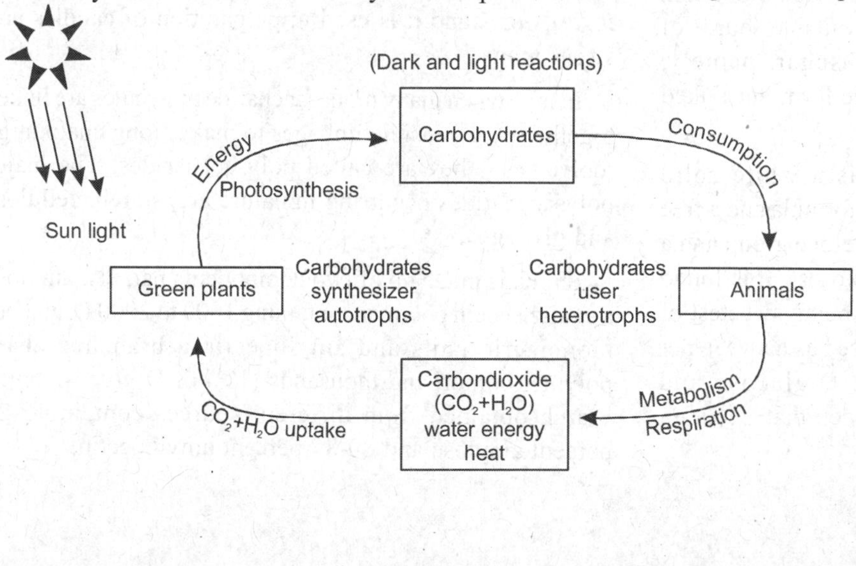

Fig. 2.1: Energy cycle in autotrophic and heterotrophic organisms

of photosynthesis, they are mostly present in plants as starch and cellulose. Animals (including human beings), on the other hand, have small token amount of carbohydrates, obviously because of their inherent inability to undertake carbohydrate synthesis. Chemically, carbohydrates are defined as aldehyde or ketone derivatives of the polyhydric (having more than one hydroxyl groups) alcohols, or as compounds that yield such derivatives on hydrolysis.

CLASSIFICATION

Carbohydrates have been classified into two, viz. simple and complex, groups. The former includes natural and refined sugars and the latter, starch, glycogen, cellulose, dextrins and dietary fiber.

Simple carbohydrates or sugars, chemically referred to as monosaccharides and disaccharides, being small molecules and water soluble, are rapidly absorbed by the digestive tract of the body. In nutritional parlance, they are known as single and double sugars respectively.

The members of the simple carbohydrates category have a single unit–monosaccharide (mono or one, saccharide or sugar containing). Glucose is an example of this class. The disaccharides contain two sugars linked together to form a chain. Cane or beet sugar (sucrose), milk sugar (lactose), and maltose (malt sugar) are members of this class. Complex carbohydrates, made up of long chains of sugars are called polysaccharide (poly-many). Among them are starch, dextrins, glycogen, cellulose, hemicellulose, pectins, plant gums and mucilages.

Glucose, the most common monosaccharide, is present in fruits, honey, and corn syrups. After absorption of food in the digestive tract, it is transported through blood and hence is present in blood as an easily available source of energy. Another single aldohexose sugar, namely, D-galactose, occurs in nature not in free form but linked to glucose in disaccharide—lactose.

Fructose, another single sugar, is a white solid ketohexose, having the same molecular formula and a free active keto group (sugar having a free ketone group and a chain of six carbons are called keto-hexoses). It is found in sweet fruits and honey. By virtue of being sweetest of all the natural sugars, it is commonly used as a sweetener in soft drinks and syrups. In fact, D-glucose and D-fructose are the two monosaccharides that occur in nature in free forms.

Lactose is the double sugar abundantly present in mammalian milk. It comprises D-galactose and D-glucose linked through glycosidic linkage. This sugar also has the distinction of being the disaccharide of animal origin. However, it is least sweet among all the commonly occurring sugars.

Lactose yields glucose and galactose on hydrolysis by the enzyme lactase present in the digestive tract. It is also less soluble than sucrose and maltose. Persons having lactase insufficiency cannot digest and metabolize lactose and hence have to refrain from taking milk and milk products. Children, who are born without the liver enzyme lactase, cannot digest milk and have to be fed soya milk instead.

Maltose is also a disaccharide that does not occur freely in nature to an appreciable extent. It is formed in sprouting seeds during the process of germination. During beer manufacturing, a large amount of maltose is formed in the 'malting' of barley.

Another disaccharide, sucrose occurs richly in nature. It contains glucose and fructose, again linked by glycosidic linkage. Commonly called cane sugar, table sugar or, simply sugar; sucrose is extracted from sugarcane or sugar beats and is mainly used to sweeten foods.

Sucrose is the common sugar of consumption and used in milk beverages and other food preparations as a sweetener. In the tropical areas, it is mainly manufactured from cane sugar and from sugar beets in the temperate regions. It is also present in honey, molasses, fruits and vegetables. Sucrose is hydrolysed to a blend of equal amounts of glucose and fructose by the action of digestive enzymes or by the acid present in foods at boiling temperatures. This mixture of glucose and fructose is called *invert sugar* and it is used in preparation of candies and sweet icings.

In fact, when many monosaccharide molecules are linked together by glycosidic linkages to make 'long chain large molecules', they are called polysaccharides. The major polysaccharides occurring in nature are, starch, cellulose and glycogen.

Starch is made up of two components namely, amylose a straight chain polymer containing 1000 to 2000 D-glucose monomeric units and amylopectin a branched chain polymer comprising thousands (10^5) of D-glucose units. Starch obtained from different sources contain 15-20 percent amylose and 80-85 percent amylopectin.

Starch occurs in plants as stored form of energy and is present in fruits, vegetables, cereals, pulses and legumes. It is the major carbohydrate present in our diet. It is mostly eaten in cooked form, in order to enhance its taste palatability and digestibility.

Just as starch is the storage polysaccharide in plants, a similar form present in animals is named 'glycogen'. It is also, therefore, known as 'animal starch'. Both, starch and glycogen are digestible polysaccharides.

Structurally, glycogen is a branched amylopectin type of polysaccharide. However, glycogen has more branching points in its structure as compared to amylopectin of starch. Energy stored in the form of glycogen, can be quickly utilized in times of 'flight or fight' situations, when a person is either scared to run away (flee) or ready to take on his opponents (fight).

Cellulose is the most abundantly occurring polysaccharide present in living tissues. It contributes almost half of the total organic carbon of the biosphere. It is a structural polysaccharide that imparts strength and toughness to the plant. Each cellulose molecule is formed by the joining together of 3000 D-glucose molecules through glycosidic linkages. However, these glycosidic linkages are different from those present in starch and glycogen. That precisely is the reason why cellulose cannot be digested by human gastrointestinal tract since the latter lacks the enzyme needed to hydrolyze glycosidic linkages of cellulose.

Hence cellulose is not used as a nutrient by human species. Ruminants (cow, buffalo, sheep, goat etc.), on the other hand, have a large four chambered stomach and the microorganisms present in the first chamber (rumen) produce enzymes that hydrolyze cellulose into glucose which is used as a nutrient by the cattle. Some other products derived from cellulose are cotton textile (cellulose), rayon (cellulose xanthate) and explosives (cellulose nitrate).

Cellulose and hemicelluloses, pectins, gums and mucilages are indigestible polysaccharides. Pectins are present in fruits and gums. Mucilages are part of plant exudates and seeds. A small proportion of cellulose and other indigestible carbohydrates, when present as one of the components of dietary fiber in diet proves beneficial for human health.

Dietary fiber is most simply defined as the residue of plant food resistant to hydrolysis by the enzymes of human gastrointestinal tract. Chemically, dietary fiber comprises cellulose, hemicellulose, pectin and gums, all carbohydrates; and a non-carbohydrate lignin. They all are present in plant foods. Though dietary fiber has little nutrient value, it promotes health by preventing constipation, hyperglycemia (high blood glucose levels—a symptom of diabetes mellitus), hyper-cholesterolemia (high blood cholesterol level—a possible causative factor in atherosclerosis and coronary heart disease), and above all, colon cancer (Table 2.1).

Table 2.1: Major types of fiber and their properties

Types of fiber	*Major source in diet*	*Chemical properties*	*Physiological effects*
Cellulose	Unrefined cereals	Non-digestible	↑ Stool bulk
	Bran	Water insoluble	↓ Intestinal transit time
	Whole wheat	Absorbs water	↓ Intracolonic pressure
Hemicellulose	Unrefined cereals	Partially digestible	↑ Stool bulk
	Bran	Usually water insoluble	↓ Intestinal transit time
	Whole wheat	Absorbs water	↓ Intracolonic pressure
Lignin	Vegetables	Non-digestible	↑ Stool bulk
		Water insoluble	Binds cholesterol
		Adsorbs organic substances	Binds carcinogens (Probably)
Pectin	Fruits	Digestible	↓ Rate of gastric emptying
		Water soluble	↓ Rate of sugar uptake
		Mucilaginous	↓ Serum cholesterol
Gums	Legumes	Digestible	↓ Rate of gastric emptying
		Water soluble	↓ Rate of sugar uptake
		Mucilaginous	↓ Serum cholesterol

In addition to these, another type of polysaccharides—mucopolysaccharides or acidic polysaccharides—having structural functions are present in human tissues. They do not make a part of our dietary carbohydrates but, nevertheless, are important as intercellular cementing materials and as blood group substances. Hyaluronic acid and chondroitin sulfates are prominent among them. Simple sugar mono-saccharides, glucose and galactose, act as the precursor substances for the repeating monomeric units (N-acetyl glucosamine, N-acetyl-galactosamine and N-acetyl glucuronic acid) of these polysaccharides.

CARBOHYDRATES AS SWEETENERS

In Table 2.2 there are relative sweetness values of the various sugars as well as artificial sweeteners.

Table 2.2: Relative sweetness of sugars and artificial sweeteners

S. No.	*Sugar/Artificial sweetener*	*Sweetness (Compared with sweetness of sucrose)*
1.	Sucrose (S)	100
2.	Lactose (S)	15
3.	Galactose (S)	30
4.	Maltose (S)	32
5.	Glucose (S)	73
6.	Invert sugar (S) (1:1 mixture of glucose and fructose)	124
7.	Fructose (S)	172
8.	Sodium cyclamate (AS)	3,000
9.	Aspartame (AS)	15,000
10.	Saccharin (AS)	40,000

Carbohydrates can be ranked according to their sweetness. Fructose is the sweetest and the most soluble sugar. It is followed by sucrose, glucose, dextrin and lactose. Starches are not sweet, but bland in flavour. Tender corn is sweet, as it matures it becomes less sweet as sugars are converted to starch. Raw fruits contain starch, which changes to sugars during the ripening process with development of sweet taste.

CARBOHYDRATES AS BODY NOURISHERS

Our body uses carbohydrates in a number of ways, the most important being as a food source. It is no surprise, therefore, that carbohydrates contribute 60 to 65 percent of the caloric value of the normal diet. Of the important functions carbohydrates perform in the human body, the most vital one is to act as energy providing fuel to the body tissues. In addition, certain carbohydrates also perform specific functions, for example D-ribose and D-deoxyribase as a component of nucleic acids structure, and lactose as a constituent of milk. Besides this, carbohydrates also act as a source of carbon atoms for the synthesis of important compounds like glycerol, non-essential amino acids, fatty acids etc. Further, they make meaningful contributions in the structural organization of cell membranes, blood groups substances and connective tissues. They are also the major players in the energy cycle of animal and plant kingdoms. Human beings are largely utilizing carbohydrates for shelter and clothing, apart from being food sources. Since carbohydrates as foods are cheap and easily available, they most easily become the major contributors towards the caloric intake to an almost 80 percent of the world population that depends mainly on plant food.

CARBOHYDRATE RICH FOODS AND GLYCEMIC RESPONSE

Researchers have found that the increase in blood glucose levels produced by different carbohydrate containing foods vary considerably from one another. For example, isocaloric amounts of carbohydrate from potato cause a higher increase in post prandial (after consuming the concerned foodstuff as a meal) blood glucose as compared to that from bread or rice. The information about the glycemic response of foods has a value for diabetics in planning their meals. Table 2.3 provides this information for common foods.

ROLE OF DIETARY FIBER AS HEALTH PROMOTER

Eating whole cereals, leafy vegetables, fruits, etc., has been found to ensure smooth, regular elimination and avoiding constipation. Intake of refined foods, on the other hand, becomes the cause of constipation. With regular elimination of softer stools, the formation of haemorrhoids is reduced and diverticulosis is prevented and controlled. Pectins and gums bind bile acids and cholesterol and thus reduce their blood levels. Dietary fiber, by increasing bulk and needing more chewing, may reduce the food intake. It helps obese persons in reducing their energy intake to

Table 2.3: Glycemic index[a] of some selected foods[b]

Grain and cereal products		*Root vegetable*	
Bread (white)	69±5	Beets	64±16
Bread (whole wheat)	72±6	Carrots	92±20
Rice (white)	72±9	Potato (white)	70±8
		Potato (sweet)	48±6
Breakfast cereals			
		Beans (kidney)	29±8
Cornflakes	80±6	Beans (soy)	15±5
Oatmeal	49±8		
Shredded wheat	67±10		
Vegetable		*Fruits*	
Sweet corn	59±11	Apple (golden delicious)	39±3
Frozen peas	51±6	Banana	62±9
		Oranges	40±3
Dairy products		*Sugars*	
Ice cream	36±8	Fructose	20±5
Milk (whole)	34±6	Glucose	100
Yoghurt	36±4	Honey	87±8
		Sucrose	59±10

a Glycemic index is defined as the area under the blood glucose response curve for each food expressed as a percentage of the area after taking the same amount of carbohydrate as glucose (mean of 5-10 individuals).

b Data from Jenkins. David A. *et al.* Glycemic index of foods: A physiological basis of carbohydrate exchange. Am J. Clin. Nutr. 34:362, 1981.

lose weight. One needs to take some 10-20 g of fiber daily in the diet. As a matter of fact, dietary fiber is of two types—water insoluble and soluble.

Structural parts of plant cell walls (cellulose, hemicellulose and lignin), which are not soluble in water, are classified as insoluble fiber. Water insoluble fibers are found in whole wheat, wheat bran, seeds, nuts and vegetables. Viscous plant fibers are soluble in water. These include pectin, gums and mucilages. Soluble fibers are found in legumes, fruits, oat and barley.

- Since human body does not have enzymes capable of breaking down cellulose, hemicellulose and pectins and so fiber is not digested in the body. However, these indigestible substances serve a useful purpose in helping with the elimination of intestinal wastes. Due to their property to absorb water, they stimulate the peristalitic (rhythmic) movements of the gastrointestinal tract by adding bulk to the intestinal contents.
- The insoluble fiber requires long chewing and thus improves mastication of food. In general, dietary fiber absorbs water, swells and thus increases surface area of the mass. As a result, there is increased contact between the food mass and enzymes which improves digestion. This also causes an early feeling of fullness and makes one eat less. The sponge like swollen mass of fiber ensures smooth elimination of faeces.
- Fiber reduces transit time and binds some minerals such as calcium, iron, zinc, etc. Soluble fiber binds bile salts and cholesterol and helps carry these out of the body. This spares the oxidation of bile salts by microorganisms of colon, the oxidized products can become potentially carcinogenic and cause colon cancer.
- The carbohydrates absorption is slowed by dietary fiber, which helps to regulate blood sugar and lower insulin need of diabetics. Large soft stools with reduced microbial activity almost rules out the formation of potential carcinogens saving the person from the occurrence of colon cancer. However, an obsession with dietary fiber may cause a decrease in the absorption

of some vitamins and minerals. Thus moderation in fiber intake is the key to its positive role in health.

ARTIFICIAL SWEETENERS OR SUGAR SUBSTITUTES

They are beneficial for diabetics and overweight obese people. Two most common artificial sweeteners are saccharin and aspartame.

Chemically, saccharin is o-sulphobenzimide. It is 400 times as sweet as sucrose and passes through the body unchanged. It has been used as a sugar substitute for about hundred years without any adverse effects. It is used in beverages and desserts. The only drawback is, it leaves a bitter aftertaste, if used in large amount. Some studies made on animals castigate saccharin as being carcinogenic when consumed in substantial amount over a long period.

Aspartame, on the other hand, is a dipeptide of two amino acids, aspartic acid and phenylalanine. It is marketed as Equal and NutraSweet. As dipeptides are heat labile, its sweetness bears off in cooked or baked foods. Persons suffering from phenylketonuria should avoid use of aspartame due to the presence of phenylalanine as its component.

STUDY QUESTIONS

1. Justify the statement 'carbohydrates are readily available source of energy'.
2. Classify carbohydrate and furnish the nutritional importance of important members of each class.
3. Elaborate upon the statement 'dietary fiber promotes health'.
4. Define the term 'glycemic index' and explain the importance of 'low glycemic index' carbohydrate rich foodstuffs.
5. Explain what sugar substitutes or artificial sweeteners are along with the role they play in diet.

CHAPTER 3

Fat and Extra Fat Lipids

Chapter Outlines

- Fats as part of both, diet and body tissues
- Occurrence
- Classification
- Oils and fats
- Fatty acids
- Other lipids
- Lipoproteins
- Refining and hydrogenation of oils
- Rancidity of oils and fats
- Intake levels of oils and fats
- Study questions

FATS AS PART OF BOTH, DIET AND BODY TISSUES

Fats are the major members of another family of biomolecules known as lipids. Lipids are a heterogeneous group of water insoluble, oily or greasy organic substances that can be extracted from tissues by nonpolar solvents, such as carbontetrachloride, chloroform and ether. Since fats act as major storage form of chemical energy for most of the organisms (including humans) and they occur widely in plants and animals, it is but natural that they make substantial portions of our diet. Most of the times, the term 'fat' is used to refer to both fats and oils. However, the two (oils and fats) can be differentiated by the fact that fats are normally solid at room temperature, in contrast to oils, that are liquid. Secondly, fats are mostly obtained from animal tissues, again in contrast to oils that are mostly of plant origin and occurrence. Being organic substances, fats are composed of carbon, hydrogen and oxygen. Since fats quantitatively constitute the major part of the food lipids (95-98 percent) and in human body too, they are present to a similar extent, nutritionists mostly use the terms 'food fat' and 'body fat' almost synonymously with 'food lipids' and 'body lipids' respectively.

In human body, fat and other lipids account for 15-18 percent body weight in healthy non-obese men and 18-20 percent in healthy non-obese women. The fat content of body increases in sedentary individuals, especially in adults and elderly, if they do not have active and exercise based life styles.

OCCURRENCE

Sources of fat include vegetable oils that are used as cooking media in food preparation. They are extracts of oil seeds and nuts.

Butter and ghee are animal fats extracted from milk.

Plant oils are hydrogenated to form almost a solid fat known as *vanaspati.*

Vanaspati is usually fortified with vitamin A and D, as it is used in place of *ghee*. Oils, butter, ghee and *vanaspati* contribute the visible fats in the Indian dietary. The amounts of oils and fats in the diet vary with the region. As these are expensive foods, the amount and kind used in the diet, vary with the socio-economic status of the family.

The animal foods, milk, egg, meat and liver, which contain fat, are sources of hidden fat in the diet. Nuts, oilseeds, milk, egg and meat supply not only fat but also protein, minerals and vitamins of B-complex group. Ghee, butter, eggs and liver are good sources of vitamin A. Some refined oils and *vanaspati* are fortified with vitamin A.

Vegetable oils contain poly-unsaturated fatty acids such as linoleic and arachidonic acid. Linoleic and arachidonic acids are required for growth and maintenance of integrity of the skin. It may be noted that vegetable oils are a fairly good source of essential fatty acids.

It is easier to control visible fats in the diet than those that are hidden. Invisible fats include the cream in the milk and curd, nuts used in the preparation and fat present in red meat, egg to a lesser extent, in other foodstuffs.

CLASSIFICATION

Chemically, lipids are either esters of fatty acids or as substances capable of forming such esters. Their occurrence is widespread ranging from animal to vegetable matter. Diversity in chemical structures of different lipids makes their rational classification difficult. That is why, a number of classifications have been proposed for lipids. However, the one devised by Bloor is most simple and convenient. As per this classification, lipids have been divided into three categories, namely simple, complex and derived. Simple lipids are the ester of fatty acids and alcohol (mostly glycerol) and include fats, oils and waxes. Oils and fats are thus triacylgycerols (triglycerides), the difference between the two arises because of the comparatively large presence of unsaturated fatty acids in oils vis-à-vis fats.

Compound lipids also contain fatty acids and glycerol or any other alcohol but also contain, in addition, other substances like phosphorus (glycero-phospholipids), nitrogenous base (sphingo phospholipids), carbohydrates (glycolipids) and proteins (lipoproteins). Derived lipids, the third category, mostly comprise lipid monomers, obtained by the hydrolysis of lipids of the other two classes. Fatty acids, higher aliphatic alcohols and all the members of the group 'sterols', including the all important cholesterol, are included in it.

In a nutshell, lipids are classified into three groups on the basis of their chemical structure:

1. Simple lipids, which include fats and oils.
2. Compound lipids, consisting of phospholipids and lipoproteins.
3. Derived lipids such as fatty acid and sterols.

OILS AND FATS

Oils and fats, the major lipid components (95 to 98 percent) of human diet, are chemically triacylgycerols (triglycerides). They are triesters of glycerol (a trihydric alcohol having three hydroxyl groups) and fatty acids (unsaturated or saturated or mixed).

As food components (Table 3.1), oils and fats perform many important functions ranging from enhancing the food taste and palatability by absorbing flavors and aromas, becoming dense sources (their energy value per unit weight is more than double than that of carbohydrate or protein) and stored forms of energy (fats stored in the body during favorable, nourishing conditions and utilized during times of starvation or insufficient energy intakes), becoming the source of essential fatty acids and solvent carriers for fat soluble vitamins. However, a high fat diet when consumed over a long period of time may result in the incidence of obesity, coronary heart disease, hyperlipidemia and cancers of breast and bowel.

Table 3.1: Fat content of certain foods

Product	*Average fat content (gram percent)*
Rice	0.5
Coconut	34
Groundnut	40
Soybean	19
Milk (cow's)	4.1
Butter	80
Cheese	25
Ghee	100
Oil	100
Almond	58.9
Cashew	46.9
Egg (Hen)	13.3
Goat's meat	3.6

FATTY ACIDS

Fatty acids are obtained from the hydrolysis of oils and fats. These are acid components of fats and mostly occur as straight chain carbon atoms joined end to end, like links of a chain having acidic (carboxylic) group at the end. Fatty acids of natural fats mostly contain even number of carbons because they are synthesized from acetic acid (two carbon carboxylic acid) units. Fatty acids differ from each other in the length of carbon chain and the presence of double bonds or unstauration in their structure. Generally, fatty acids with six carbons or less are termed as 'short chain' and those between eight to twelve and fourteen to twenty carbon atoms are called 'medium' and 'long chain' fatty acids respectively. Most of the oils and fats (triglycerides) have long chain fatty acids in their structures. Table 3.2 gives the names of saturated fatty acids that occur in natural fats.

Among unsaturated fatty acids, the most common occurring in natural fats are listed in Table 3.3.

Polyunsaturated fatty acids (PUFA) have two or more double bonds in the molecules. Corn oil contains polyunsaturated fatty acids.

The methyl end of the fatty acid molecule is called the *omega* end. If the first double bond in the fatty acid is in the third carbon atom from the methyl end, it is called *omega-3* fatty acid; if it is in the sixth carbon from the methyl end, it is called *omega-6* fatty acid, when it is in ninth carbon, it is called *omega-9* fatty acid. Examples given below will illustrate the point:

Oleic acid is an omega-9-fatty acid and is a MUFA with a total of 18 carbons.

Linoleic acid is an omega-6-fatty acid and is a PUFA with a total of 18 carbons.

Linolenic acid is an omega-3-fatty acid and is also a PUFA with a total of 18 carbons.

Table 3.3: Unsaturated fatty acids

Name	*Sources*	*Shorthand notation*
Oleic acid	All vegetable oils	18:1;9
Linoleic acid	All vegetable oils	18:2; 9:12
Linolenic acid	Soyabean and sunflower oils	18:3; 9, 12, 15
Arachidonic acid	Fresh water fish oils	20:4; 5, 8, 11, 14

Mammals, including human beings, are not able to synthesize linoleic and linolenic acids, since body tissues lack the enzymes needed to introduce double bonds beyond carbon nine in saturated fatty acids. These two fatty acids along with a third one namely, arachidonic acid (formed from linoleic acid in the body); play vital roles in metabolism and maintain the functional integrity of cell membranes. Arachidonic acid acts as a precursor of prostaglandins

Table 3.2: Saturated fatty acids of natural fats

Name	*Sources*	*Shorthand notation*
Acetic acid (C_2)	Major products of carbohydrate fermentation by rumen microorganisms in the cattle	2:0
Butyric acid (C_4)	Minor end product of carbohydrate fermentation by rumen microorganisms in the cattle	4:0
Caproic acid (C_6)	Minor end product of rumen microorganisms Small amounts in butter fat	6:0
Caprylic acid (C_8)	Small amounts in fats of plant origin Small amount in butter fat	8:0
Capric acid (C_{10})	Small amounts in fats of plant origin Small amount in butter fat	10:0
Lauric acid (C_{12})	In coconut oil, palm kernel and cinnamon	12:0
Myristic acid (C_{14})	In cotton seeds, palm oil	14:0
Palmitic acid (C_{16})	Common in all animal and plant fats	16:0
Stearic acid (C_{18})	Common in all animal and plant fats	18:0
Arachidic acid (C_{20})	Small amount in groundnut oil	20:0
Behemic acid (C_{22})	Small amounts in seed fats, groundnut oil	22:0
Lignoceric acid (C_{24})	In groundnut oil	24:0

and thromboxanes as substances of immense physiological value and therapeutic potential. These three fatty acids (or at least two, linoleic and linolenic acids) have to be essential components of the diet. They are essential for general growth in the young and maintenance of normal healthy skin at all stages. Their other functions are as components of membranes to ensure their permeability to water and other small molecules. They are precursors of eicosanoids, a group of important metabolites which regulate vascular function, one of these are prostaglandins.

The omega fatty acids, DHA (decosa hexenoic acid) and EPA (eicosa pentenoic acid) have an important role in fetal brain and eye development. These acids also protect against rheumatoid arthritis and cardiovascular diseases. Certain varieties of fish are the richest food sources of these fatty acids. Common plant oils with the exception of coconut oil are good sources of linoleic acid.

Green leafy vegetables, cabbage and lettuce, are good sources of omega-3 fatty acids. Soyabean and rapeseed are also good sources of omega-3 fatty acids. Fatty fish, such as tuna, sardines and salmon are good sources of omega-3 fatty acids and a weekly consumption of any of these fish can help to meet the need.

Dietary recommendations for essential fatty acids stipulate that linoleic acid (omega-6) should provide at least one percent and linolenic acid (omega-3) at least 0.2 percent of the dietary energy so as to satisfy human requirements in general for all age groups.

As it is well known that fat is a major nutrient and it has several functions. Oils and fats are concentrated sources of energy. Each gram supplies 9 calories. Besides providing energy, oils and fats have several functions in the body. Food fats are a source of two groups of essential nutrients– essential fatty acids (EFA) and fat soluble vitamins; A, D, E and K and their precursors. Food fats also aid the transport and absorption of fat soluble vitamins. Cholesterol is an essentially derived lipid synthesized in the liver. Some important hormones and bile acids are formed from cholesterol. Fats stored in various parts of the body are known as adipose tissue. The vital organs in the body are supported and protected by the cushion like padding of this tissue. Thus, fats of the adipose tissue also act as a cushion for certain vital organs. Nerve fibers are protected by a fat covering and it aids in the relay of nerve impulses. Since fat is a poor conductor of heat, a layer of fat beneath the skin helps to conserve body heat and regulate body temperature (Tables 3.4 and 3.5).

Table 3.4: Melting points of important fatty acids

Name	*Melting point (Celsius)*
Lauric acid	44
Myristic acid	58
Palmitic acid	63
Stearic acid	70
Oleic acid	4
Linoleic acid	-5
Linolenic acid	-11
Arachidonic acid	-49.0

Table 3.5: Iodine values of certain fats and oils

Name	*Iodine value*
Butter fat	50
Human fat	68
Lard	59
Coconut oil	10
Corn oil	122
Cottonseed oil	106
Linseed oil	179
Olive oil	81
Palm oil	54
Peanut oil	93
Safflower	144
Soyabean	130

The flavour, palatability and satiety value of foods is increased by fats. The slower rate of digestion of fat as compared to carbohydrates results in a feeling of satisfaction.

Iodine values are indices of degree of unsaturation of oils and fats.

OTHER LIPIDS

Since oils and fats constitute 95-98 percent of the total dietary lipids, the other lipids being present in small proportion include phospholipids and cholesterol. Cholesterol, a derived lipid, is a sterol chemically, it acts as the starting material for the synthesis of bile salts and adrenal cortical and reproductive hormones, besides being a constituent of membrane structures of all cells and myelin sheaths of nerve cells. However, high cholesterol levels have also been found to be one of the causative factors in atherosclerosis and coronary heart disease (CHD).

LIPOPROTEINS

Lipoproteins are a cluster of lipids associated with proteins that serve as transport vehicles for lipids in blood and lymph. The four main types of lipoproteins are:

1. *Chylomicrons*: A type of lipoproteins (very low in density) made by the cells of the intestinal wall; serve as a means of transporting newly digested fat from the intestine through lymph and blood. Chylomicrons donate lipids to all body cells, and the remnants are ultimately cleared from the blood by liver cells.
2. *VLDL*: Very low density lipoproteins carry fat made by liver to various tissues in the body.
3. *LDL:* Low density lipoproteins, mainly carry cholesterol from the liver to the blood vessels and other cells of the body tissues. A high blood cholesterol level usually reflects high LDL.
4. *HDL:* High density lipoproteins scavenge cholesterol from the blood vessels and tissues and transport it back to the liver for recycling or disposal.

Of these types, two have a greater significance to the health of the heart and blood vessels. They are the LDL and HDL. Both LDL and HDL carry similar lipid around in the blood, but there is a functional difference between them. Raised LDL concentrations in the blood are an indication of high risk of heart attacks, because LDL in the blood tend to deposit cholesterol in the arteries and is hence referred to as 'bad cholesterol'. Evevated HDL concentrations are associated with a low risk of heart attacks because HDL tend to carry cholesterol out of the arteries, therefore, the name 'good cholesterol'. Elevated blood level of triglycerides is also an independent risk factor for heart diseases.

REFINING AND HYDROGENATION OF OILS

Crude olive oil is exceptional in that it can be used for edible purposes without refining. Most vegetable oils, however, contain a number of impurities such as moisture, free fatty acids, colouring matter, resins, gums and sometimes vitamins. These impurities affect flavour, odour and clarity, and are removed during refining. The refining process is carried out in a number of stages as detailed below:

1. *Degumming*: Crude oil, often contains impurities in suspension which in the presence of water form gums. The impurities are removed by adding hot water to the warm oil, which is then transferred to a centrifugal separator. The separator revolves at a high speed and the gum particles, which have a higher density than the oil, are thrown to the bottom of the vessel leaving an upper layer of clarified oil.
2. *Neutralizing*: Owing to spoilage, all crude oils contain a small proportion of free fatty acids and low-grade oils may contain considerable quantities. The fatty acids are removed by neutralizing the oil with a solution of caustic soda, which converts the fatty acid into an insoluble soap. The soap is then removed by allowing it to settle to the bottom of the neutralizing tanks. It the acid impurity is palmitic acid, for example, insoluble sodium palmitate is formed:

   $$C_{15}H_{31}COOH + NaOH \rightarrow C_{15}H_{31}COONa\downarrow + H_2O$$

   Palmitic acid   Sodium palmitate
3. *Washing and drying:* In order to remove the last traces of soap from the oil, it is washed with warm water. Two layers form and the lower water layer is run off, leaving the oil layer, which is then vacuum dried.

   In modern plants these separate stages are being replaced by a continuous automatic process in which the neutralizing stage is carried out much more quickly in a centrifugal separator.

   The oil is now clear and free from fatty acids, but it is usually yellowish in colour and still has a distinct odour. It is, therefore, bleached and deodorized.
4. *Bleaching*: The oil is warmed and fuller's earth and activated carbons are added. Both these materials have a large capacity for adsorbing colored matter. The mixture is stirred and a partial vacuum is maintained. When all the coloured matter has been adsorbed, the oil-earth mixture is passed through filter presses, from which the oil emerges as a clear, colorless liquid.
5. *Deodorizing*: The oil is heated under vacuum in a tall tank and steam injected so that the liquid mixture is violently agitated. In one method, it is sprayed upwards as an umbrella-shaped fountain, so that a large surface area of liquid is continually exposed, and the volatile odoriferous substances and remaining free fatty acids are stripped from the oil.

The oil is now pure and ready for use, or, as is usually the case, ready for blending. It is desirable that the oil should not come in contact with air once it has been refined, as this leads to deterioration due to oxidation. In some modern plants, therefore, the oil is stored under an inert atmosphere of nitrogen.

Hydrogenation is the process whereby an oil is converted into a fat, i.e., by which it is hardened. This important process has resulted in a considerable increase in the use of hardened vegetable oils at the expense of animal fats which were once such a staple feature of the diet.

Hydrogenation is the simple addition of hydrogen to the double bonds of unsaturated fatty acids combined with glycerol in oil. During hydrogenation one molecule of hydrogen is absorbed by each double bond.

$$—CH{=}CH— + H_2 \rightarrow —CH_2—CH_2—$$

The most commonly occurring unsaturated fatty acids found in combination with glycerol in vegetable oils, namely oleic, linoleic and linolenic acids, contain one, two and three double bonds respectively. As they all contain 18 carbon atoms, complete hydrogenation converts them all into stearic acid. It has a much higher melting point (70°C) than any of the other three, so the hydrogenated oil is harder than the original. The equation below illustrates the conversion of liquid triolein into solid tristearin which takes place when a molecule of triolein absorbs three molecules of hydrogen.

$$\begin{array}{lcl} CH_2OCO_{17}H_{33} & & CH_2OCOC_{17}H_{35} \\ | & & | \\ CHOCOC_{17}H_{33} + 3H_2 & \rightarrow & CHOCOC_{17}H_{35} \\ | & & | \\ CH_2OCOC_{17}H_{33} & & CH_2OCOC_{17}H_{35} \end{array}$$

Triolein (Oil) Tristearin (Saturated Fat)

Hydrogenation only proceeds at a reasonably fast rate in the presence of a catalyst, finely divided nickel being used industrially. The nickel is usually made by reducing finely divided nickel carbonate or nickel formate. The catalyst is added in small quantities to the oil, which is contained in large closed steel vessels called converters, operating at a temperature of about 170° C and high pressure. The oil is stirred and hydrogen gas is pumped in. The oil is heated to start the reaction, but as the reaction is exothermic, further heating is not necessary. After hydrogenation, the oil is collected and filtered to remove the nickel which can be reused.

The way in which a catalyst affects a reaction can be summed up in the fact that catalysts reduce the energy required for a reaction to proceed, i.e., the energy of activation. Nickel, like enzymes, catalyses this reaction by providing a surface upon which the reaction can take place, and converts a single-step high energy mechanism into one involving several low energy stages.

The first stage of hydrogenation is the adsorption of reactants, in this case hydrogen and oil, come on to the nickel surface. Adsorption takes place only at certain preferred parts of the surface known as active centres and results in the adsorbed hydrogen oil molecules being brought close to each other. Exchange of energy between the nickel and the reacting molecules weakens the internal bonds of the latter and activates them sufficiently to provide them with the necessary energy of activation. Reaction occurs, after which the hydrogen that oil molecules absorb, i.e., they leave the nickel surface which is then available to catalyse further reaction. Thus hydrogenation of oils is accomplished in several stages.

Surface catalysts, such as nickel, are easily poisoned by substances which are adsorbed in preference to the hydrogen and oil molecules. Carbon monoxide and sulphur compounds, if present in even minute amounts, poison nickel. This means that the hydrogen gas, which is often produced from water gas (a mixture of carbon monoxide and hydrogen), must be most carefully purified before use and that the oil to be used must be carefully refined before hydrogenation.

Hydrogenation is a selective process, some triglycerides becoming saturated more rapidly than others. The most unsaturated triglycerides are partially hydrogenated before the less unsaturated ones react, so that in terms of the fatty acids combined in the triglycerides, more linolenic acid is converted into linoleic in a given time than linoleic into oleic. The relative rates of reaction of oleic, linoleic and linoleic acids are in the ratio 1:20:40. The fact enables the hydrogenation to be controlled, and food oils are only partially saturated with hydrogen.

Hydrogenation of oils not only converts unsaturated fatty acids into saturated ones, but it also converts naturally occurring cis forms of unsaturated fatty acids into their trans forms. Such trans forms are treated by the body in the same way as saturated fatty acids. Trans forms have adverse health effects.

Careful control of the hydrogenation process is important. For health reasons, it may be desirable to retain a degree of unstauration in the partially hardened oil. In addition, complete hydrogenation would make fats too hard and lacking in plasticity for use in food preparation. Apart from its hardening effect, hydrogenation is advantageous in that it also bleaches the oil and increases its stability.

RANCIDITY OF OILS AND FATS

Oils and fats are liable to spoilage which results in the production of unpleasant odours and flavours; such spoilage is usually described by the general term rancidity. Different types of oil and fat show varying degrees of resistance to spoilage; thus most vegetable oils deteriorate only slowly whereas animal fats deteriorate more rapidly and marine oils, which contain a relatively high proportion of combined highly unsaturated fatty acids deteriorate so rapidly that they are useless for edible purposes unless they have been refined and hydrogenated.

Spoilage may occur in many ways, but two important types of rancidity may be distinguished, namely hydrolytic rancidity and oxidative rancidity.

Hydrolytic Rancidity: Hydrolytic rancidity occurs as a result of hydrolysis of triglyceride molecules to glycerol and free fatty acids and it is brought about by the presence of moisture in oils. The rate of hydrolysis in the presence of water alone is negligible, but it is hastened by the presence of enzymes and microorganisms. Oils and fats that have not been subjected to heat treatment also contain lipases which catalyse hydrolysis. They may also contain moulds, yeasts and bacteria present in the natural oil or they may become contaminated with them during processing. Such microorganisms hasten hydrolytic breakdown.

The nature of the unpleasant flavours and odours produced by hydrolysis depends upon the fatty acid composition of the triglycerides. If the triglycerides contain combined fatty acids of low molecular weight containing 4-14 carbon atoms, hydrolysis yields free acids having characteristically unpleasant odours and flavours. For example, hydrolysis of butter yields the rancid-smelling butyric acid, while palm kernel oil yields considerable amounts of lauric and myristic acids. Oils containing combined fatty acids with more than 14 carbon atoms are not liable to hydrolytic rancidity as the free acids are flavorless and odorless.

Oxidative Rancidity: Oxidative rancidity is the most common and important type of rancidity and it results in the production of rancid or 'tallowy' flavours. It is caused by the reaction of unsaturated oils with oxygen and its occurrence does not depend, therefore, on the presence of impurities or moisture in an oil; it can consequently affect pure and refined oils. The actual mechanism of the oxidation is complex and not completely elucidated, but the main features are known and are as follows.

The oxidation of oils takes place by means of a chain reaction which is a type of reaction that is characterized by extreme speed. A chain reaction takes place in three stages known as initiation, propagation and termination. In the initiation stage, which is slow to occur, a hydrogen atom is removed from an unsaturated triglyceride molecule with the production of a free radical (R). Free radical, which are groups containing an 'unpaired' electron, are extremely unstable and immediately react with another molecule to form a more stable substance. This initiation stage only occurs under the influence of catalysts in the form of minute traces of metals, particularly copper, and in the presence of heat and light.

The slow initiation stage is followed by a fast propagation stage in which free radicals from the initiation stage, combine with atmospheric oxygen to form an unstable peroxy free radical which reacts with molecules of unsaturated oil to form another free radical and an unstable hydroperoxide. It can be seen from the sequence shown below, that for every free radical R• used up another is generated with the result that the reaction is self-generating. The site of the reaction in the unsaturated oil is a methylene ($-CH_2-$) group adjacent to a double bond and one can represent such molecules by RH, H being the hydrogen atom of the methylene group adjacent to a double bound.

Initiation Initiator $\longrightarrow$ R (Free radical)

Propagation $R^{\bullet} + O_2 \longrightarrow RO^{\bullet}_2$ (Peroxy free radical)

$RO^{\bullet}_2 + RH \longrightarrow R^{\bullet} + ROOH$ (Hydroperoxide)

As the reaction proceeds, hydroperoxide is continually formed and, being unstable, it breaks down to form ketones and aldehydes, which are responsible for the off-flavours of rancid fats. The reaction continues either until all the oxygen (or oil) is used up or until the free radicals which are responsible for maintaining the reaction are removed. Many fats, particularly vegetable oils, contain natural substances, such as vitamin E, known as antioxidants which help to retard rancidity by reacting with peroxy free radicals ($RO^{\bullet}_2$) so that they are not long available for the propagation stage. Synthetic antioxidants are also added to fats to control rancidity.

INTAKE LEVELS OF OILS AND FATS

The fat requirement is based on two factors, namely to meet energy and the essential fatty acids needs. About 10 percent of the total energy need is met by invisible fat in the diet. Around 10 percent of total energy needs to be provided as visible fat in the diet. This amounts to about 20 g of fat per day for adults to provide energy, palatability characteristics, essential fatty acids and fat soluble vitamins. At least, half of this should be derived from oils of vegetable origin.

STUDY QUESTIONS

1. Define lipids and explain the role of fat as the major nutritional lipid.
2. Classify lipids, giving the composition of each class.
3. Explain the terms saturated, unsaturated and omega fatty acids by giving suitable examples.
4. What are lipoproteins? Write their different types.
5. Explain rancidity along with its various types.

CHAPTER 4

Proteins

Chapter Outlines

- Introduction
- Proteins
- Classification
- Importance of proteins
- Food sources of protein
- Study questions

INTRODUCTION

The term 'protein' has a Greek origin. Derived from 'proteios', it means 'primary' or 'first place'. Appropriately, thus proteins occupy distinguished place as biomolecules that perform vital functions in living organisms. For the same reasons, they have immense significance as a macronutrient component of the diet. The fact that half of the dry weight of most organisms is contributed by proteins is also a testimony to their paramount importance in living species. In fact, proteins are the means through which genetic information stored in thousands of genes is manifested.

It is also amazing that all the fifty thousand proteins present in human body are made from the same basic set of twenty amino acids, which on their own, do not have intrinsic biologic activity. It is only when these amino acids join themselves in a specific sequence (dictated by a particular gene on DNA) that a protein with a specific biological function results. Hence proteins of various types differ from each other in the sequence of their building block amino acid units.

PROTEINS

Proteins are one of the most abundant and important components of the body. It accounts for about 16 percent of the body weight, one third of the total protein content is found in the muscles. One fifth of them in the bones and cartilage, a tenth in the skin and the remaining in other tissues and fluids. There are thousands of different proteins in the body, each having a unique structure and specific function. For this reason, the term protein connotes a large group of complex compounds, diverse in structure and functions. Proteins are present in all living tissues of both plants and animals. Proteins are essential to life as they are components of every subcellular component such as nucleus, mitochondria and cell membrane of every cell in the body.

Proteins are organic compounds or macromolecules with large molecular size. Being organic compounds, they contain carbon, hydrogen and oxygen like carbohydrates and fats. In contrast to other macromolecules in the body, namely carbohydrates and fats, they contain about 16 percent nitrogen, making them unique in this aspect. Some proteins also contain sulphur, and at times, phosphorus, iron and cobalt. In fact, proteins are more complex than fats and carbohydrates, as there is great variation in the sequence of amino acids from which they are formed.

Plants are the primary sources of proteins in nature. They synthesize proteins from the nitrates and ammonia in the soil. Herbivorous animals use plant proteins to meet their protein needs. Human beings, on the other hand, use plant as well as animal foods (meat and milk) to meet their protein needs. Nitrogen is returned to the soil through degradation of products of protein metabolism, excretion of nitrogen compounds in excretory materials and decomposition of organic compounds of body tissues after death, to make the nitrogen in different forms available for protein resynthesis and to complete the nitrogen cycle in nature.

All proteins in animals and plants are built from basic units of their structure known as amino acids. Amino acids join with each other, combining a carboxylic carbon of one amino acid with amino nitrogen of the next. The resulting chemical joint is called peptide bond and the structure, a peptide. The resulting peptide has a free amino group at one end and a free carboxyl group at the other, permitting addition of other amino acids at the carboxyl end. The proteins are amphoteric in nature due to presence of free amino and carboxylic acid groups, one each at the two ends of the chain in their molecules. Polypeptides formed by the condensation of amino acids thus make the primary structure of proteins. The secondary structure formed due to the H-bond interactions occurring within or between polypeptide chains. It may be helical, pleated sheet or random coil. Proteins also have a tertiary structure in which the polypeptide chain is wound and coiled into a globular form.

As a matter of fact, proteins exist in fibrous and globular forms. Fibrous proteins are generally insouble and make structural elements, e.g., collagen of connective tissue, myosin of muscle tissue and keratin of hair. Globular proteins, on the other hand, are soluble and occur in tissue fluids. These include casein, albumins and globulins of blood plasma, egg—white albumin and haemoglobin. In free or conjugated forms, globular proteins also function as intracellular enzymes (Table 4.1).

Table 4.1: Structure of amino acids, $H_2NCHRCOOH$

Name (E=essential)		*Abbreviation*	*R*	*Isoelectric point*
Neutral				
Glycine		Gly	H	6.0
Alanine		Ala	CH_3	6.0
Valine	(E)	Val	$(CH_3)_2CH$	6.0
Leucine	(E)	Leu	$(CH_3)_2CHCH_2$	6.0
Isoleucine	(E)	Ile	$CH_3CH_2CH(CH_3)$	6.0
Phenylalanine	(E)	Phe	$C_6H_5CH_2$	5.5
Tyrosine		Tyr	$C_6H_4(OH)CH_2$	5.7
Serine		Ser	$HOCH_2$	5.7
Threonine	(E)	Thr	$CH_3CH(OH)$	5.6
Cysteine		CySH	$HSCH_2$	5.1
Cystine		CySSCy	$HOOCCH(NH_2)CH_2S_2CH_2$	4.8
Methionine	(E)	Met	$CH_3SCH_2CH_2$	5.7
Tryptophan	(E)	Trp	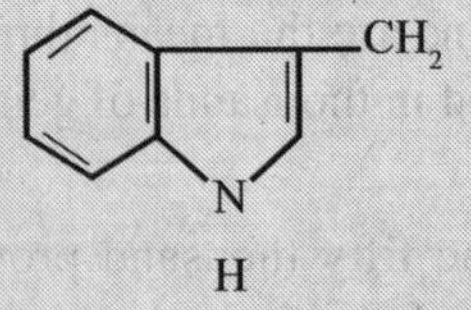	5.9
Basic				
Ornithine		Orn	$H_2N(CH_2)_3$	9.7
Arginine		Arg	NH_2 $HN{=}CNH(CH_2)_3$	10.8
Lysine	(E)	Lys	$H_2N(CH_2)_4$	10.0

Contd.

Contd.

Histidine	His	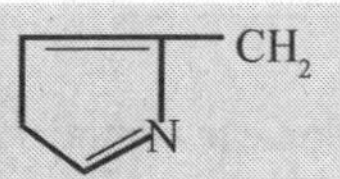	7.6
Acidic			
Aspartic acid	Asp	$HOOCCH_2$	2.8
Glutamic acid	Glu	$HOOC(CH_2)_2$	3.2

CLASSIFICATION

Chemically, proteins are high molecular weight, nitrogen containing organic compounds or amino acids linked through peptide bonds in specific sequences to make long polypeptide chains. Simple proteins are polypeptide chains and they do not contain any non-protein substances, conjugated proteins, in comparison, contain non-protein components–commonly called prosthetic groups in addition to the polypeptide chain. Prosthetic groups of conjugated proteins can be carbohydrate, lipid, nucleic acid, colored groups and metal ions. Derived proteins, as the third groups are named, are formed from denaturation and partial hydrolysis of native proteins. Simple proteins yield only amino acids on hydrolysis. Albumins, globulins glutelins, prolamins and albuminoids are simple proteins. Albumins and globulins, which are soluble in water and salt solution, are present in animal fluids (milk, blood, plasma). Those which are less soluble are present in tissues (muscle, protein, myosin).

Conjugated proteins are combinations of simple proteins with non-protein substances. The combinations result in formations, which are functionally very important to the body. Conjugated proteins include:

- Nucleoproteins (proteins + nucleic acids) found in cells (RNA, DNA).
- Phosphoproteins (proteins + phosphoric acid) found in milk, e.g., casein.
- Lipoproteins (proteins + lipids) found in blood plasma (HDL, LDL, VLDL, etc).
- Mucoproteins and glycoproteins (proteins + polysaccharides) found in gastric secretion (mucin).
- Metalloproteins (proteins + metals), found in ferritin and hemosidirin.

Derived proteins are proteoses, peptones and peptides formed in the various stages of protein metabolism.

As discussed earlier too, that on the basis of shape and other characteristics too, proteins can be divided into two groups, viz. fibrous and globular proteins. The former being insoluble in water and long sheet like in appearance, have structural functions in the body tissue and the latter being compact, spherical and water soluble, perform catalytic and other functions.

To perform its specific biological function, each protein possesses a unique yet complex three dimensional structural organization which can be divided into primary, secondary, tertiary and quaternary levels, overall referred to as protein conformation. However such a structural organization is the outcome of specific amino acid sequence. A small change in the order of amino acids in a protein chain may alter the protein conformation with an attendant loss of biological activity (Tables 4.2 to 4.4).

Table 4.2: Simple classification of proteins

Type	*Solubility/Function*	*Examples/Source*
Animal		
Fibrous	Insoluble, elastic proteins forming structural part of tissues	Keratin (hair) Collagen (connective tissue) Elastin (tendons, arteries) Myosin (muscle)
Globular	Relatively soluble, part of fluids of all body cells, many food proteins	Enzymes, protein hormones, albumins, globulins (blood), casein (milk), albumin (egg—white)

Contd.

Contd.

Plant		
Glutelins	Insoluble in neutral solutions, soluble in acids and alkalis	Glutenin (wheat) Hordenin (barley) Oryzenin (rice)
Prolamines	Insoluble in water, soluble in alcohol	Gliadin (wheat) Zein (maize)

Table 4.3: Classification of conjugated proteins

Type	*Prosthetic group*	*Examples*
Nucleoproteins	Nucleic acid	DNA combined with protamines RNA combined with ribosomes
Lipoproteins	Lipid	Distinguished by density e.g. LDL (Low density)
Chromoproteins	Coloured group containing a metal	Haemoglobin (blood)
Glycoproteins	Carbohydrate	Some enzymes and hormones Mucins (egg-white)
Phosphoproteins	Phosphate	Casein (milk)

Table 4.4: Molecular weights and isoelectric points of some food proteins

Protein	*Source*	*Molecular weight*	*Isoelectric point*
Casein	Milk	34,000	4.6
Lactoglobulin	Milk	35,000	5.1
Ovalbumin	Eggs	44,000	4.6
Gliadin	Wheat	27,000	6.5
Gluten	Wheat	39,000	4.0
Gelatin	Bones	Variable	4.9
Myosin	Meat	8,50,000	5.4

IMPORTANCE OF PROTEINS

Proteins occupy pride of place and importance in living beings. It can be better appreciated by having a look into plethora of functions that they perform in them (living beings) to realize their significance from nutritional standpoint. There are many proteins stored in the seeds of many plants for their prospective role in the growth of embryonic plant during germination. Prominent among these are glutenin and gliadin of wheat, oryzenin of rice, zein of corn, hordein of barley, phaseolin of beans, legumienin and legumin of peas, arachin of groundnut and amandin of almonds. Proteins of animal origin include ovalbumin of egg white, ovaglobulin of egg yolk and casein of milk. They are also storage proteins for the prospective use of newborn in birds and animals. Human beings are also using them for their nutrition because of their ingenuity and heterotrophic disposition.

In fact, primary function of proteins is tissue building. Proteins are the main solid matter in the muscles, they are also the major constituents of blood, matrix of bones, teeth, skin, nails and hair. Our body, which consists of about 60-62 percent water and 16-18 percent fat, has a structural framework laid by 16 percent proteins and 4 percent minerals in animal tissues. They not only build but also maintain the tissues. For example, proteins are the chief constituents of skin, bones, hair, finger nails, muscles and tendons. Whereas collagen is the protein present in skin, cartilage and bone, keratins' hard and insoluble nature is reflected in the construction of hair, finger nail and feathers. Elastin, another structural protein is present in ligaments.

Apart from structural role, catalysis is another one of the most vital functions of proteins as most of the chemical reactions taking place in cells are catalyzed specifically by highly specialized proteins, the enzymes. So far more than two thousand enzymes, each catalyzing a different chemical reaction, have been discovered in different forms of life.

Living beings' (animals') motility or movement has also been made possible by those proteins that have the ability to contract and to change shape. Actin and myosin are the proteins that make us move our fingers, climb stairs or even blink our eyes. The heart itself is a muscular organ, contracting some 70 to 80 times in a minute, largely because of the ability of its protein to undergo contraction relaxation cycles.

Another aspect of tissue survival and functioning, that is well taken care of by proteins is transport of various nutrients and metabolites to the tissue cells and removal of waste products. For this purpose, they are present in the blood as the transport proteins, e.g., haemoglobin, lipoproteins and transferrin, transporting oxygen carbon-dioxide, lipids and iron respectively. Other proteins, localized in the plasma membranes of the cell, are instrumental in the transport of glucose, amino acids and other nutrients across membrane barriers.

Proteins are also doing a yeomen's service to the body by providing defence or protection against invading micro-organisms and injuries. When foreign substances (microbes or other toxic substances, generally called antigens) gain entry into the body, there is a quick reprisal reflected in the synthesis of certain specific proteins (antibodies or immunoglobulins) to counteract against bacteria, virus or foreign substances. Likewise, other proteins, viz, blood clotting proteins such as prothrombin, fibrinogen and other coagulation factors prevent the loss of blood at the level of a body injury.

To cap it all, some proteins have another distinguishing function to perform, namely regulating many physiological and biochemical activities contributing towards body's health and physiological functioning. These proteins are termed as regulatory proteins. Prominent amongst such proteins are hormones; insulin, glucagon, oxytocin and human growth hormone or somatostatin.

This apart, proteins of blood plasma also play roles in the maintenance of osmotic pressure and water balance by virtue of their colloidal nature, and in the acid base balance by acting as protein buffers. Not to be left behind their macronutrient brethren carbohydrates and fats. Proteins also have the potential to act as energy sources, though they actually do so only when carbohydrates and fats become scarce under conditions of prolonged starvation or other such stress evoking events. This, however, is a costly affair as it amounts to taking proteins away from their vital function and is resorted to only when survival of the organism is at stake for want of energy.

Since our body tissues have a very elaborate and efficient protein synthesizing machinery which require amino acids as the precursor or raw materials or functional units of protein structure, the dietary protein are required by the human body not as such, but as the source of certain (essential) amino acids, as also the source of nitrogen for the synthesis of non-essential amino acids and other nitrogen containing compounds of biologic importance. Incidentally, the human body has the metabolic wherewithal to make twelve amino acids from the carbon and nitrogen sources available in the body and the rest have to be supplied in the diet and hence called essential amino acids. Since they cannot be dispensed with in the diet. However, for the synthesis of protein in the tissues, all the twenty amino acids are needed in right proportion.

That probably is the reason for nature tuning human metabolic clock in such a way that proteins are spared metabolic breakdown to provide energy as long as carbohydrates and fats are abundant in the diet and accessible to metabolizing tissues in the body. The phenomenon is known as *protein sparing action.* Thus eight essential amino acids (Table 4.5) are the hallmark determinants of protein quality and nutrition. Histidine, another amino acid becomes essential in the diet in case of infants and children in growth phase. However, all the essential amino acids should be present in the diet in proportions in which they are required for the synthesis of body proteins in the tissues.

Hence protein quality of a food is defined as the concentration of essential amino acids in it vis-à-vis their concentration in tissue proteins being synthesized. That is the reason for the better nutritional quality of animal proteins, animals being nearer to humans in phylogenetic scale than plants.

Table 4.5: Approximate daily requirement (mg/kg body wt.) for each indispensable (essential) amino acid in adult man

S. No.	*Amino acid*	*Symbol*	*Requirement (mg/kg body wt)*
1.	Isoleucine	Ile (I)	0.70
2.	Leucine	Leu (L)	0.98
3.	Lysine	Lys (K)	0.84
4.	Methionine	Met (M)	0.90†
5.	Phenylalanine	Phe (F)	0.99*
6.	Threonine	Thr (T)	0.50
7.	Tryptophan	Trp (W)	0.24
8.	Valine	Val (V)	0.69
		Total	5.84 (mg/kg body wt)

† About 75 percent of the requirement can be met by cystine.

* About 75 percent of the requirement can be met by tyrosin.

Plant proteins can be upgraded nutritionally by judicious blending of proteins from two or more sources. Since deficiency of one or two essential amino acids (limiting essential amino acids) in one protein source can be made up by their abundance in the other and vice versa. Egg protein is one of the best quality protein and is widely used as a standard for comparison of protein quality from other animal and plant sources. Cereal proteins are mostly deficient in lysine and threonine (Table 4.6); soyabean, a high protein bean, is abundant in lysine but contains very little of methionine. Cotton seed proteins on the other hand, are deficient in lysine and ground nut protein in both methionine and lysine. Potato, never a very good source of protein quantitatively, nevertheless has excellent quality protein matching with the protein quality that of whole egg.

Table 4.6: Limiting amino acids (essential) in grains/proteins

Name	*Limiting amino acids*
Rice	Lysine, Threonine
Wheat	Lysine, Threonine
Corn	Lysine, Tryptophan
Sorghum	Lysine, Threonine
Millet	Lysine, Threonine

FOOD SOURCES OF PROTEIN

Plant foodstuffs are the primary source of proteins (Table 4.7). Plants synthesize proteins combining nitrogen and water from the soil and carbon dioxide from the air. Animals depend on plants to fulfill their essential amino acid requirement for protein synthesis.

Milk, pulses, nuts and oilseeds, meat, eggs, fish and poultry are the main sources of protein in the diet. With plant-based diets prevalent in India, cereals are the major source of protein in the Indian dietaries. In India, cereals are consumed in large quantities and are included in almost all the meals. Therefore, these contribute a large part of the day's need for protein in the Indian dietaries. Secondly, as mentioned earlier, addition of pulses in most of the meals, along with the cereals, results in mutual amino acid supplementation and improvement in the protein quality in the diet. Proteins from leafy vegetables also act excellent supplements to the cereal diet.

Milk is a foodstuff, which is partaken in vegetarian, non-vegetarian menus as well as in feasting and fasting alike. The quantity of milk included depends on the availability and cost. In all, cereals, pulses, milk and milk products contribute most of the proteins in the Indian dietaries. Dry, salted or smoked fish and meat are concentrated sources of protein, especially in the diet of people from coastal regions. Eggs, fish, meat and poultry are other sources of proteins. As a matter of fact, importance of any food as a source of protein depends on how often and how much of it is consumed.

Table 4.7: Protein content of some selected foods

Product	*Protein (g/100 g)*
Egg (hen's)	13.3
Goat meat	21.4
Chicken meat	23.1
Goat liver	20.1
Fish	18.5
Milk (cow's)	3.2
Wheat flour (whole)	12.1
Wheat flour (refined)	11.0
Rice (raw, milled)	6.8
Corn (dry)	11.1
Bread	8.7
Bengal gram (whole)	17.1
Soyabeans (dry, raw)	43.2
Groundnut	25.3
Almond	20.8
Potato	2.0

It is a fact that the type and amount of amino acids in the food proteins in a meal are efficiently utilized if their content and proportions are in keeping with the body's needs. For example, when cereals and pulses are included in the same meal, the essential amino acid content of the combination is more in tune with the body's needs than that of each of these taken individually.

Any additional foods such as products like butter milk, curd, vegetables, fish/meat and soyabean products that may be included in the meal, improve the quality of the protein by virtue of the essential amino acids they supply. Thus including two or more sources of protein in each meal helps in improving the quality of protein and its utilization. Most of the traditional dietary patterns are based on this principle.

In fact, a large part of our heritage and food ethos can be scientifically relied upon and thus needs to be retained; though some aspects may need to be modified in the light of emerging scientific realities and changing times.

STUDY QUESTIONS

1. Write the various foods as sources of proteins.
2. Explain the importance of proteins in the human body.
3. Define the term essential amino acids. Write their names.
4. Write a detailed note on protein classification.
5. What are 'proteins'? How are they classified? What is the special importance of proteins in human nutrition?

CHAPTER 5

Macronutrients: Utilization and Functions

Chapter Outlines

- Introduction
- Carbohydrates
- Lipids
- Proteins
- Study questions

INTRODUCTION

One of the fundamental attributes of life is essentiality for food and nourishment. Organisms, simple as single celled microbes to the most evolved of all the species—humans; have to obtain a supply of raw materials and energy. Whereas raw materials are needed for building up of biosynthetic processes so vital for growth and maintenance; energy is the ingradient required to accomplish biosynthesis as well as other activities, such as muscle contraction, motility and other muscular activities, and osmotic work.

As we look discerningly at the nutritional requirement of different species, it baffles us to find that nutritional requirements of certain micro-organism types and all green plants are simple, in a sharp contrast to higher animals (the term 'higher animals' used throughout this book includes farm animals, laboratory rodents and the human organism, since the basic metabolic machinery is the same in all these species).

A number of bacterial species and green plants only require carbondioxide, water and ammonia and some mineral elements to build the complex molecules. Thus they synthesize the intricate cellular structures to support and sustain life using a remarkable capacity vested in them by nature–the ability to utilize sunlight as a source of energy for this purpose. Such a mode of nourishment is called autotrophic, and organism subscribing to this strategy autotrophs.

However, the higher organisms, or the evolved ones, thrive on autotrophic organisms, utilizing their complex organic substances for obtaining energy and raw materials to sustain vital activities of survival, growth and maintenance. This type of nourishing mode is known as heterotrophic and organisms heterotrophs (most evolved ones devouring the simple, just as big fish eating the small fry is, curiously, the law of nature). As a matter of fact, in the process of evolution, the evolved species had lost the ability to use simple compounds for nourishment, replacing it with requirements for complex mixture of organic compounds. Obviously, simple substances could not be used as the raw materials for biosynthesis, for higher organisms had lost the capacity to extract energy from sunlight.

Liver, being the key player in nutrient processing and metabolism, performs these functions with alacrity and efficiency, funneling nutrients from food for usage or storage in varying proportions dictated by their demand and supply situations. Whereas non fat nutrients, e.g., glucose, amino acids and water soluble vitamins reach liver through the portal vein traversing a shorter distance, the fat (triglycerides) and fat soluble vitamins take to a circuitous route via lymphatic channels emptying into the blood circulation. The latter group being hydrophobic in nature, travels through the blood stream as lipoprotein named chylomicrons. That precisely is the reason why blood plasma acquires a whitish tinge after a fat rich meal. In fact, chylomicrons entering into the blood circulation in abundant amounts impart it a milky appearance.

CARBOHYDRATES

Bulk of the sugar monosaccharides that reach liver after absorption are comprised glucose. Depending upon the starvation or satiety status of the individual, the glucose is channelized into the tissues for satisfying their energy needs of basic house keeping (basal metabolism) and activity or used up for conversion into storage polysaccharide (glycogen) in liver and muscle and energy reserve fat (triglycerides) in adipose tissue. In addition, a part also transformed into the other monosaccharides (ribose and deoxyribose) and their derivatives (glucosamine and glucuronic acid) (Fig. 5.1) for synthesizing biomolecules that make subcellular structures; nucleic acids and mucopolysaccharides respectively. Hence one can say that the major role of carbohydrates is in furnishing energy either for usage or storage. However, apart from this, they also play a major role in the structure building.

Glucose, as the carbohydrate currency of the body, yields energy on being metabolized by glycolytic pathway and tricarboxylic cycle (Fig. 5.2). Energy released in the stepwise oxidation reactions is trapped in the form of high-energy phosphate bond of ATP–the energy currency–by the mitochondrial enzymatic machinery of respiratory chain and oxidative phosphorylation with an efficiency of 40 percent. Rest of the energy gets dissipated steadily serving another function of body temperature maintenance. That is precise the reason why do we feel warm after an hour or two of the carbohydrate rich meal digestion. Glucose remaining in excess after satiating the energy needs of the body tissues is stored as a reserve polysaccharide (glycogen) mainly in the liver and to a lesser extent in the muscle by the process of glycogenesis. The stored glycogen can be ploughed back into the blood, through its conversion into glucose by 'glycogenolysis' during fasting. However, there is a limit to the storage of glycogen by the liver and muscle. The glucose still in excess is converted into fats and stored in the adipose tissue beneath the skin as fat folds and around vital internal organs as fat pads or cushions. All this glucose management takes place under the influence of a number of hormones of which insulin, epinephrine and glucagon are prominent. Whereas insulin promotes the utilization and storage of glucose as energy, glycogen and fat respectively in fed state, the other two (glucagon and epinephrine) work in the direction of glycogen and fat mobilization to fulfil energy needs during fasting and starvation.

Apart from metabolic functions of energy generation and storage, carbohydrates may also play meaningful roles in structure building by providing sugar moieties (groups) to proteins and lipids (glycoproteins and glycolipids) to enable them perform their biological functions. Such

Glucose (The chief sugar)

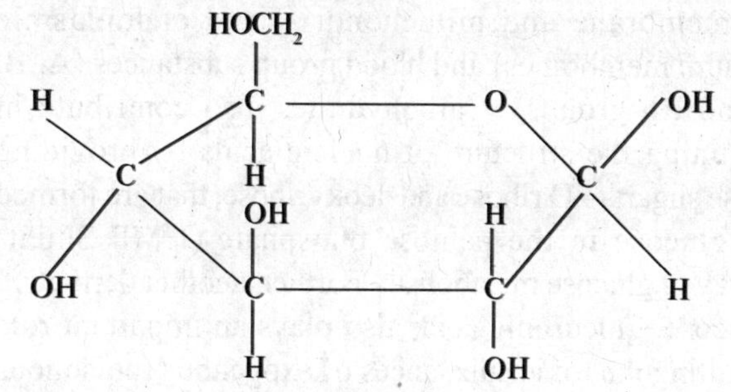

Palmitic acid (A saturated fatty acid)

$CH_3 \cdot CH_2 \cdot CH_2 \cdot CH_2 \cdot CH_2 \cdot CH_2 \cdot CH_2 \cdot CH_2 \cdot CH_2 \cdot CH_2 \cdot CH_2$
$\cdot CH_2 \cdot CH_2 \cdot CH_2 \cdot CH_2 \cdot COOH$

Fig. 5.2: The carbons of glucose are already partially oxidized, but most of those of fatty acid palmitic acid are fully reduced

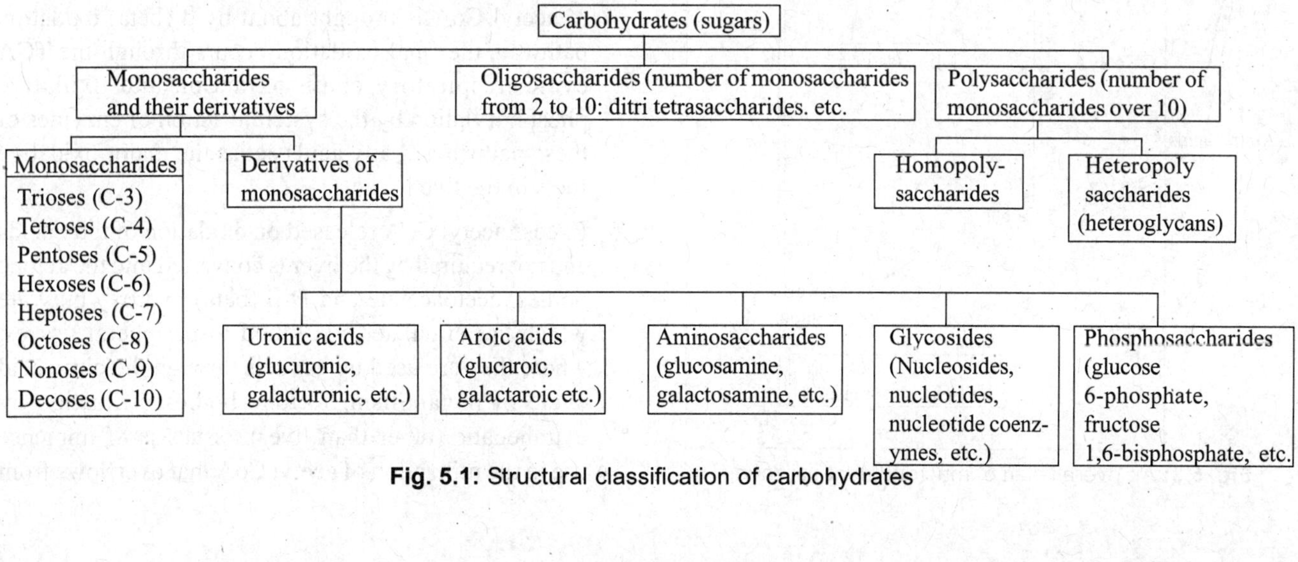

Fig. 5.1: Structural classification of carbohydrates

molecules are present in cellular and subcellular membranes (cell membrane and mitochondrial and endoplasmic reticulum membranes) and blood group substances (A, B, AB and Rh groups). Carbohydrates also contribute in constituting the structure of nucleic acids by providing pentose sugars—D ribose and deoxyribose, that are formed from glucose in the pentose phosphate (HMP Shunt) pathway of glucose metabolism. Further, another derivative of glucose, glucuronic acid, also plays an important role in handling the toxic substances of exogenous (poisonous substances of the environment entering into the body) and endogenous (toxic substances formed within the body) nature by making glucuronide conjugates with them (glucuronides of bilirubin and other toxic substances). Such conjugates have lower toxicity and higher solubility and thus can be easily excreted out of the body through urinary route.

Most of the carbons of a fatty acid are in a fully reduced state. Thus fatty acids can potentially undergo a greater number of oxidative steps of each carbon than can carbohydrates. Thus they are an ideal substance of use as an energy store. Glycogen (a polymer of glucose) is, on the other hand stored as an immediate reserve of blood glucose (Fig. 5.3).

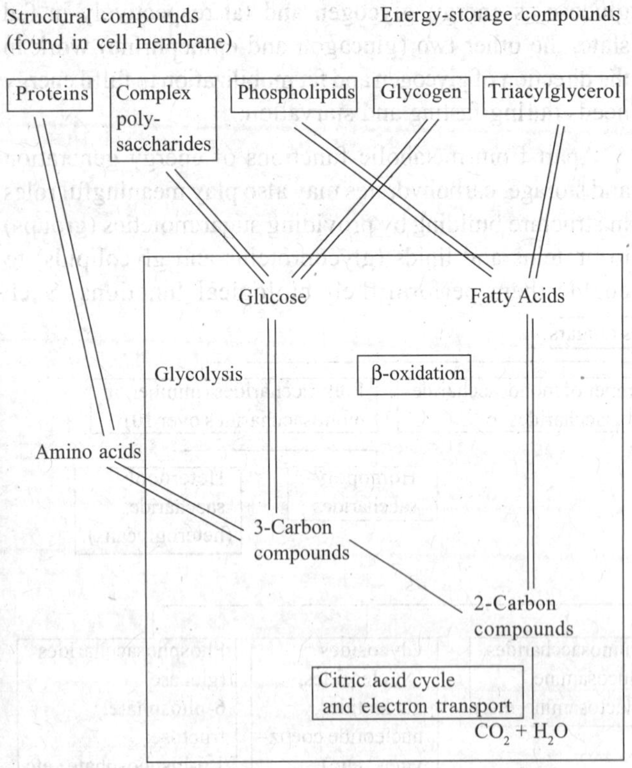

Fig. 5.3: An overall plan of macronutrient utilization

Carbohydrates also exercise supporting functions as structural polysaccharides, as evidenced by the supportive role played by chondroitin sulphate in bone. Besides this certain acidic polysaccharides (hyaluronic acid) also act as lubricating material and thereby protect the cell surface of blood vessels, urinogenital tracts, digestive tract and mucous membranes of the nose, bronchus, trachea and joints and protect them against mechanical damage. Interestingly, certain polysaccharides, like heparin and dermatine sulphate also act as cofactors in anticoagulation (prevention of blood coagulation) and antilipaemic (decrease in the level of blood lipids) processes. That is the reason why heparin and other synthetic heparin like polysaccharides (heparinoids) are used widely as anticoagulants and anti atherosclerotic (preventing blood coagulation and deposition of lipids respectively in the blood vessels) drugs.

LIPIDS

Major functions of lipids are summarized in (Table 5.1).

Intestinal absorption products of dietary lipids, the chylomicrons, enter into venous blood from lymph causing the blood to assume a milky appearance known as absorptive lipaemia. Though most of the lipids of the chylomicrons are made available to the liver and adipose tissue, small parts are also delivered to the lungs, heart and other organs. The fatty acid components of the lipids entering the liver also have five pathways for their metabolic disposal.

1. Free fatty acids are oxidized to yield CO_2 and ATP through intermediate formation of acetyl CoA. Whereas oxidative conversion of activated fatty acid (acyl CoA) to acetyl CoA is brought about by β (beta) oxidation pathway, the final oxidation occurs through the TCA cycle, respiratory chain oxidation and oxidative phosphorylation by the systemic action of enzymes of these pathways. Fatty acids act as the major oxidative fuels in the liver.
2. Excess acetyl CoA released on oxidation of fatty acids and not required by the liver is converted into the ketone bodies, acetoacetate and D-β (beta) hydroxy butyrate which are circulated via blood to peripheral tissues, where they are used up as fuels through the citric acid cycle of metabolism. Ketone bodies utilization by extrahepatic (other than liver) tissues is of immense use in the utilization of acetyl CoA that overflows from

Table 5.1: Main biological functions of lipids

Function	*Characterization of the function*	*Lipids exercising the function*
Substrate-energetic	The oxidation of lipids in the organism is accompanied by a release of energy greater than from other energetic substrates (proteins and carbohydrates). Energy generated by combustion of 1 g of lipid amounts to 39.1 KJ	Acylglycerides, free fatty acids
Structural	Lipids are components of the cell membranes and form a lipid basis thereof	Phospholipids (phosphoglycerides, sphingomyelins), cholesterol and its esters
Transporting	Participation in the transport of materials (for example, cations) across the lipid layer of biomembranes	Phospholipids
Electric insulating	Lipids serve as a specific electro-insulating material in the myelin sheath of nerve tissues	Sphingomyelins, glycosphingolipids
Emulsifying	Amphipathic lipids are emulsifiers. They are located at the oil/water interface surface stabilizing thereby emulsions and preventing their separation into layers	Phosphoglycerides, bile acids (sterols) are emulsifiers of the intestinal acylglycerides. Phosphoglycerides stabilize the solubility of cholesterol in the blood
Mechanical	Protection of internal organs from eventual damage on exposure to mechanical action (lipids of connective integumental tissues of internal organs and lipids of the adipose tissue)	Triacylglycerides
Heat-insulating	Conservation of heat by the lipids of subcutaneous adipose tissue owing to their low heat conduction	Triacylglycerides
Dissolving	Dissolution of certain lipid materials in other lipids under physiological conditions	Bile acids (sterols) are solvents for fat-soluble vitamins in the intestine
Hormonal	Regulation of a large variety of physiological functions with the involvement of steroid hormones (lipids) and prostaglandins (hormone-like lipids)	Steroids (sex hormones, corticosteroids). Derivatives of unsaturated fatty acids
Vitaminogenic	Special function with the participation of fat-soluble vitamins	Isoprenoids, unsaturated fatty acids

the liver. They can supply a good part of the energy to the peripheral (other than liver) tissues as in the case of heart muscle, they supply as much as 30 percent of the total energy requirements.

3. Biosynthesis of cholesterol and bile salts occurs when some of acetyl CoA derived from fatty acids is also used up for making cholesterol, a part of which is converted into bile salts.

4. Fatty acids are also used as the main starting material for the synthesis of the lipid part of the plasma lipoproteins, which carry lipids in adipose and fat tissue for storage as triglycerides.

5. Some fatty acids become complexed with serum albumin and are carried via blood to the heart and skeletal muscle, which consume a significant amount of them to satisfy their fuel requirements.

In a nutshell, liver tissue is a small sophisticated laboratory, where a number of different processes occur depending upon the nutritional and physiological states of the individuals, the body's specific requirements in such states being signalled by hormones and enzymes that regulate the lipid metabolic processes.

An overall look on the functioning of liver reveals that fat (triglycerides) is synthesized in liver from fatty acids and the process is known as lipogenesis. These are normally transported out of the liver by the lipoproteins (VLDL), which carry them to adipose tissue for storage. Lipogenesis and subsequent storage are triggered by lipotropic factors such as choline and methionine, thereby preventing excessive accumulation of fat in the liver.

However, this is not to say that lipolysis (breakdown of fat) doesn't occur in liver. Since reactions associated with triglycerides turn over are reversible and occur in the direction that is dictated by the fuel needs of the individual at a particular time. If there is an over supply of fat to the liver it will be converted into transport and storage forms by lipogenesis. If energy needs of the person require fat fuels, lipolysis will occur to furnish products of fat (as indicated in the preceding paragraphs explaining lipid utilization).

Adipose tissue, on its part, coordinates closely with liver. It is in essence, a reserve of stored energy and is located not only under the skin but also in the abdominal cavity around vital organs. Stored forms of lipids in the adipose tissue are triglycerides (fat). However adipose tissue is not an inert store but metabolically dynamic one. Fat cells (adipocytes) of adipose tissue contain both lipogenic and lipolytic enzymes, whereas the former are active (in response to insulin) when energy intake exceeds energy usage to take the pendulum of metabolism towards lipogenesis and the latter are activated (mediated by epinephrine, glucagon etc.) when organism is in negative energy balance and the pendulum swings towards lipolysis.

PROTEINS

Liver, being the major nutrient distribution tissue in humans, receives and processes the amino acids brought to it by the portal vein and thereafter channelizes these to the other tissues. This is an arduous job as the liver has to contend with sharp fluctuations in the supply of amino acids in consonance with the quantity and frequency of meals.

However, the stoic liver lives up to its importance as the supreme metabolic organ by keeping the amino acids levels of various tissues in dynamic equilibrium. This is made possible by the ability of hepatic tissue to funnel amino acids through five metabolic routes in varying proportions depending upon the physiologic and life span conditions of the body. Firstly and most importantly, amino acids pass from liver into the systemic blood and therefrom to the various tissues for utilization as building blocks in the biosynthesis of tissue proteins.

Secondly, liver keeps constantly renewing its own intrinsic proteins (mostly enzymes of a number of metabolic pathways operating in liver) as almost all of them have a very high turnover rate and a short half life. Besides this, the liver is a major site of synthesis for most of the proteins present in blood plasma.

The third major channel of amino acid utilization is the deamination and degradation of the amino acids not used up in protein biosynthesis, to yield TCA cycle intermediates for energy generation.

In addition to these three major routes, the liver also participates in the metabolism of amino acid alanine, which it gets from skeletal muscle via blood. Alanine is deaminated into pyruvate and subsequently converted into glucose via gluconeogenesis. The same glucose may return to skeletal muscle in a bid to replenish its glycogen content (glucose-alanine or cori cycle). The main purpose of such cyclic interplay is to smoothen out fluctuations in blood glucose level in the periods intervening between two meals.

Lastly, small amount of amino acids is also utilized in the biosynthesis of purine and pyrimidine nitrogenous rings of nucleic acids (nucleotides constituting DNA and RNA), and other important specialized products like porphyrine (heme) and hormones (epinephrine, norepinephrine etc).

Synthesis of new protein molecules by the body cells is a hallmark of life. Each cell synthesizes only those proteins that are needed by it and that too in amounts in which they are needed, though biosynthesis of a far larger number of protein types is possible. Hence the concept of cellular economy, though true for every living form, be it a bacterium or bat, is highly manifested in human organism—the most evolved one of all species. As a matter of fact, behind all this need-supply synchronization lies the fine tuning of cellular chemical activities dictated by a meticulously programmed expression of genes that lie unassumingly within the chromosomes inside every cell nucleus. Table 5.2 summarizes the functions performed by proteins in the body.

Table 5.2: Biological functions of proteins

Protein function	*Characterization of protein function*	*Illustrative proteins exercising the function*
Enzymatic or catalytic	A most essential protein function exercising acceleration of chemical conversion (synthesis and degradation of materials; transfer of electrons, atoms and molecules from one compound to another)	*Fumarate hydratase:* Catalyzes the reversible conversion fumarate + $H_2O \leftrightarrow$ malate. *Cytochrome oxidase:* Participates in the transfer of electrons onto oxygen.
Hormonal or regulatory	Regulation of intracellular metabolism and integration of cellular metabolism throughout the whole organism	*Insulin:* Participates in the regulation of metabolic processes involving carbohydrates, proteins, fats and other materials. *Lutropin:* Participates in the regulation of progesterone synthesis in the corpus luteum.
Receptory	Selective binding of various regulators (hormones, mediators and cyclic nucleotides) on the surface of cell membranes or inside the cells (cytosolic receptors)	Cytosolic receptor of estradiol: Binds estradiol inside the cells, for example, those of endometrium. *Glucagon receptor:* Binds the hormone glucagon on the surface of a cell membrane, for example, that of liver. *Regulatory subunit of protein kinase:* Binds cAMP inside the cells.
Transport	Binding and transport of materials between tissues and through the cell membranes	*Lipoproteins:* Responsible for the transport and distribution of lipids in the organism tissues. *Transcortin:* Responsible for the transport of corticosteroids (hormones secreted by the adrenal cortex into the blood). *Myoglobin:* Responsible for the transport of oxygen in muscle tissues.
Structural	Involvement in the buildup of various membranes	*Structural proteins* of mitochondria, cytoplasmic membranes etc.
Supportive or mechanical	Functionally close to the structural function. Provide for the strength of supporting tissues and intervene in the formation of extracellular structures	*Collagen*, as a structural element of supporting framework of osseous tissues and tendons. *Fibroin*: Intervenes in the formation of silkworm cocoon capsule. *β-Keratin:* Structural basis for wool, nail and hoof.
Reserve or trophic	Utilization of proteins as reserve material for nutrition of developing cells	*Prolamines and glutelins:* As reserve material in wheat grains. *Ovalbumin:* As reserve protein of hen's egg (consumed in developmental growth of foetus).
Substrato-energetic	Functionally close to the trophic function. Protein is used as a substrate (in degradation) for energy supply. On degradation, 1 g of protein releases 17.1 kJ of energy	All proteins (dietary or intracellular): Decompose to end products (CO_2, H_2O, urea).
Mechano-chemical, or contractile	Contraction (mechanical process), by making use of chemical energy	*Myosin*: Fixed filaments in myofibrils. *Action:* Movable filaments in myofibrils.
Electroosmotic	Involvement in the buildup of electric charge, difference in electrochemical gradient and ion concentration gradient across the cell membrane	*Na^+, K^- AT Pase:* An enzyme mediating in the buildup of Na^+ and K^+ ion concentration gradient and electrochemical gradient across the cell membrane.

Contd.

Contd.

Energy converting	Conversion of electric and osmotic energy to chemical energy	*ATP-synthetase:* Performs the synthesis of ATP owing to the electric potential difference or ion osmotic concentration gradient across inner mitochondrial membrane.
Cogenetic	Auxiliary genetic function of proteins (the latin prefix 'co' implies a cooperative action). The proteins themselves are not genetic (hereditary) material, but assist the nucleic acids in the accomplishment of self-reproduction and genetic information transfer	*DNA-polymerase:* An enzyme participating in the replication of DNA. *DNA-dependent RNA-polymerase:* An enzyme involved in the information transfer from DNA to RNA.
Gene-regulatory	Ability of certain proteins to participate in the regulation of template functions of nucleic acids and genetic information transfer	*Histones:* Proteins participating in the regulation of replication and partly in the transcription of certain portion of DNA. *Acidic proteins:* Participate the regulation of transcription of certain portions of DNA.
Immunological or antitoxic	Antibodies participate in the defence reaction against foreign antigens of microorganism (toxins produced by them) via formation of antigen-antibody complexes	Immunoglobulins IgA, IgM, IgG etc. perform defense functions. *Complement:* A complex series of proteins that interact to combine with antigen-antibody complex.
Toxigenic	Certain proteins and peptides produced by organisms (primarily, by microorganisms) are poisonous for other living organisms	*Botulinum toxin:* A peptide secreted by botulism causing bacteria.
Detoxicating	Proteins, owing to their functional groups, are capable of binding toxic compounds (heavy metal ions and alkaloids) rendering them harmless	*Albumins:* Binding agents in heavy metal ions and alkaloids.
Hemostatic	Participation in thrombosis and arrest of bleeding (homeostasis)	*Fibrinogen:* A protein of blood serum, polymerizable area network (structural basis for thrombus formation).

STUDY QUESTIONS

1. How do carbohydrates play a key role in furnishing energy to the body tissues?
2. Give a brief description of lipid functions. Why do we call lipids as the concentrated and stored source of energy?
3. Evaluate critically the functional properties of proteins that make them occupy the first place in living entities.
4. Explain briefly how macronutrients are utilized in human body.
5. What functions—other than energy yielding—do carbohydrates and lipids perform? Explain briefly.

CHAPTER 6

Micronutrients: Vitamins and Minerals

Chapter Outlines

- Discovery of Vitamins
- Water soluble vitamins as coenzymes
- Thiamine
- Riboflavin
- Nicotinic acid (Niacin)
- Pyridoxine
- Biotin
- Folic acid
- Cyanocobalamin (B_{12})
- Vitamin C (L-ascorbic acid)
- Preserving vitamins in food
- Life, an organized state of elements
- Minerals and trace metals
- Other trace metals
- Study questions

Vitamins and minerals are essential for good nutrition as it was found that animals maintained on diets containing sufficient carbohydrates, fats and proteins and provided with an ample water supply couldn't survive. They also needed the essential organic components, called vitamins and inorganic ions, called minerals.

DISCOVERY OF VITAMINS

The name "vitamin" comes from a mistaken generalization. Casimir Funk (1884-1967) discovered that certain diseases such as beriberi, scurvy and pellagra are caused by lack of certain nutrients. He found that the 'anti-beriberi factor' compound is an amine and mistakenly thought that all such nutrients are amines. Hence he coined the term 'Vitamine'. It was later changed to 'vitamin' by Sir Jack Drummand.

Vitamins are thus organic compounds that are needed in trace amounts by the body and perform one or more essential metabolic functions. They must be provided in the diet, for human body cannot synthesize them. Much of the understanding of the role of vitamins in the physiologic functioning of the animals, including human beings, has come from the study of deficiency diseases.

Vitamins have been classified according to their solubility in water or fats. Obviously, solubility affects a number of characteristics: distribution in foods, absorption, metabolism, excretion, and even toxicity. The fat soluble vitamins (A, D, E and K) are all absorbed into the body in the same manner as fat from the intestine, requiring bile. Any factor or condition that affects bile secretion or the absorption of fats, influences the absorption of these vitamins. Unlike water soluble vitamins, the human body tends to retain fat soluble vitamins more readily. That explains the potential toxicity of excessive fat soluble vitamins as their high concentrations in tissues hampers normal tissue functioning.

Vitamin A

Vitamin A or retinol is present in some animal foods like butter and ghee, whole milk, curds, egg yolk, liver etc. The liver oils of certain fish like cod, halibut and shark and saw fish are some of the richest known natural sources of the vitamin. Vitamin A is not present as retinol in vegetable foods. These foods contain yellow pigments called carotenes which are converted into vitamin A in the body.

Carotenes are therefore termed provitamin A. Since these pigments were isolated from carrots, they are called carotenes. There are different types of carotenes, α, β and γ. Of these β-carotene has such a chemical structure that on a unit weight basis it can yield equal amount of vitamin A. But when β-carotene is converted into retinol in the body, the efficiency of conversion is less, i.e., 1 µg of carotene yielding only 0.5 µg of retinol. However, other carotenes yield even less amount of vitamin A. Further, while preformed vitamin A is completely absorbed, carotene present in vegetable foods is not completely absorbed. For practical purpose only about fifty percent of β-carotene in foods is considered to be absorbed. The rich source of β-carotene is green leafy vegetables, spinach, amaranth, coriander, drum-stick leaves, curry leaves, mint, raddish leaves etc. Ripe yellow fruits such as mango, papaya and tomato are also rich in carotene. Among other vegetables, carrots and yellow pumpkin are good sources. It can be said that in general the greener the leafy vegetables, higher the content of carotene, and thus the outer green leaves of cabbage have more carotene than inner white leaves. Most of the Indian diets have β-carotene as the main source of vitamin A. The availability of β-carotene from these diets vary from 25-50%, depending on the fat content of the diet. Thus taking into consideration the physiological conversion of β-carotene to retinol and the absorption of β-carotene, one unit of β-carotene in food is assumed to yield only 0.25 units of retinol. The requirement of β-carotene will be therefore 4 times the requirement of retinol or vitamin A (Fig. 6.1).

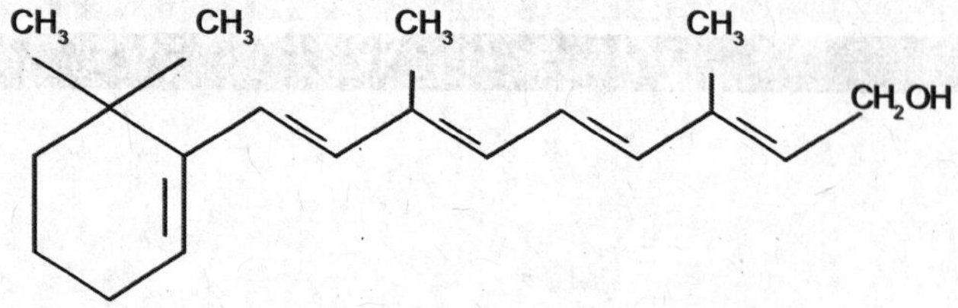

Fig. 6.1: Retinol

A well understood function of retinol is in the visual process. Vitamin A is necessary for clear vision in dim light. Lack of vitamin A thus leads to night blindness (Fig. 6.2). *Another function of vitamin A is to maintain the integrity of epithelial tissues. For example, in the absence of adequate vitamin A intake, the outer lining of the eye ball loses its usual moist white appearance and becomes dry and wrinkled. Redness and inflammation of the eye and gradual loss of vision may follow.* The central portion of eye (cornea) may lose its transparency and become opaque and soft and if not treated may lead to total blindness. Its function in vision and eye is well understood but not its other functions. Although its function in growth and in maintaining the integrity of other epithelial tissues is known the manner in which these functions operate is not understood clearly. Recently, it has become known that vitamin A also helps in the cellular differentiation of epithelial tissue. Provitamin, β-carotene acts as an antioxidant and offers protection against atherosclerosis and certain types of cancer.

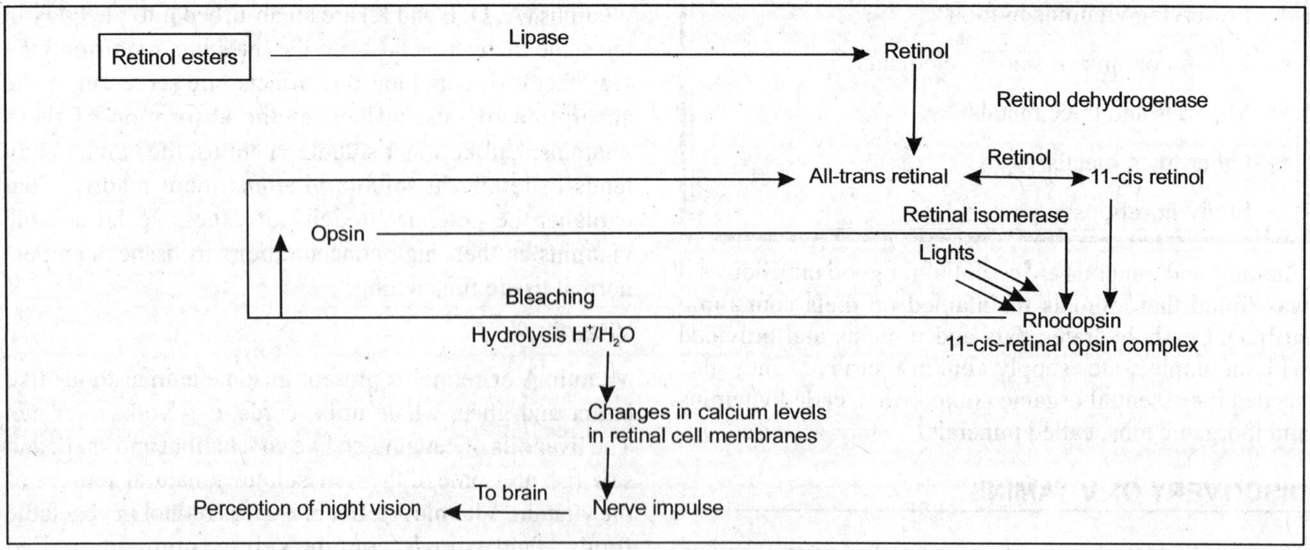

Fig. 6.2: Role of vitamin A in visual cycle

The daily requirement of vitamin A for an adult is estimated to be in the neighbourhood of 750 μg (or about 2500 IU) of vitamin A. This amount of retinol or vitamin A can be derived from vegetable foods in the form of β-carotene. To derive the same amount of vitamin A, i.e., 750 μg, β-carotene intake should be about 3000 μg taking into account the efficiency of conversion of β-carotene to retinol (which is only 50%) and its absorption from vegetable sources (which is about 50%). The requirement of vitamin A is greater during pregnancy, lactation and during growth. Animal foods rich in vitamin A (retinol) are expensive and hence the most inexpensive and convenient way of ensuring adequate intake of vitamin A is to include green leafy vegetables (GLV) in the daily diet. About 50 g of the common leafy vegetables like amaranth will provide adequate β-carotene to meet the vitamin A requirement of an adult. Preschool children upto 6 years may have to take daily about 20 g of GLV. But in the case of infants and very young children, who cannot eat and digest leafy vegetables, can be given carotene rich fruits like papaya, mangoes (50-100 g) or animal foods like milk, liver, egg etc. Vitamin A can also be given in the form of a dose of cod or shark liver oil and medicinal concentrates derived from such oils or synthetic vitamin A.

Intake of large amount of vitamin A for prolonged periods can lead to toxic symptoms which include irritability, headache, nausea and characteristic forceful vomiting. The symptoms subside on stoppage of the intake.

Vitamin D

It is chemically stable vitamin and is often present in two primary biologically active forms. Ergocalciferol, the first form, is derived from irradiation of a plant precursor (Ergosterol D_2), and cholecalciferol (D_3) from irradiation of 7-dehydrocholesterol found in the skin of animals. Vitamin D_2 (Ergocalciferol) is also metabolized to its biologically active form exactly like vitamin D_3 (Cholecalciferol) (Fig. 6.3).

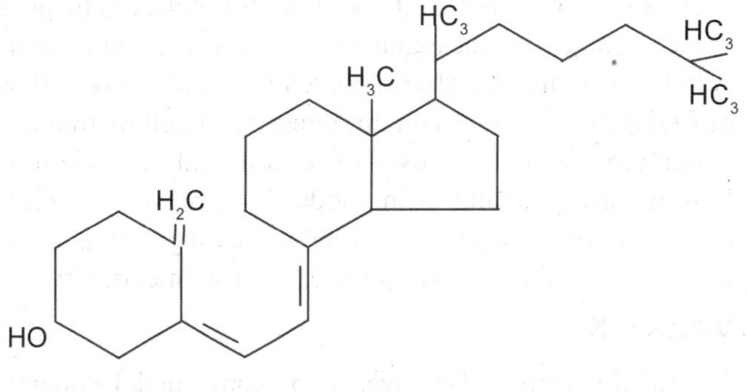

Fig. 6.3: Vitamin D_3 (cholecalciferol)

Animal food sources of vitamin D include cod liver oil, cheese and eggs. Alternatively, the exposure to sun also converts precursor form of this vitamin into active form or D_3. Major circulating form of vitamin D is 25-hydroxy D_3 and this hydroxylation takes place in liver microsomes. The physiologically active form is obtained by its second hydroxylation into 1-α, 25-dihydroxy D_3 by the kidney mitochondria. This metabolite acts like a hormone derepressing the gene for calcium binding protein in the intestinal mucosal cells. Active form of vitamin D (1–α, 25–$(OH)_2$ D_3) serves chiefly to maintain optimum blood levels of calcium and phosphorus by acting at three levels, viz intestine, bone and kidney. Parathyroid hormone closely cooperates in this process.

Vitamin D is required for bone growth and calcium metabolism. Lack of vitamin D leads to rickets and osteomalacia. As vitamin D plays an important role in the absorption of dietary calcium from the intestine and its deposition in bone, gross deformities of bone may, therefore, result if enough vitamin D is not available to the body.

Osteomalacia manifests itself initially as pain in bones, usually starts during pregnancy when the demand for Ca is raised to meet the increased need of the growing foetus in the womb. After the child birth, the disease may regress but it may recur in a more severe form in the subsequent pregnancies. Ultimately, the bone of the victim may become so bent that the woman is unable to stand upright and the distortion of the pelvis may cause child birth very difficult. A good supply of vitamin D during pregnancy benefits the mother and helps satisfactory development of the infant. Vitamin D requirement of children is placed between 200-400 IU. This requirement may be obtained in great measure in tropical countries through exposure to adequate sunlight. Since vitamin D cannot be easily obtained through diets by majority of Indians who can obtain it through exposure to sunlight, the recent Expert Group of ICMR has not recommended dietary intake of vitamin D for Indians. Only in those cases where vitamin D requirement is not met through adequate exposure to sunlight or due to metabolic or genetic reasons, therapeutic supplementation of vitamin D may be necessary. One gm of pure vitamin D is equivalent to 40 million IU, i.e. (400 IU =10 μg) of the vitamin. Approximate daily allowance for adults is 10 μg.

As in the case of vitamin A, intake of excessive amounts of vitamin D can also lead to toxic symptoms, which include irritability, nausea, vomiting and constipation. The margin of safety for vitamin D appears to be much smaller than that for vitamin A. Cases of toxicity as children have been reported vitamin D toxicity even with prolonged daily intakes of a dose as low as 1000 IU (Fig. 6.4).

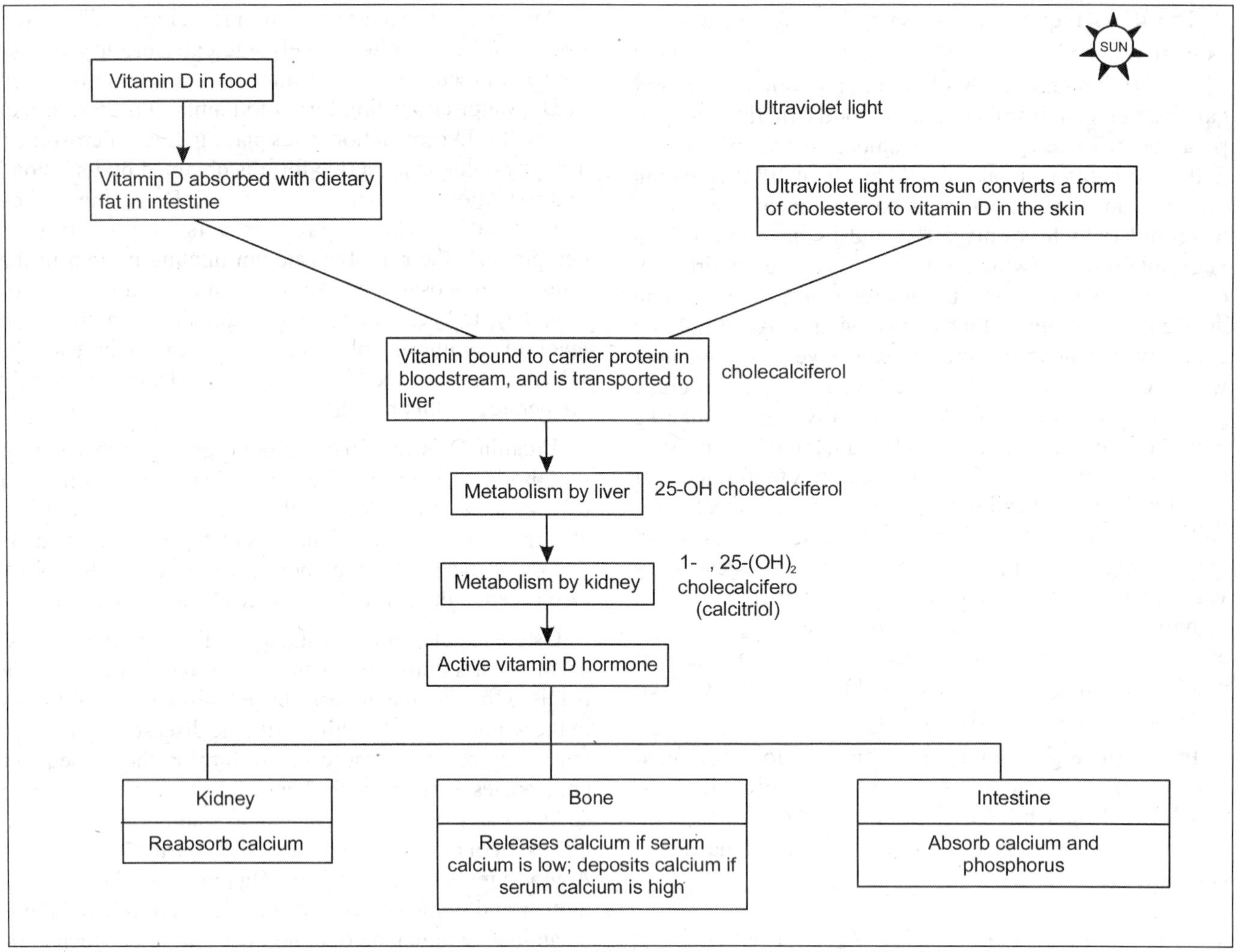

Fig. 6.4: Summary of vitamin D metabolism and functioning (It acts more like a hormone)

Vitamin E

Vitamin E is the general term used to denote a group of closely related lipid soluble chemical compounds, the tocopherols and tocotrienols, that possess varying degree of vitamin activity. α-tocopherol is most active of all these compounds.

The best known function of vitamin E is its antioxidant activity. Vitamin E reacts with compounds that have an unpaired electron. They are, therefore, highly reactive as oxidizing agents. Such compounds are known as free radicals. By reacting with them, vitamin E prevents the radicals from oxidizing polyunsaturated fats, vitamin A, various enzymes, and cell membrane constituents. Thus by preventing oxidative damage, vitamin E increases the stability of cellular and intracellular structures, especially membranes. By preventing free radical activity, vitamin E is also thought to retard the ageing process as free radicals are also believed to participate in the formation of ageing pigments which may contribute to the ageing process in various tissues. It, therefore, plays an all important role of a protective antioxidant. Vitamin E is readily available from dietary sources such a spinach, potatoes, vegetable oils and nuts. The only known deficiency condition is hemolytic anemia in premature infants. Vitamin E is believed to have a role in preventing the oxidation of β-carotene and vitamin A in the intestine and also in preventing lipid peroxidation of PUFA in cells and maintain integrity of cell membrane which are largely composed of unsaturated fats. Vitamin E is widely distributed in foods. It is present in high concentration in vegetable oils and in cereal grains. Human requirement of vitamin E is not known with certainty.

Vitamin K

Vitamin K is a group of relatively stable compounds belonging to the chemical family of substances called quinones. Vitamin

K (Phylloquinone) is the only form synthesized by plants. About half of the amount of vitamin K in the body is in the form of K_2 (Menaquinone) synthesized by intestinal bacteria. Dietary sources like spinach, potatoes, cauliflower and liver supply the rest. Primary function of vitamin K is to act as a factor for the enzyme involved in the synthesis of proteins essential to blood clotting, namely coagulation factor II (Prothrombin), VII (Pro convertine), IX (Christmas factor) and (Stuart Rower factor) (Fig. 6.5).

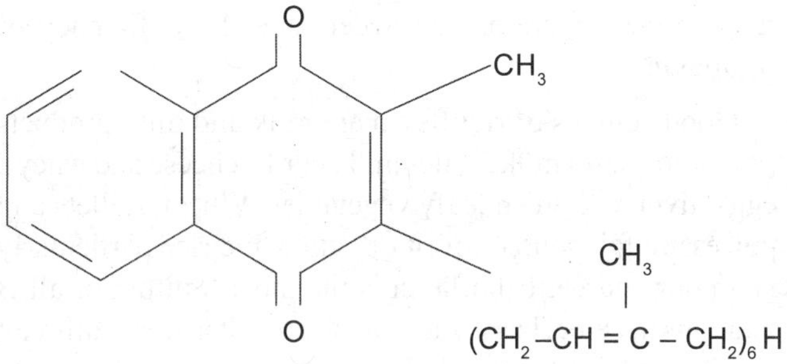

Fig. 6.5: Phylloquinone (Vitamin K)

Vitamin K acts as a cofactor in the carboxylation of glutamic acid residues in these proteins.

WATER SOLUBLE VITAMINS AS COENZYMES

Coenzymes are molecules that cooperate in the catalytic action of an enzyme. A coenzyme may be tightly bound to the protein or it may in other cases be free to diffuse away from the enzyme, acting essentially as an additional substrate (e.g., NAD^+ in many dehydrogenase reaction). If tightly bound to the enzyme, it may sometimes be referred to as a prosthetic group. The term cofactor refers rather non-specifically to the various materials required for full enzyme activity, including cations (e.g., Zn^{2+} or Mg^{2+}).

Water-soluble vitamins function as coenzymes, or as components of coenzyme molecules.

THIAMINE (Fig. 6.6)

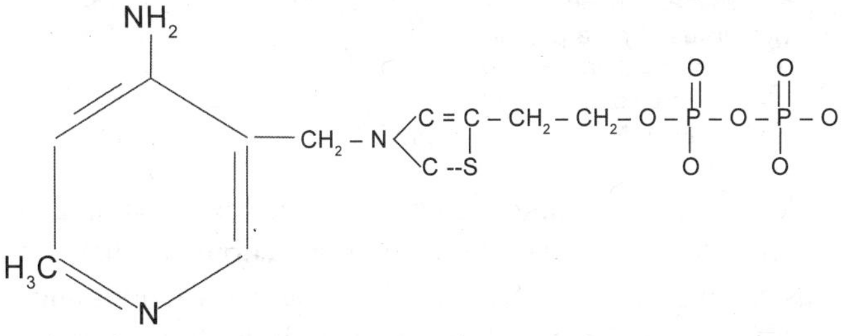

Fig. 6.6: Thiamine pyrophosphate (Vitamin B_1)

Vitamin B_1 or 'thiamine', as it is most commonly referred to, is the first of the vitamins to be discovered. It was also known formerly as the 'anti beriberi' or 'anti neuritic' vitamin. Prolonged deficiency of thiamine in the diet is one of the main factors leading to the disease beriberi which may manifest in one of the two forms. In the 'dry beriberi', there is a loss of appetite, tingling and numbness in the legs and hands and a dropping of the feet. In 'wet beriberi', on the other hand, there is dropsy, palpitation and breathlessness and weakness of heart muscle leading to heart failure. Thiamine is concerned in the proper utilization of carbohydrates in the body and in the absence of adequate amount of thiamine, full utilization of sugars and starches for meeting the energy needs is adversely affected.

The richest source of thiamine is yeast and the outer layers of cereals like rice, wheat and millets. The commonly consumed food which contain a high level of thiamine are unmilled cereals, pulses and nuts, particularly groundnut. Fruits, vegetables and animal foods like meat, fish, eggs and milk are poor sources of this vitamin. It would appear in general that foods which contain carbohydrates as a major source of energy contain a higher level of thiamine which is required for the metabolism of carbohydrates. In typical diets consumed in India, cereals contribute a major portion of daily thiamine intake and hence the need for using whole cereals rather than highly polished cereals like rice. Removal of the outer bran layers of grain results in removal of thiamine and therefore diets largely based on highly milled raw rice contain insufficient thiamine and can cause beriberi.

This disease used to be common in certain parts of India particularly in costal districts of Andhra Pradesh since diets consumed in these areas used to consist mainly of highly polished rice. In recent years, however, the incidence of this disease has declined presumably due to use of less polished rice and diversification of diets consumed. Now-a-days, the government has restricted through legislative act the extent of polishing of rice during milling.

Thiamine requirement of an individual depends upon a number of factors among which the composition of diet is one. Since thiamine is essentially concerned in the utilization of carbohydrates, the need for thiamine increases when the proportion of carbohydrates in the diet is high as in the case of Indian diets. Conversely, the presence of fat in the diet reduces the need for the vitamin and hence fat is said to have thiamine sparing action.

Thiamine requirements are closely related to energy intake and hence its requirement is usually expressed in terms of energy intake and it is about 0.5 mg of the vitamins per 1000 kilo calories. Whenever thiamine requirements of certain groups like infants and children are not directly determined experimentally, they are computed on the basis of their calorie needs. Daily thiamine requirement ranges between 0.5-2.0 mg/day depending upon age, physiological status and level of daily physical activity. It is not difficult to plan a diet containing enough thiamine. Diets based on whole wheat, any of the millets, raw hand pounded rice or parboiled rice (hand pounded) usually supply adequate amounts of thiamine. The greatest danger of thiamine deficiency arises when highly milled (polished) raw rice is consumed as the main component of a diet with practically negligible amounts of other thiamine rich foods like pulses. Inclusion of pulses in the diet can improve the thiamine content of this diet. The greater the proportion of energy derived from cereals, the more important it becomes to avoid preponderance of milled raw rice in diets. An easy and effective means of preventing thiamine deficiency is to have recourse either to parboiled rice or under milled raw rice or partial replacement of milled raw rice by wheat or any of the millets to the extent of about 100 g/day. This can also be achieved by including 60-70 g pulse in the diet based exclusively on raw milled product.

RIBOFLAVIN (Fig. 6.7)

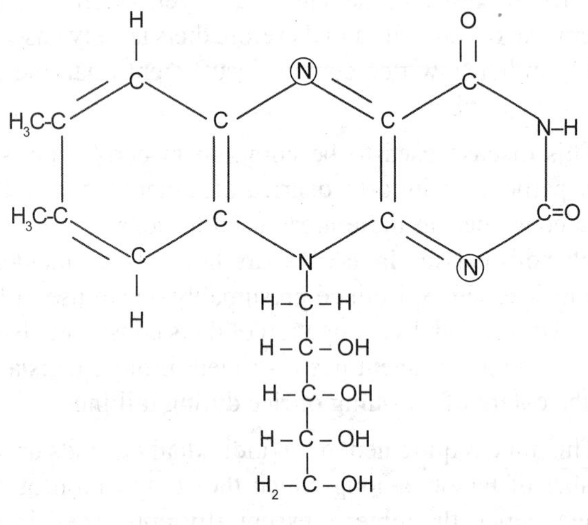

Fig. 6.7

Riboflavin, as part of a coenzyme, is essential for several oxidation processes inside the cell and is concerned with energy and protein metabolism. Some of the clinical symptoms attributed to inadequate intake of this vitamin in the diet are the soreness of tongue (glossitis), cracking at the angles of the mouth (angular stomatitis), redness of the eye and burning sensation in the eyes, scaliness of the skin in the region between the nose and angles of the lips (seborrheic dermatitis). Scrotal dermatitis can also be a result of riboflavin deficiency. Recent studies indicate that psychomotor development in children may be impaired in riboflavin deficiency. Among the several B-complex vitamins, riboflavin deficiency is the most widespread, particularly among children and women in our country. Recent studies indicate that common infections like respiratory infections can accentuate the deficiency of riboflavin.

Good sources of riboflavin are milk and milk products (including skim milk, butter milk, curds, cheese and whey), eggs, liver and green leafy vegetables. Wheat, millets and pulses are fair sources of riboflavin while rice particularly is a poor source. Riboflavin is the most limiting of all B vitamins in cereal based diets of the poor. It is rather difficult to ensure adequate supply of this vitamin in a predominantly vegetarian diet. Inclusion of milk, greens and pulses in a cereal diet will improve the dietary supply of this vitamin.

Dietary requirement of this vitamin has been established in recent years. Its requirement is also related to energy intake, it being about 0.6 mg per 1000 kilo calories. The daily safe requirement of this vitamin ranges from 0.7 to 2.2 mg/day depending upon age, physiological status and level of activity. There is good evidence that poor Indian diets which contain little milk are generally deficient in riboflavin.

NICOTINIC ACID (NIACIN) (Fig. 6.8)

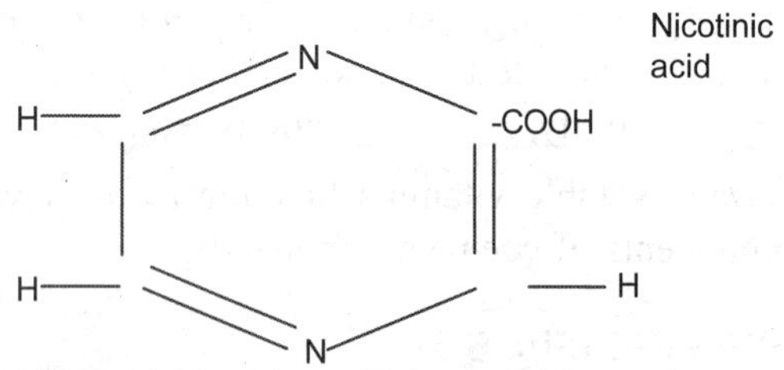

Nicotinic acid (niacin) is a vitamin used as a precursor of the nicotinamide moiety of the nicotinamide nucleotides - NAD^+ and $NADP^+$

Fig. 6.8

Nicotinic acid (also called niacin) is a vitamin intimately connected with several metabolic reactions. It takes part as a component of coenzyme in oxidative reactions and is concerned with metabolism of carbohydrate, fats and proteins. This vitamin can be formed in the body from the amino acid tryptophan, which is present in all dietary proteins. Part of the dietary tryptophan is converted into niacin. Sixty mg of this amino acid can give rise to 1 mg of nicotinic acid in the body. Hence body requirement of this vitamin is met partly from the vitamin present in foods and partly by conversion from tryptophan present in dietary proteins. Hence in the assessment of requirement of this vitamin, the contribution from both is to be considered. Similarly, in the assessment of content of diets, both are considered and total niacin content are expressed in terms of niacin equivalents (mg) which is

$$(\text{Niacin content} + \frac{1}{60}\ \text{Tryptophan content}).$$

Since this vitamin takes part in many reactions of energy metabolism, its requirement has also been related to energy requirement. The safe level of this vitamin has been estimated as 6.6 mg niacin equivalents per 1000 kcal. The daily requirement of this vitamin varies from 8-26 mg niacin equivalents for various physiological activity groups.

Lack of this vitamin in the diet leads to the disease pellagra, which is characterized by soreness of tongue, pigmented skin and diarrhea. The dermatitis appears most often over areas of skin which is exposed to sun such as the back of hands and feet and symmetrically distributed. Although pellagra is essentially due to deficiency of nicotinic acid, in some countries of southern part of America (USA) and Mexico where some population groups used to consume maize as the main cereal with no other supplement, pellagra was commonly seen because maize is a poor source of both nicotinic acid and tryptophan. Further, a part of nicotinic acid present in maize is in a bound form and not physiologically available. In Southern Peninsula of India, pellagra has been observed in areas where jowar (sorghum vulgarae) is the main cereal consumed. Pellagra in these areas is seen among the poor who eat mostly sorghum based diet without much protective foods. Pellagra among jowar eaters is attributed to the presence of excessive amounts of the amino acid leucine in the protein of jowar and to the resultant imbalance between leucine and the other related amino acids, particularly isoleucine. Such an imbalance has been shown to interfere with the conversion of tryptophan to nicotinic acid in the body thus causing a deficiency of nicotinic acid.

Whole cereals, pulses, nuts and meat are good sources of nicotinic acid. Groundnut is particularly rich in nicotinic acid. Although poor in nicotinic acid milk is also effective in preventing pellagra because it is rich in tryptophan.

PYRIDOXINE (Fig. 6.9)

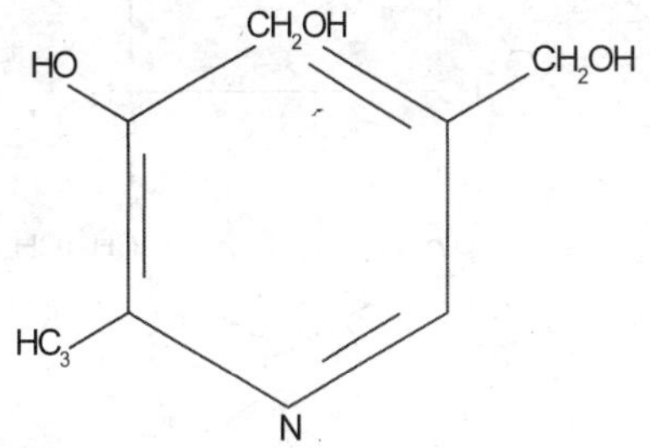

Fig. 6.9: Pyridoxine (Vitamin B_6)

This vitamin also known earlier as vitamin B_6 exists in three forms–pyridoxal, pyridoxamine and pyridoxine. These are interchangeable in the body.

Some of the important functions of vitamin B_6 in the body are the metabolism of proteins and fats. Pyridoxal phosphate, the coenzyme form of this vitamin is required for the metabolism of amino acids and conversion of tryptophan to nicotinic acid. It is also associated with the metabolism of essential fatty acids. Although the need for the vitamins in humans is clearly established, clinical symptoms of B_6 deficiency have not been clearly defined. Some types of angular stomatitis (cracking at the corners of the lips) and certain type of anaemia have been shown to be cured by the administration of pyridoxine. Inadequate intake of the vitamin by infants has been reported to cause convulsions.

Although vitamin B_6 requirement of Indians have not been established, it would appear that a daily intake of 0.6 to 2.5 mg B_6 would meet the requirement of different age groups. The B_6 content of Indian foods have not been systematically studied. However, available information indicated that meat, liver, vegetables and whole cereal grains are good sources of pyridoxine.

BIOTIN (Fig. 6.10)

Biotin is an essential food factor and is a coenzyme for carboxylation reactions (e.g., pyruvate carboxylase). Cereals, legumes, egg yolk and organ meats are good sources of biotin. Eating raw egg white causes antagonism of this vitamin because avidin, a protein present in raw egg white binds biotin and inhibits its bioavailability. Deficiency of biotin causes dermatitis, anorexia and nausea.

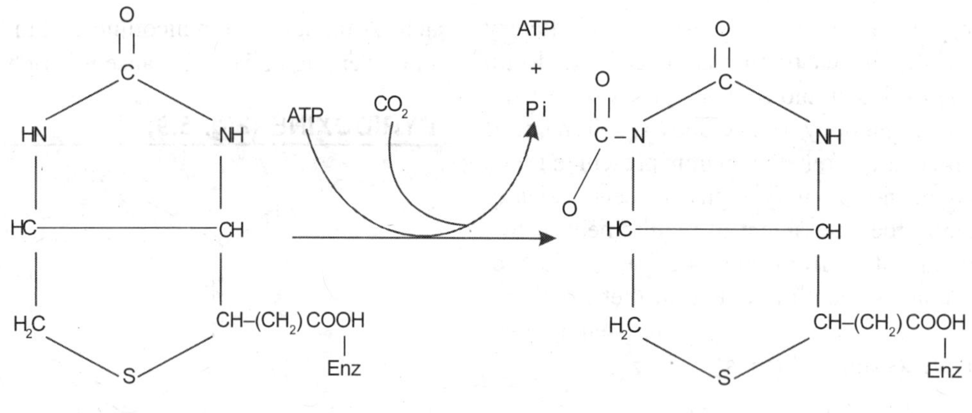

Fig. 6.10: Biotin and carboxybiotin

FOLIC ACID (Fig. 6.11)

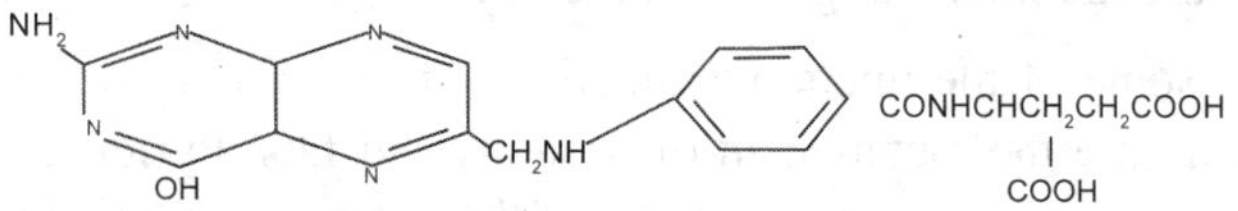

Fig. 6.11: Folic acid

This is one of the two vitamins associated with certain type of anaemia (megaloblastic anaemia). Folic acid is required for the multiplication and maturation of red cells. Its deficiency results in megaloblastic anaemia which is often seen in children and pregnant women. The actual requirement of folic acid ranges between 50–100 µg depending on the age. However, in pregnancy, the requirement of this vitamin is increased to 150–300 µg. Some data are available on the folic acid content of Indian foods. Folic acid is present both in animal and plant foods. Fresh green vegetable, liver, pulses are good sources of this vitamin.

CYANOCOBALAMIN (B_{12})

Vitamin B_{12} was first isolated as the factor in raw liver that would alleviate the symptoms of pernicious anaemia. Four pyrrole rings form a porphyrin-like structure around a cobalt atom. The vitamin is known to act as coenzyme in the methylation of homocysteine, and in a reaction in which methylmalonyl CoA is converted to succinyl CoA. Both of these reactions involve a methyl group transfer (Fig. 6.12).

Like folic acid, vitamin B_{12} is also involved in the maturation of cells and deficiency of this vitamin will also result in megaloblastic anaemia. This vitamin is also required for proper functioning of the central nervous system and also required for metabolism of folic acid. This vitamin is required for DNA synthesis and methyl group transfer.

The human requirement of this vitamin is placed at about 1 µg/day. Vitamin B_{12} is synthesized by bacteria and is present only in animal foods. Although a majority of Indians live on a diet predominantly based on foods of vegetable origin, B_{12} deficiency per se is not widespread. The manner in which the people get their vitamin B_{12} is not clear. There are various explanations offered, one is the bacterial contamination due to poor hygienic practice which is believed to provide small quantities of B_{12}.

VITAMIN C (L-ASCORBIC ACID)

The action of L-ascorbic acid in preventing poor wound healing in scurvy be explained by its involvement in the hydroxylation of proline.

Deficiency of L-ascorbic acid, found in fresh vegetables and fruit, causes scurvy, a disease characterized by defective connective tissue, with bleeding gums and loss of teeth.

Proline is hydroxylated to hydroxyproline after being incorporated into collagen precursor peptides.

–Pro–Gly–+α-oxoglutarate→

–Hydroxypro–Gly–+CO_2+succinate +H_2O

Fe^{3+} and L-ascorbic acid appear to be required in this reaction. In the absence of L-ascorbic acid, abnormal and non-functional collagen is formed (Fig. 6.13).

L-ascorbic acid, that is vitamin C, is an essential nutrient for humans as they lacks the capacity to synthesize it like many other animal species. L-ascorbic acid is a strong reducing agent. It is involved in collagen synthesis, bone and teeth calcification and many other reactions in the body as a reducing agent. Vitamin C deficiency causes

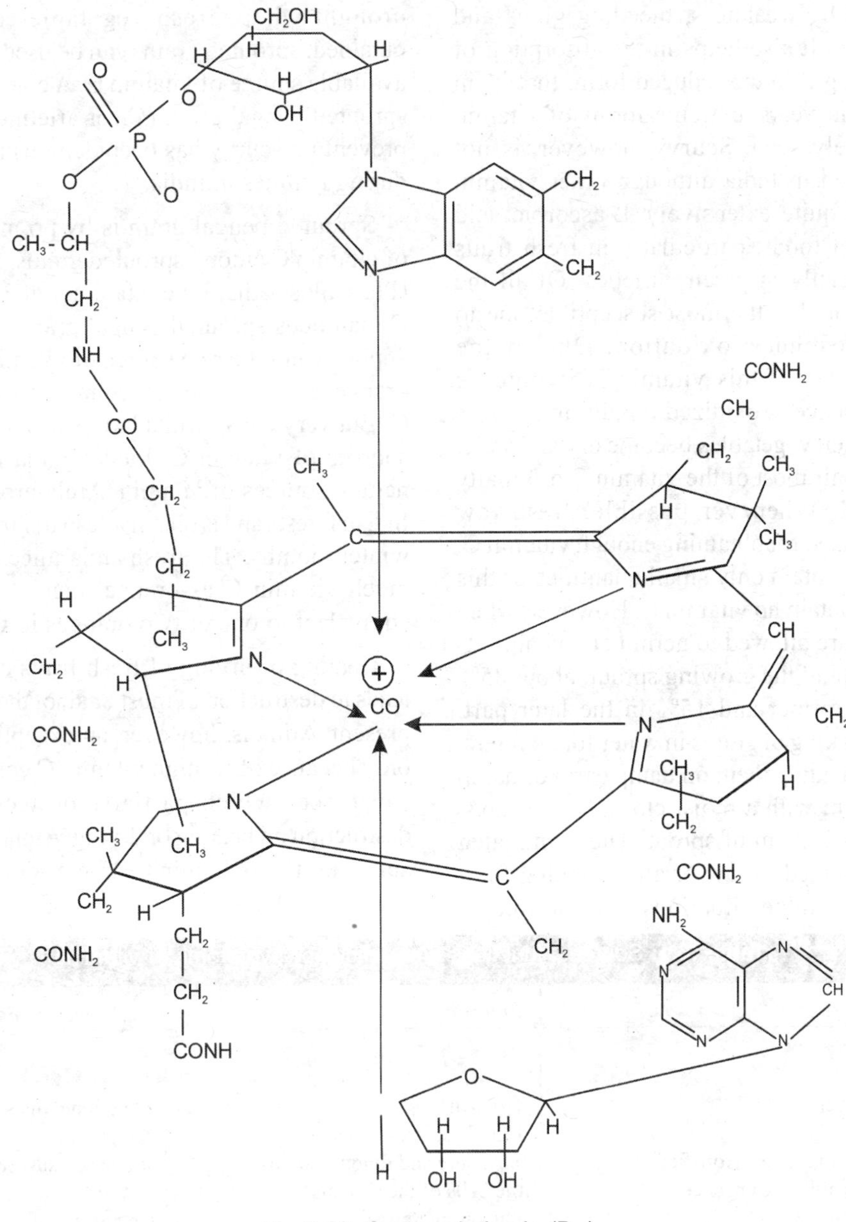

Fig 6.12: Cyanocobalamin (B_{12})

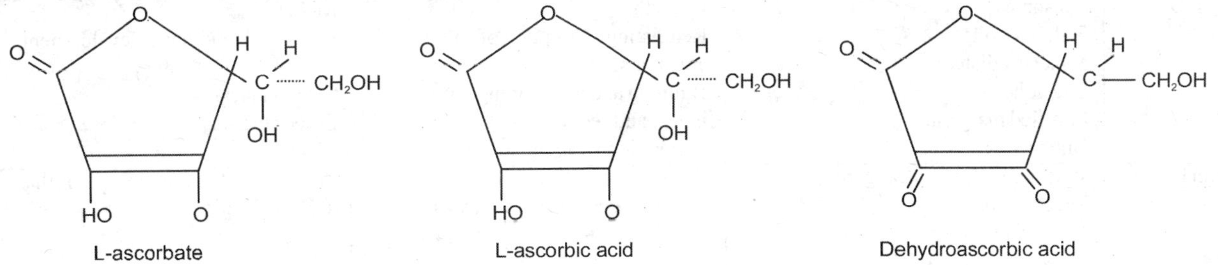

Fig 6.13: L-ascorbic acid undergoes ionization and can act as a reducing agent being oxidized to dehydroascorbate

scurvy characterized by weakness, bleeding gums and defective bone growth. It also helps in the absorption of dietary iron by keeping it in the reduced form, that is, in ferrous form. In recent years, extreme forms of vitamin C deficiency are rarely seen. Scurvy, however, is not commonly encountered in India although other vitamin deficiencies are seen quite extensively. L-ascorbic acid occurs widely in plant foods, particularly in fresh fruits and vegetables, especially in green varieties. Of all the vitamins, L-ascorbic acid is the most susceptible one to destruction by atmospheric oxidation. One of the characteristic properties of this vitamin is its intense reducing action and hence is oxidized rapidly in air. It is for this reason that when vegetables become dry and stale, or cut and exposed to air most of the vitamin C originally present is destroyed. Whenever possible, fresh raw vegetables should be used for obtaining enough vitamin C. Fresh meat and milk contain only small quantities or this vitamin. Dry grains contain no vitamin C. However, when dry pulses and beans are allowed to germinate, vitamin C is formed in the grain and the growing sprout, about 85% being present in the former and 15% in the later part. Sprouting involves soaking of grains in water for 24 hours, draining them and spreading them on damp earth or damp blanket. Covering them with a moist cloth, in 2–3 days, the grains sprout with 1–2 cm of sprout. The germinated grains should be consumed as raw or after cooking for a short period. During famine situations, viz, prolonged drought where fresh vegetables or fruits cannot be obtained, sprouted grains can be used as a cheap and easily available source of vitamin C. A commonly used source is sprouted bengal gram (Cicer arietinum); its efficiency in preventing scurvy has been demonstrated more than once during famines in India.

Sprouted bengal gram is by no means the best source of vitamin C among sprouted grams. Sprouted green gram (Phaseolus radiatus) contain about 3 times more vitamin C than does sprouted bengal gram. Expensive fruits like apple are not the rich source of vitamin C. Fresh fruits like orange, grapes, lime etc. contain good amount of vitamin C. But very cheap fruits like amla and guava are very rich sources of vitamin C. Indeed amla is one of the richest natural sources of vitamin. Amla grows abundantly in all Indian forests and is obtainable in unlimited quantities during winter months. The fresh amla juice contains 20 times as much vitamin C as orange juice. A single amla fruit is equivalent to one or two oranges in vitamin C content.

Heating or drying of fresh fruits or vegetables usually leads to destruction of most or all of the vitamin C originally present. Amla is, however, an exception among fruits not only because of its high vitamin C content, but also due to substances which partially protect the vitamin from destruction on heating or drying. Amla juice which is highly acidic protects vitamin C. Use of dried amla is an ancient practice and has much nutritional relevance (Table 6.1).

Table 6.1: Sources, functions and deficiency symptoms of vitamins

Names	*Sources*	*Functions*	*Deficiency symptoms*
Fat-soluble vitamins			
Vitamin A	Fish liver oils Liver Butter, margarine (fortified) Whole milk, cream, cheese Egg yolk Vegetable (leafy green and yellow) Fruits (yellow)	Growth Health of eyes and skin Structure and functioning of the cells of the skin and mucous membranes Immune system	Functional disorders of the eye (night blindness) Increased susceptibility to infections Changes in skin and membranes Xerophthalmia Blindness
Vitamin D	Sunshine Fish liver oils Milk (irradiated) Egg yolk Fortified margarine Butter	Growth Regulating absorption of calcium and phosphorus Building and maintaining normal bones and teeth Prevention of tetany	Rickets Poor tooth and bone development Osteomalacia Osteoporosis
Vitamin E	Wheat germ and wheat germ oils Vegetable oils Margarine Nuts Dark green, leafy vegetables	Considered essential for protection of cell structure, especially of red blood cells	Increased rate of hemolysis of the red blood cells

Contd.

Contd.

Vitamin K	Spinach Kale Cabbage	Normal clotting of blood	Defective blood clotting
Water-soluble vitamins			
Thiamine (B_1)	Wheat germ Lean pork Yeast Legumes Whole grain and enriched cereal products Liver Heart Kidney	Metabolism of carbohydrates and some amino acids	Loss of appetite Irritability Fatigue Constipation Beriberi
Riboflavin	Milk, cheese Enriched bread and cereals Green, leafy vegetables Liver, kidney, heart	Carbohydrate, fat and protein metabolism Health of the mouth tissue Healthy eyes	Cheilosis Eye sensitivity Dermatitis
Niacin	Meats (especially organ meats) Poultry and fish Enriched breads and cereals Legumes	Prevention of pellagra Carbohydrate, fat and protein metabolism	Skin eruptions Diarrhea Nervous disorders Anorexia Pellagra
Vitamin B_6	Fish Poultry Whole gram cereals Liver, kidney Pork Eggs Legumes	Metabolism of proteins	Anemia Dermatitis Confusion Depression Convulsions Nausea
Vitamin B_{12}	Liver, kidney Muscle meats Milk, cheese Eggs Poultry Fish	Metabolism Healthy red blood cells Treatment of pernicious anemia	Anemia Sore mouth and tongue Anorexia Neurological disorders Pernicious anemia
Folic acid	Dark green, leafy vegetables Liver Legumes Fruits	Metabolism Formation of hemoglobin	Anemia Impaired cell division and protein synthesis
Biotin	Organ meats Egg yolk Cereals Legumes	Metabolism	Nausea Anorexia Dermatitis Increased serum cholesterol
Vitamin C (L-ascorbic acid)	Citrus fruits, pineapple Melons Berries Tomatoes Cabbage Broccoli Green peppers	Maintaining collagen Healthy gums Aids in wound healing Aids in absorption of iron	Sore gums Tendency to bruise easily Scurvy

PRESERVING VITAMINS IN FOOD

Substantial amounts of vitamins in foods can be lost from the time the fruit or vegetable is picked until we eat it. The water-soluble vitamins, particularly thiamine, vitamin C, and folate, can be destroyed with improper storage and excessive cooking. Heat, light, exposure to the air, cooking in water, and alkalinity are all factors that can destroy vitamins. Sooner the food is eaten, the less chance of nutrient loss.

In general, if the food is not to be eaten within a few days, freezing is the best method to retain nutrients. In fact, frozen vegetables and fruits are often better than supermarket fresh ones. Frozen foods are often processed immediately after harvesting. As part of the freezing process, vegetables are quickly blanched in boiling water. This destroys the enzymes that would otherwise degrade the vitamins. Given hereunder are some tips to aid in preserving the vitamins in food:

1. Keep fruits and vegetable cool. Enzymes in foods begin to degrade vitamins once the fruit or vegetable is picked. Chilling reduces this process, so refrigerating these foods until they are consumed is important.
2. Refrigerate foods in moisture-proof containers. Nutrients keep best at temperatures near freezing, at high humidity, and away from exposure to air.
3. Avoid trimming and cutting fruits and vegetable into small pieces as much as possible. The greater surface area speeds up vitamin breakdown by oxygen. Keep in mind the outer leaves of lettuce and other greens have higher values of vitamins and minerals than the inner, tender leaves or stems. The skins of potatoes, apples and carrots for example, are higher in vitamins and minerals than the central part.
4. To retain the high levels of nutrients in vegetables, microwave cooking steaming, or using a pan with very small amounts of water and a tight-fitting lid are best. The less contact with water and the shorter the cooking time, the more nutrients retained. Whenever possible, cook fruits or vegetables in their skins.
5. Minimize reheating food. This reduces the vitamin content.
6. Don't add baking soda to vegetable to enhance the green color. The alkalinity destroys much of vitamin C, thiamine and other vitamins.
7. Keep milk cold, covered, and away from strong light. Riboflavin may be lost in direct light. Pasteurizing raw milk does not destroy the main nutrients that milk products provide – protein, riboflavin, and calcium, among others.

Microwave cooking provides many advantages as far as preserving nutrients including vitamins, during cooking. When cooking vegetables in a microwave a little water is needed, decreasing the amount of vitamins that can be lost into the surrounding fluid. Also, microwave cooking exposes food to heat for shorter period of time than conventional ovens or stoves.

LIFE, AN ORGANIZED STATE OF CERTAIN ELEMENTS

Living cells and tissues are made up of molecules, and molecules in turn, of elements. Thus life is an organized state of certain elements. Most of the solid matter of living organisms consists of organic compounds covalently bound to C, H, O, N, S and P. Carbon appears to have been selected in the course of biological evolution because of a number of desirable properties. Among them is its ability to form single and double bonds with each other, making possible formation of linear, branched and cyclic backbone structures in great variety which are attached to different kinds of functional groups so as to make building block molecules, i.e., nucleic acids, proteins, carbohy drates (Polysaccharides) and lipids. The building block molecules appear to have been selected by nature during early biological evolution as the most fit for their biological function.

In addition to six foundation elements (C, H, N, O, S and P) that make the building block molecules, many other elements are known to be required in the nutrition of humans. These elements are grouped into bulk and trace elements, also known as macro minerals and micro minerals. The bulk elements are required in excess of 100 mg/day, and the trace elements in amounts not greater than a few mgs per day. Hence Ca, Cl, Mg, P, K and Na are designated as bulk elements and Cu, F, I, Fe, Mn, Mo, Se and Zn as trace elements.

Other trace elements known to be essential for animals and not proved yet to be essential for humans are As, Cr, Ni, Si, Sr, Vn.

There are still other elements, like Pb and Hg that are patently toxic in all forms of life and have to be avoided at all costs.

MINERALS AND TRACE METALS

A large number of minerals and trace metals are present in the body. Some of these form part of body structural components and some others act as catalytic agents in many body reactions. Bones and skeleton are made up mainly of calcium, magnesium and phosphorus, and iron is a component of blood. Minerals like zinc, molybdenum, copper, manganese and magnesium are either structural part or activate a large number of enzyme systems. Iodine is a part of hormone and thyroxine. Sodium, potassium are important elements present in fluids within and outside the cells and along with ions like chloride, bicarbonate and carbonate keep water and acid base balance. On an average man excretes daily 20-30 g of mineral salts consisting of Na, K, Mg, Ca, chloride, sulphate and phosphates and this must be made good by an adequate intake of these mineral salts through our food. In the case of growing infants and children intake of additional amounts of several minerals are essential to ensure adequate growth of tissues.

Sodium and potassium are important constituents of fluids present outside and within the cell respectively. Proper concentration of these electrolytes inside and outside the cell is essential to maintain osmotic balance and keeps cells in proper shape. Sodium and potassium are present in all foods, particularly so in fruits and vegetables. In plant foods, potassium is present in higher concentrations than sodium by a factor of 10 to 50 fold. Plant foods are indeed the rich source of potassium. The exact requirement of K is not known, but potassium present in a vegetarian food is probably adequate to meet the daily requirement.

Sodium is lost in urine and particularly in sweat as sodium chloride. Sodium present in foods is not adequate to meet the requirement. Hence sodium chloride, i.e., salt has to be included in the diet. Besides imparting taste to food, salt provides necessary amount of Na required by the body. The exact amount of sodium required in a tropical country like India is not known with certainty. The daily intake of salt in our country may be as high as 20 g, the average being around 15 g per adult. In view of the association of hypertension with high salt intake, a lower intake of 8-10 g/day may be advisable, under conditions of excessive sweating as in summer and for those who work in hot environment a still higher intake may be necessary.

Calcium

Calcium is an essential element required for several life processes. As the structural component, calcium is required for the formation and maintenance of skeleton and teeth. It is also required for a number of other essential process. It is required for normal contraction of muscle to make limbs move, contraction of heart for its normal function, nervous activity and blood clotting. These later functions are carried out by ionized calcium present in the cells. The Ca levels in cells and plasma are well maintained. Ca present in bones help to maintain the Ca level in plasma in the face of dietary Ca deficiency.

Calcium is present in both animal and plant foods. The richest source of Ca among animal foods is milk (butter milk, skim milk and cheese) and among the vegetable sources is green leafy vegetables. Among the leafy vegetables, amaranth, fenugreek, and drumstick leaves are particularly rich in calcium and among root vegetables tapioca is a good source. Most cereals and millets contain some amount of this element and the millet ragi is a particularly rich source of calcium. Some of the pseudocereals like grain amaranth (Rejkeera) is also an equally good source. Rice is a poor source of calcium and therefore insufficiency of calcium is one of the main defects of diets largely based on rice. Children need relatively more calcium than adults to meet the requirements of growing bones. Calcium requirements are also increased during pregnancy to meet the needs of growing foetus and during lactation to compensate for Ca secreted in breast milk. A healthy breast fed baby of 3 months, receives a large amount of Ca, all of which has been drawn from mother's milk. If the mother's diet during this period is deficient in Ca, the Ca present in mother's bones will be depleted and she, and later, infant will suffer due to poor Ca nutritional status of the mother. Since there is considerable drain of Ca during pregnancy and lactation, particularly in the latter state, adequate supply of the mineral is essential during these conditions. A generous intake of milk and green leafy vegetables is therefore recommended during these periods.

Since there are no specific signs and symptoms attributable to Ca deficiency, the Ca requirement of man is not known with certainty. Moreover, man appears to adapt himself to low intakes of Ca without any apparent deleterious effects. The currently recommended allowances for Ca should be considered only as tentative.

Based on the available information on retention of Ca by the human body in long term balance studies, the suggested level of intake for an adult man and growing children is between 0.4 and 0.6 g/d. In the case of pregnant and lactating mothers, the Nutrition Expert Group of the Indian Council of Medical Ressearch has suggested a daily allowance of 1.0 g. In recommending these dietary allowance of Ca, the fact that part of Ca in cereal based diets is unavailable duc to the presence of phytate and oxalic acid, has been taken into account.

Certain foods like leafy vegetables (viz. amaranth) are rich in oxalates which bind Ca to form insoluble calcium oxalate and thus render Ca unavailable to the body. Similarly, phytates present in whole cereals bind calcium. Other foods which contain oxalates are horse gram, gingelly seeds, tea and coffee, but in the case of latter beverages only small amounts of oxalates pass into infusion.

The habit of chewing betel leaves with slaked lime (calcium hydroxide), a practice quite common in India (particularly among the poor), can increase Ca intake. Calcium ingested in this way can be utilised by the body. The habit of chewing betel leaves with slaked lime several times a day by expectant and nursing mothers in India has indeed a scientific basis. Since many cereal based diets are not likely to provide enough Ca unless plenty of milk is consumed, it may be useful to supplement the diet with Ca during pregnancy and lactation.

Phosphorus

Another major element in the body, next in importance to calcium is phosphorus. Utilization of calcium is closely linked with that of phosphorus, since most of the calcium in the body is deposited as calcium phosphate in the bone and the teeth. Phosphorus is also a component of nucleic acids and phosphate esters play an important part in the cellular metabolism of other nutrients like carbohydrate, fat, etc.

The rich sources of phosphorus in our diets are cereals, pulses, nuts and oilseeds. However, much of the phosphorus (40-80%) in these foods, particularly in cereals, is present as component of phytin which is not available to the body.

It is usually considered that about a gram of phosphorus should be supplied in the diet. This amount of phosphorus is easily obtained even from a poor vegetarian (cereal based) diet and phosphorus deficiency is rarely seen.

Magnesium

Magnesium is present in small concentration in all cells and is required for cellular metabolism. It is also present in bone along with calcium. Magnesium share many of the properties of calcium so far as absorption and metabolism and tissue distribution are concerned. Magnesium is also implicated to have a role in cardiovascular diseases.

Dietary intake of magnesium to maintain balance is around 350 mg/day. Cereals, pulses and nuts contain 40-200 mg magnesium per 100 g. Magnesium contents of food is generally much higher than Ca. Green leafy vegetables are also good source of magnesium. Diets based on cereals, pulses and vegetables can provide adequate magnesium to meet the requirement.

Trace Elements

It is known now that a large number of elements are required in trace amounts for a wide range of functions in the body. Their importance has been realized in recent years when sensitive tools for the determination of trace amounts of these elements became available. Atomic absorption spectrophotometry has become a standard method for trace element analysis. After the advent of this sensitive method, it has been possible to have data on the trace element content of foods. Some of the important trace elements of relevance in human nutrition are zinc, copper, selenium, cobalt, fluoride, manganese, chromium, iodine and molybdenum. Other trace elements are arsenic, nickel, vanadium and silicon. Essentiality of some of the trace elements for humans are well established, viz. iodine, Zn, Cu, F, Mn, Cr.

Iron

Iron is an essential element for the formation of hemoglobin of red cells of blood and plays an important role in the transport of oxygen. Tissues also require iron for various oxidation reduction reactions. Most of the iron in the body is reutilized and some of the body iron is also stored in liver and spleen. The amount of iron to be absorbed from the daily diet is quite small. It is in the neighbourhood of 1-3 mg depending upon the sex and the physiological status. Since there is limited capacity to absorb dietary iron, diet should contain 10-25 fold iron required daily. Diets differ very widely in the bioavailability of their iron. Diets predominantly based on cereals permit only a low level of absorption in the range of 2-5%, while diet containing low levels of cereals and high levels of meat and fish permit 10-20% absorption. The types of diet consumed normally in India should contain 20-30 mg iron to meet the iron requirement of an adult. In considering iron requirements, availability of iron from the composite diet is more important than from the individual foods because of profound interaction between foods in influencing iron absorption.

Rich sources of iron are cereals, millets, pulses, green leafy vegetables. Of the cereal grains and millets, bajra and ragi are very good source of iron. Since these grains are contaminated with dust etc., the true content of these grains are often lower than the values obtained by analysis of the market samples. Contaminant iron, which is often not available at all, may constitute 20-30% of the total iron present in foods when purchased. Milk, a good source of several nutrients, is a poor source of iron.

Inclusion in our daily diet about 50 g of green leafy vegetables which are rich sources of iron can meet a fair proportion of iron needs besides providing Ca, beta-carotene and vitamin C.

Although diet rich in iron may be able to meet our daily iron requirement and prevent iron deficiency, they may not be effective in correcting iron deficiency anaemia as indicated by lowered level of hemoglobin in the blood. Medicinal iron in the form of iron salts and other haematinics have to be provided to correct anaemia. Pregnant woman because of her high iron requirement often suffer from anaemia even on a diet containing normal levels of iron. In such cases supplementation with iron salts may be essential at least during later half of pregnancy.

In view of widespread prevalence of iron deficiency anaemia in many parts of the world, fortification of foods with iron is advocated to prevent iron deficiency. In our country fortification of common salt with iron has been successfully developed and demonstrated to be effective in preventing iron deficiency in the population if regularly used in place of ordinary salt.

Iodine

Iodine deficiency diseases including goitre are widespread in many parts of the world and it forms a major public health problem in our country. Over 120-150 million people in the world are estimated to suffer from iodine deficiency. Iodine deficiency is characterized by swelling of thyroid gland in the neck. Iodine deficiency during fetal stage may lead to mental retardation and in later life retardation of body growth. The daily requirement of iodine is reported to be 100-150 μg. In a non-endemic area 60-75% of the iodine needs are met by the iodine present in the diet and the rest through iodine content of water. In an endemic goitre area, there is iodine deficiency in the soil, water and locally grown foods. Besides, certain compounds present in foods, particularly vegetables of brassica species interfere with iodine utilization and lead to goitre. They are known as goitrogens.

Till recently, there were no reliable figures for iodine content of Indian foods, to enable assessment of dietary intake of iodine. This was mainly due to difficulties with establishing a reliable micro method for the estimation of trace amount of iodine in foods. Recently an improved micro method for estimation of iodine in foods has been standardized at National Institute of Nutrition and used for analyzing commonly consumed foods for their iodine content both from the endemic and non-endemic areas. It would appear that at least in the non-goitre area, diet provides daily nearly 200 μg iodine which should meet the entire day's requirement.

One of the well tested approaches to control iodine deficiency disease in the population is the distribution of iodised salt to the affected population. On the basis of daily salt consumption, iodised salt containing atleast 15 μg of iodine per g could easily meet the daily iodine requirement. In India goitre is endemic in sub-Himalayan regions affecting nearly 120 million population. In recent years, several pockets of goitre have been identified in other parts of the country which were traditionally considered as the non-endemic area. These pockets are mostly in the tribal areas.

A programme of distribution of iodised salt in the endemic area is in operation in India. For salt iodization, potassium iodate, a more stable compound, is used. Notwithstanding this, in actual practice there is considerable loss of iodine during transportation and storage under prevailing conditions. Hence a higher level of initial iodization upto 30 ppm has been recommended to take care of these losses. A new process has also been developed to improve the stability of iodine in iodized salt.

Zinc

Zinc is an important element performing a range of functions in the body as it is a cofactor for a number of enzymes. Zinc deficiency leads to growth failure and poor development of gonadal function. Dwarfism and hypogonadism seen in Egypt and Iran are attributed to dietary zinc deficiency. Althouth zinc intake and zinc absorption is low on diets of poor income population in India suggesting a possible dietary zinc deficiency. No clinical abnormality attributable to zinc deficiency is seen in our country. However, sub-clinical deficiency of zinc does exist in our population, but the functional significance of this is not as yet clear.

Copper

Copper is an essential element for man. It plays an important role in iron absorption. It is also involved in cross linking of connective tissues, neurotransmission and lipid metabolism. Part of body copper circulates in plasma as ceruloplasmin. Copper is also present in oxidative enzymes like cytochromes. Copper metabolism in the body is under homeostatic regulation, in case of inadequate intake, excretion is reduced. The estimated dietary intake of copper from a typical Indian diet is around 2 mg/day. A daily intake of 2-3 mg through diet may satisfy these requirements. Absorption of copper from poor diet is lower than that from well balanced diets, absorption varying from 5 to 33%. Copper content of Indian diets of poor income groups is just marginal and some level of dietary deficiency of copper may exist. However no clinical abnormality attributable to copper deficiency is recognized. Clinical symptoms due to copper deficiency either nutritional or genetic lead to pathological symptoms in organs rich in connective tissue. Central nervous system disorders may also result from copper deficiency with impaired myelination and catecholamine metabolism.

Chromium

Chromium is essential for animals and probably for man. Chromium deficiency has been shown to lead to impaired glucose tolerance. The factor responsible for this property has not yet been isolated. Because of its role as glucose tolerance factor, chromium has been much studied in relation to diabetes. However, clear cut disease or abnormality attributable to chromium deficiency has not been identified so far. Because of its low content in foods, chromium content of foods was not determined till recently for want of reliable method. Use of atomic absorption spectrometer with graphite furnace has helped in estimating chromium content of a number of foods consumed in India. Chromium content of cereal based Indian diets ranges between 70-150 µg/day; low income group diets have generally a lower (25%) content. Absorption of inorganic chromium is quite low, i.e., 1-2%, chromium present in our diets is absorbed to an extent of 70-80% or more. This is presumably due to the fact that chromium in foods is present in organically bound form which facilitates greatly its absorption. Chromium requirement has been estimated to be around 70 µg/day and most of our diets consumed by rich or poor are able to provide this amount of chromium. Dietary chromium deficiency is not likely to occur in our population.

Manganese

Manganese is established as an essential element as it participates in a number of reactions as a component of metaloenzyme or as enzyme cofactor. Its function in glycosyltransferase is well recognized and its deficiency leads to abnormality in skeletal bone mineralization. It also participates in lipid and carbohydrate metabolism. A large number of foods consumed in India have been analyzed for manganese. Manganese content of diets consumed in India varies from 4-10 mg/day. Absorption of manganese from these diets vary from 5-20%. Surprisingly, diets of poor income groups have a better absorption of manganese than diets of high income groups. The basis for these differences in absorption is not known. The estimated manganese requirement on these diets based on human balance studies is 5 mg/day. Most of our diets can provide this amount. Hence manganese deficiency is not likely to occur in our population. Excess of manganese is toxic, a situation that may be encountered in manganese mines and other industries.

Molybdenum

Molybdenum is an essential constituent of xanthine and aldehyde oxidases and is involved in uric acid metabolism. Since molybdenum deficiency in humans is unknown, current dietary intakes must be adequate. The daily requirement for an adult may range from 0.15 to 0.5 mg. Molybdenum content of several Indian foods have been estimated. Dietary deficiency of Mo is unlikely in our population. However, excess Mo intake may increase the risk of gout. High Mo and low copper intakes has been implicated in the etiology of endemic genuvalgum and bone disorders which occurs in certain endemic flurosis areas.

Fluoride

Fluoride is also an important element in human health. It is an essential element, a minimum amount being required for prevention of dental caries. However, its presence in high concentration in the environment, particularly in water (> 2-3 ppm) leads to fluorosis resulting in hardening of bone. Fluorosis occurs as an endemic disease in India in parts of Andhra Pradesh (Nalgonda district) and Punjab (Patiala district). In the endemic area of Andhra Pradesh, another clinical manifestation of fluoride toxicity called 'Genu valgum' has been identified in recent years. In the development of genu valgum apart from fluoride toxicity, other environmental factors appear to have contributed to its emergence, viz., high levels of Mo and low levels of Cu. One important strategy to control fluorosis in these areas is to supply low fluoride water. Different approaches to achieve this have been suggested.

While high intake of fluoride is a health hazard a minimum level of fluoride in water (< 1 ppm) is essential to protect against dental caries. Dental caries may be caused by excess intake of sticky sweets among children. This situation is more prevalent in the West than in our country. However, the practice of brushing the teeth and washing the mouth after food should be inculcated among children to reduce the risk of caries. Because of health implication of F, there has been some interest to obtain reliable data on F content of foods. It is estimated that by food alone, 0.3-0.8 mg F may be supplied. Daily intake of F upto 2 mg through foods has been reported from some areas. Fifty to 80% of food fluoride is absorbable. It is suggested that in assessing the benefits and risks of fluoride ingestion, that apart from water, F derived from foods also needs to be considered.

OTHER TRACE METALS

Other trace metals of significance in human nutrition are selenium, cobalt, silicon, arsenic, nickel and vanadium. Selenium is an essential element and along with vitamin E, it is required for maintaining liver integrity. Selenium deficiency leads to liver necrosis. An endemic disease of cardiomyopathy in children (Keshan syndrome) is attributed to low Se in the environment. Selenium deficiency is also implicated as a risk factor in cancer. Selenium being a cofactor of an antioxidant enzyme–glutathione peroxidase can spare us some of vitamin E intake. Cobalt is important trace element as it forms part of the vitamin B_{12}. It is also reported that cobalt is required for optimum utilization of low doses of iodine. The possible role of low Co in iodine deficiency disorders (Goitre) is however not known. The nutritional significance of the other trace elements like Si, As, Ni and V in man is uncertain although their essentiality for animals have been established (Table 6.2).

Table 6.2: Sources, functions and deficiency symptoms of minerals

Names	*Best sources*	*Functions*	*Deficiency symptoms*
Calcium	Milk Cheese Some dark green, leafy vegetables	Normal development and maintenance of bones and teeth Clotting of the blood Nerve irritability Normal heart action Normal muscle activity Activates enzymes	Retarded growth Poor tooth and bone formation Rickets Slow clotting time of blood Tetany
Phosphorus	Milk and cheese Lean meat Poultry Fish Whole grain cereals Legumes Nuts	Normal development and maintenance of bones and teeth Maintenance of normal acid-base balance of the blood Constituent of all body cells Necessary for effectiveness of some vitamins Metabolism of carbohydrates, fats and proteins	Poor tooth and bone formation Rickets Weakness Anorexia Pain in bones General malaise
Magnesium	Avocados Nuts Milk Whole grains Green, leafy vegetables Legumes Bananas	Constituent of bones, muscles and red blood cells Necessary for healthy muscles and nerves Metabolism	Mental, emotional and muscle disorders
Sodium	Salt Meat Poultry Eggs Milk and cheese	Fluid balance Acid-base balance Osmosis Regulates muscle and nerve irritability Glucose absorption	Nausea Exhaustion Muscle cramps
Potassium	Vegetables Fruits, especially oranges, bananas and prunes	Osmosis Fluid balance Regular heart rhythm Cell metabolism	Muscle weakness Apathy Abnormal heartbeat
Chloride	Salt Meat Milk Eggs Seafood	Osmosis Fluid balance Acid-base balance Formation of hydrochloric acid	Nausea Exhaustion

Contd.

Contd.

Sulfur	Meat Poultry Fish Eggs	For building hair, nails and all body tissues Constituent of all body cells Metabolism	Unknown
Trace Minerals			
Iron	Liver Muscle meats Legumes Dried fruits Whole grain or enriched breads and cereals Dark green and leafy vegetables Potatoes	Essential for formation of hemoglobin of the red blood cells and provision of oxygen to cells Constituent of cellular enzymes	Anemia characterized by weakness, dizziness, loss of weight and pallor
Copper	Liver Kidney Shellfish Legumes Nuts Whole grain cereals	Essential for formation of hemo-globin and red blood cells Component of enzymes	Anemia Bone disease
Iodine	Seafood Foods grown in soil bordering salt water Iodized salt	Formation of hormones in thyroid gland	Goiter Myxedema Cretinism
Manganese	Whole grains Nuts Vegetables Fruits	Component of enzymes	Unknown
Zinc	Seafood especially oysters Liver Meat Eggs Milk	Component of insulin and enzymes Wound healing Taste acuity Essential for growth	Dwarfism, hypogonadism, anemia Loss of appetite Skin changes Impaired wound healing Decreased taste acuity
Fluoride	Fluoridated water Seafood	Increases resistance to tooth decay	Tooth decay Possibly osteoporosis
Chromium	Yeast Cheese Wheat germ	Associated with glucose metabolism	Possibly disturbances of glucose meta-bolism
Molybdenum	Milk Cereal Legumes	Enzyme functioning Metabolism	Unknown
Selenium	Seafood Kidney Liver Muscle meats	Constituent of most body tissue cofactor for the antioxidant enzyme Glutathione peroxidase	Unclear

STUDY QUESTIONS

1. How do you classify vitamins? What role does retinol play in visual cycle, skin and mucosal membranes?
2. Why is vitamin D branded more a hormone and less a vitamin? What role does it play in calcium homeostasis?
3. Why is vitamin E considered an antidote for lipid peroxidation? Explain briefly.
4. Comment critically on the statement 'Vitamin K keeps blood coagulation click quickly'.
5. What general function do B complex vitamins perform in the body? Enumerate briefly the coenzyme forms of B complex vitamins along with a brief mention of the role that each coenzyme play in the body.
6. Explain briefly the role of vitamin C:
   a. As antioxidant.
   b. In wound healing.
7. Explain the special importance of calcium for the children and expectant mothers.
8. Why is selenium said to spare vitamin E?
9. Differentiate heme and non-heme iron as a source of iron.
10. What is goitre and what causes it?

CHAPTER 7

Blood and Its Role

Chapter Outlines

- Functions of blood
- Constituents of blood
- Blood coagulation
- Blood as a carrier of oxygen
- Transport of carbon dioxide through blood
- Common blood related disorders
- Blood buffers
- Blood filtration: Role of kidneys
- Urine examination and disease diagnosis
- Study questions

Blood is a tissue which circulates in what is virtually a closed system of blood vessels. It consists of solid elements–the red and white blood cells and the platelets–suspended in liquid medium, the plasma.

FUNCTIONS OF BLOOD

1. *Respiration:* Transport of oxygen from the lungs to the tissues and of CO_2 from the tissues to the lungs.
2. *Nutrition:* Transport of absorbed food materials.
3. *Excretion:* Transport of metabolic wastes to the kidneys, lungs, skin and intestines for removal.
4. Maintenance of normal acid-base balance in the body.
5. Regulation of water balance through the effects of blood on the exchange of water between the circulating fluid and the tissue fluid.
6. Regulation of body temperature by the distribution of body heat.
7. Defense against infection in the white cells and the circulating antibodies.
8. Transport of hormones; regulation of metabolism.
9. Transport of metabolites.

Table 7.1 depicts the composition of blood.

Table 7.1: Blood components and the names of diseases associated with their abnormal occurrence in blood

Whole blood		
Cellular elements	*Plasma*	
	Fibrinogen	*Serum*
Erythrocytes (high: polycythemia, low : Anemia) Leukocytes (high: leukemia; low: typhoid fever) Platelets (low: thrombocytopenia)	Water (high: edema; low: dehydration) Albumin (low: edema) Globulin (high: transplant rejection; low: infection) Clotting factors (low: hemophilia) Glucose (high: diabetes mellitus, hyperglycemia; low: hypoglycemia) Cholesterol (high: gallstones, atherosclerosis) Urea Inorganic salts Gases (N_2, O_2, CO_2) Enzymes, hormones, vitamins	

CONSTITUENTS OF BLOOD

Whole blood is a complicated mixture. It contains several types of cells and a liquid, non-cellular portion called plasma, in which many substances are dissolved. A healthy adult weighing 70 kg has about 6 litres of blood, 50 to 60 percent of which is plasma. There are three main types of cellular elements of blood, erythrocytes, leukocytes and platelets.

1. Erythrocytes

The most prevalent cells of blood are the red blood cells which are called erythrocytes. There are about 5 million red blood cells in every cubic millimeter of blood, or roughly 100 million in every drop. Erythrocytes are very specialized cells. They have no nuclei and hence no DNA. Their main function is to carry oxygen to the cells and carbon dioxide away from the cells. Erythrocytes are formed in the bone marrow. They stay in the blood stream for about 120 days. Old erythrocytes are removed by the liver and spleen and destroyed. The constant formation and destruction of red blood cells maintain a steady number of erythrocytes. In an adult male, there are approximately 30 trillion erythrocytes.

2. Leukocytes

Leukocytes (white blood cells) are relatively minor cellular components (minor in numbers, not in function). For each 1000 red blood cells, there are only one or two white blood cells. Most of the different leukocytes destroy invading bacteria or other foreign substances by devouring them (phagocytosis). Like erythrocytes, leukocytes are also formed in the bone marrow. Specialized white blood cells formed in the lymph nodes and in the spleen are called lymphocytes. They synthesize immunoglobulins (antibodies) and store them.

3. Platelets

When a blood vessel is cut or injured, the bleeding is controlled by the third one of cellular elements: The platelets, or thrombocytes. They are formed in the bone marrow and spleen, and are more numerous than leukocytes but less numerous than erythrocytes. There are about 300,000 platelets in each cubic millimeter of blood or one for every 10 or 20 red blood cells.

4. Plasma

If we remove all the cellular elements from whole blood by centrifugation, the resulting liquid is the plasma. The cellular elements, mainly red blood cells, which settle at the bottom of the centrifuge tube, occupy between 40 to 50 percent of the blood volume. The measured volume percentage of cellular elements, known as the hematocrit value or the packed cell (PCV) volume, is used for diagnosis.

Blood plasma is 92 percent water. The dissolved solids in the plasma are mainly proteins (7 percent). The remaining 1 percent are glucose, lipids, enzymes, vitamins, hormones, and such waste products as urea and CO_2. Of the plasma proteins, 55 percent is albumin, 38.5 percent globulin and 6.5 percent fibrinogen. If plasma is allowed to stand, it forms a clot, a gel-like substance. We can squeeze out a clear liquid from the clot. This fluid is the serum. It contains all the components of the plasma except the fibrinogen. This protein is involved in the complicated process of clot formation.

As for the other plasma proteins, most of the globulins take part in the immune reactions, and the albumin provides proper osmotic pressure. For example, if the albumin concentration drops (due to malnutrition or kidney disease, say), the water from the blood oozes into the interstitial fluid and creates the swelling of tissues called edema. A normal plasma albumin level is a crucial factor for maintaining tissue osmotic pressure.

BLOOD COAGULATION

When blood is drawn and allowed to clot, clear liquid (serum) exudes from the clotted blood. Plasma, on the other hand, separates from the cells only when blood is prevented from clotting.

The blood clot is formed by a protein (*fibrinogen*) which is present in soluble form in the plasma and which is transformed to an insoluble network of fibrous material (*fibrin,* the substance of the blood clot) by the clotting mechanism.

According to the original *Howell theory* of blood-coagulation, the change of fibrinogen into fibrin is caused by *thrombin,* which in fluid blood exists as prothrombin. The conversion of prothrombin to thrombin depends on the action of *thromboplastin* and calcium. These stages in the clotting process may be diagrammed as follows:

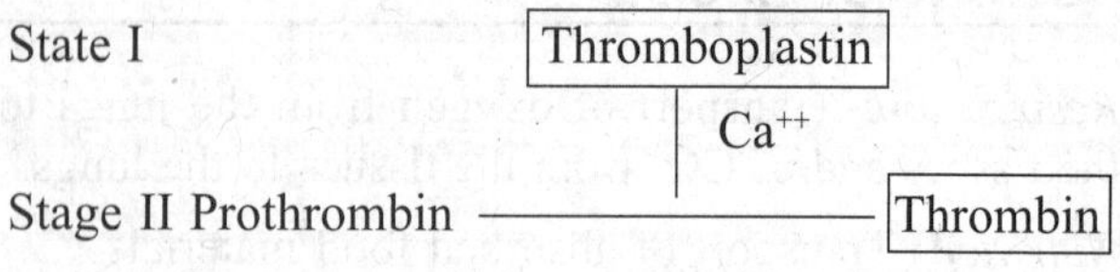

The many continuing studies on the details of the coagulation process have served to indicate how complex the system actually is. Lack of knowledge of the chemical nature of many of the factors involved has also resulted in much confusion in terminology. In an effort to introduce uniformity in nomenclature, the International Committee for the Standardization of the Nomenclature of Blood Clotting Factors has recommended a numerical system to designate the various factors presently accepted as involved in the clotting process. This system is given in Table 7.2, and each of the 12 factors, all except factor IV, are protein in nature and are synthesized by the liver or hepatic tissue.

Although earlier a factor VI had been described but it is currently believed that no such separate factor exists; consequently it has been deleted.

Table 7.2: Numerical system for nomenclature of blood clotting factors

Factor	*Name*
I	Fibrinogen
II	Prothrombin
III	Thromboplastin
IV	Calcium
V	Labile factor, proaccelerin, accelerator (AC-) globulin
VII	Proconvertin, serum prothrombin conversion accelerator (SPCA), cothromboplastin, autoprothrombin I
VIII	Antihemophilic factor, antihemophilic globulin (AHG)
IX	Plasma thromboplastin component (PTC) (Christmas factor)
X	Stuart-Prower factor
XI	Plasma thromboplastin antecedent (PTA)
XII	Hageman factor
XIII	Laki-Lorand factor (LLF)

BLOOD AS A CARRIER OF OXYGEN

One of the most important functions of blood is to carry oxygen from the tissues. This is done by hemoglobin molecules located inside the erythrocytes. Hemoglobin is made up of two alpha and two beta protein chains, each attached to a molecule of heme.

The active sites are the hemes (porphyrins), and at the center of each heme is an iron (II) ion. The heme with its central Fe^{2+} ion forms a plane. Because each hemoglobin molecule has four hemes, it can hold a total of four O_2 molecules. However, the ability of the hemoglobin molecule to hold O_2 depends on how much oxygen is in the environment. A close look at Figure 7.1 shows how the oxygen-carrying ability of hemoglobin depends on oxygen pressure. When oxygen enters the lungs, the pressure is high (100 mm Hg). At this pressure, all the Fe^{2+} ions of the hemes bind oxygen molecules; they are fully saturated.

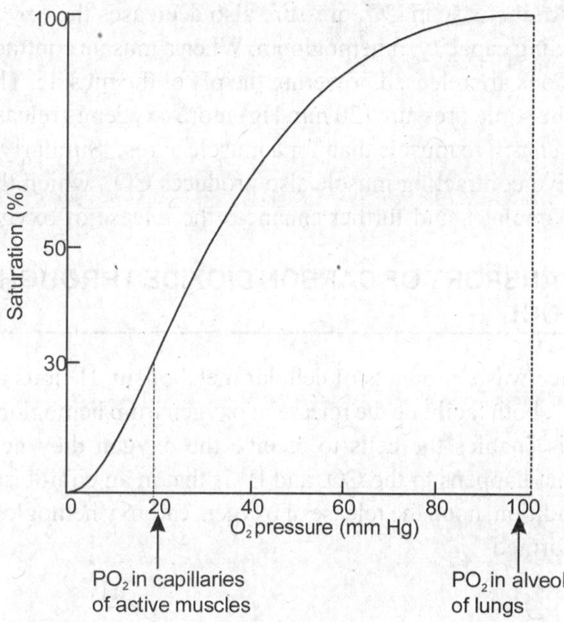

Fig. 7.1: An oxygen dissociation curve. Saturation % means percentage of Fe^{2+} ions that carry O_2 molecules

By the time the blood reaches the muscles through the capillaries, the oxygen pressure in the muscle is only 20 mm Hg. At this pressure only 30 percent of the binding sites carry oxygen. Thus, 70 percent of the oxygen carried will be released to the tissues. The S shape of the binding (dissociation) curve implies that the reaction

$$HbO_2 \rightleftharpoons Hb + O_2$$

is not a simple equilibrium reaction. Each heme binding to oxygen has cooperative effect on the other hemes. This cooperative action allows hemoglobin to deliver twice as much oxygen to the tissues as it would if each heme acted independently. The reason for this is as follows. When a hemoglobin molecule is carrying no oxygen, the four globin units coil into a certain shape. When the first oxygen molecule attaches to one of the heme subunits, it changes the shape not only of that subunit but also of the second one, making it easier for the second one to bind an oxygen. When the second heme binds, the shape changes once again, and the oxygen binding ability of the two remaining subunits is increased still more.

The oxygen-delivering capacity of hemoglobin is also affected by its environment. A slight change in the pH of the environment, changes the oxygen binding capacity. This is called the Bohr effect. Lowering the pH decreases the oxygen binding capacity of hemoglobin. This is how the body delivers more oxygen to those tissues that need it. An increase in CO_2 pressure also decreases the oxygen binding capacity of hemoglobin. When a muscle contracts, H^+ ions are released, lowering the pH of the muscle. Thus at the same pressure (20 mm Hg) more oxygen is released for an active muscle than for a muscle at rest. Similarly an active contracting muscle also produces CO_2, which then accumulates and further enhances the release of oxygen.

TRANSPORT OF CARBON DIOXIDE THROUGH BLOOD

Since waste products of cellular metabolism, H^+ ions and CO_2, both facilitate the release of oxygen from hemoglobin. This enables the cells to receive the oxygen they need. What happens to the CO_2 and H^+ is that in an equilibrium condition, upon the release of oxygen, carboxy hemoglobin is formed:

$$HbO_2 + H^+ + CO_2 \rightleftharpoons Hb\genfrac{}{}{0pt}{}{H^+}{CO_2} + O_2$$

The CO_2 is bound to the terminal $-NH_2$ groups of the four polypeptide chains so that each hemoglobin can carry a maximum of four CO_2 molecules, one for each chain. How much CO_2 each hemoglobin actually carries depends on the pressure of CO_2. The higher the CO_2 pressure, the more carboxyhemoglobin is formed.

But only 25 percent of the total CO_2 produced by the cells is transported to the lungs in the form of carboxy hemoglobin. Another 70 percent is converted in the red blood cells to carbonic acid by the enzyme carbonic anhydrase:

The remaining 5 percent of thus is transported as CO_2 gas dissolved in the plasma.

The reaction proceeds to the left because loss of CO_2 from the lungs causes this equilibrium to shift to the left (Le Chatelier's principle).

A large part of the H_2CO_3 is carried as such to the lungs, where it is converted back to CO_2 by carbonic anhydrase and released.

COMMON BLOOD RELATED DISORDERS

Anemia

Anemia is a condition in which the oxygen-carrying capacity of the blood is reduced; it is a sign, not a disease. Many types of anemia exist, all characterized by reduced numbers of RBCs or decreased level of hemoglobin in the blood. These conditions lead to fatigue and intolerance to cold, both of which are related to lack of oxygen needed for ATP and heat production, and to paleness, which is due to low hemoglobin content.

Nutritional Anemia

Nutritional anemia arises from an inadequate diet, one without enough iron, the necessary amino acids, or vitamin B_{12} and folic acid.

Pernicious Anemia

Pernicious anemia is the insufficient hematopoiesis that results from an inability of the stomach to produce intrinsic factor, which is needed for absorption of vitamin B_{12}.

Hemorrhagic Anemia

An excessive loss of RBCs through bleeding is called hemorrhagic anemia. Common causes are large wounds, stomach ulcers, and heavy menstrual bleeding. If bleeding is extraordinarily heavy, the anemia is termed *acute*. Excessive blood loss can be fatal. Slow, prolonged bleeding is apt to produce a *chronic* anemia; the chief symptom of which is fatigue.

Hemolytic Anemia

If RBC plasma membranes rupture prematurely, the cells remain as "ghosts", and their hemoglobin pours out into the plasma. A characteristic sign of this condition, called hemolytic anemia, is distortion in the shape of erythrocytes. It may result from inherent defects, such as hemoglobin defects, abnormal red blood cell enzymes, or defects of the red blood cell membrane. Agents that may cause hemolytic anemia are parasites, toxins and antibodies from incompatible blood (Rh^- mother and RH^+ fetus, for instance). Hemolytic disease of the newborn (erythroblastosis fetalis) is an example of a hemolytic anemia.

The term thalassemia (thaĺ-a-SĒ-mē-a) represents a group of hereditary hemolytic anemias resulting from a defect in the synthesis of hemoglobin, which produces extremely thin and fragile erythrocytes. It occurs primarily in populations from countries bordering the Mediterranean Sea. Treatment generally consists of blood transfusions.

Aplastic Anemia

Destruction or inhibition of the red bone marrow results in aplastic anemia. Typically, the marrow is replaced by fatty tissue, fibrous tissue, or tumor cells. Toxins, gamma radiation, and certain medications that inhibit enzymes involved in hemopoiesis are the causes. Bone marrow transplants can now be done with a reasonable hope of success in patients with aplastic anemia. Immunosuppressive drugs are given for several days before the transplant and with decreasing frequency afterward.

Sickle-Cell Anemia

The RBCs of a person with sickle-cell anemia (SCA) contain an abnormal kind of hemoglobin (Hb-S). When such an erythrocyte gives up its oxygen to the interstitial fluid, the abnormal hemoglobin forms long, stiff, rod like structures that bend the erythrocyte into a sickle shape. The sickled cells rupture easily. Even though erythropoisis is stimulated by the loss of the cells, it cannot keep pace with the hemolysis. The individual thus suffers from a hemolytic anemia that reduces the amount of oxygen that can be supplied to the tissues. Prolonged oxygen reduction may eventually cause extensive tissue damage. Furthermore, because of the shape of the sickled cells, they tend to get stuck in blood vessels and can cut off blood supply to an organ altogether.

Sickle-cell anemia is characterized by several symptoms. In young children, hand-foot syndrome is present, in which there is swelling and pain in the wrists and feet. Older patients experience pain in the back and extremities. Complications include neurological disorders (meningitis, seizures, stroke), impaired pulmonary function, orthopedic abnormalities (femoral head necrosis, osteomyelitis), genitourinary tract disorders (involuntary urination, blood in urine, kidney failure), ocular disturbances (hemorrhage, detached retina, blindness), and obstetric complications (convulsions, coma, infection).

Sickle-cell anemia is inherited. The gene responsible for the tendency of the RBCs to sickle also alters the permeability of the plasma membranes of sickled cells, causing potassium to leak out. Low levels of potassium kill the malaria parasites that infect sickled cells. Sickle-cell genes are found primarily among populations, or descendants of populations, that live in the malaria belt around the world, including parts of Mediterranean Europe and subtropical Africa and Asia.

Treatment or management consists of administration of analgesics to relieve pain, antibiotics to counter infections, and blood transfusions.

Leukemia

Clinically, leukemia is classified based on the duration and character of the disease, that is, acute or chronic. Acute leukemia is a malignant disease of blood-forming tissues characterized by uncontrolled production and accumulation of immature leukocytes. In chronic leukemia, there is an accumulation of mature leukocytes in the bloodstream because they do not die at the end of their normal life span. The *human T cell leukemia-lymphoma virus-1 (HTLV-1)* is strongly associated with some types of leukemia. Leukemia is also classified according to the identity and site of origins of the predominant cell involved, that is, myelocytic, lymphocytic or monocytic.

In acute leukemia, the anemia and bleeding problems commonly seen result from the crowding out of normal bone marrow cells by the overproduction of immature cells, preventing normal production of RBCs and platelets. One cause of death from acute leukemia is internal hemorrhaging, especially cerebral hemorrhage that destroys vital centers in the brain. Often, the cause of death is uncontrolled infection due to lack of mature, normal WBCs. The abnormal accumulation of immature leukocytes may be reduced by using X-rays and anti-leukemic drugs. Partial or complete remissions may be induced, with some lasting as long as 15 years.

BLOOD BUFFERS

The average pH of human blood is 7.4. Any change larger than 0.1 pH unit in either direction is pathological, and if the pH goes below 6.8 or above 7.8, death can result. When the pH drop below normal, the condition is called acidosis; when it rises above 7.45, it is called alkalosis. There are three buffer systems that maintain an average blood pH of 7.4. The most important is the HCO_3/H_2CO_3 buffer. The other two are the $HPO^{2-}_4/H_2PO^-_4$ buffer and the protein molecules dissolved in the plasma.

BLOOD FILTRATION: ROLE OF KIDNEYS

It has been seen that one of the functions of the blood is to carry waste products away from the cells. CO_2, one of the principal waste products of respiration, is carried by the blood to the lungs and exhaled. The other waste products are filtered out by the kidneys and eliminated in the urine. The kidney is a superfiltration machine. About 100 L of blood passes through a normal human kidney daily. Of this, only about 1.5 L is excreted as urine. Obviously, we do not have here just a simple filtration system in which small molecules are lost and large ones are retained. The kidneys also reabsorb from the urine those small molecules that are not waste products (tubular reabsorption) and also actively secrete certain other substances. The balance between filtration and reabsorption is controlled by a number of hormones.

The biological units inside the kidneys that perform these functions are called nephrons and each kidneys contains about a million of them. A nephron is made up of a filtration head called Bowman's capsule connected to tiny U-shaped tube called, tubule. The part of the tubule close to the Bowman's capsule is the proximal tubule, the U-shaped twist is called Henle's loop, and the part of the tubule farthest from the capsule is the distal tubule.

Blood vessels penetrate the kidney throughout. The arteries branch into capillaries and one tiny capillary enters each Bowman's capsule. Inside the capsule the capillary first branches into even smaller vessels, called glomeruli, and then leaves the capsule, the blood enters the glomeruli with every heartbeat and the pressure forces the water, ions, and all small molecules (urea, sugar, salts, amino acids) through the walls of the golmeruli and the Bowman's capsule. These molecules and ions enter the proximal tubule. Blood cells and large molecules (proteins) are retained in the capillary and exit with the blood.

As shown in Figure 7.2 the tubules and Henle's loop are surrounded by blood vessels; these blood vessels reabsorb vital nutrients. Eighty percent of the water is reabsorbed in the proximal tubule. Almost all the glucose and amino acids are reabsorbed here. When excess sugar is present in the blood, some of it passes into the urine, and the measurement of glucose concentration in the blood is used in diagnosing diabetes.

By the time the glomerular filtrate reaches Henle's loop, the solids and most of the water have been reabsorbed and only wastes (such as urea, creatinine, uric acid, ammonia, and some salts) pass into the collecting tubules that bring the urine to the ureter, from which it passes to the bladder, as shown in Figures 7.2a-b.

In the treatment of kidney failure, the selective elimination of waste products is done by an artificial kidney machine. The process is called hemodialysis.

URINE EXAMINATION AND DISEASE DIAGNOSIS

Normal urine contains about 4 percent dissolved waste products. The rest is water. The daily amount of urine varies greatly but averages about 1.5 L per day. The pH varies from 5.5 to 7.5. The main solute is urea, the end product of protein metabolism. Other nitrogenous waste products, such as creatine, creatinine, ammonia, and hippuric acid, are also present, though in much smaller amounts. In addition normal urine contains inorganic ions such as Na^+, Ca^{2+}, Mg^{2+}, Cl^-, PO_4^{3-}, SO_4^{2-} and HCO_3^-.

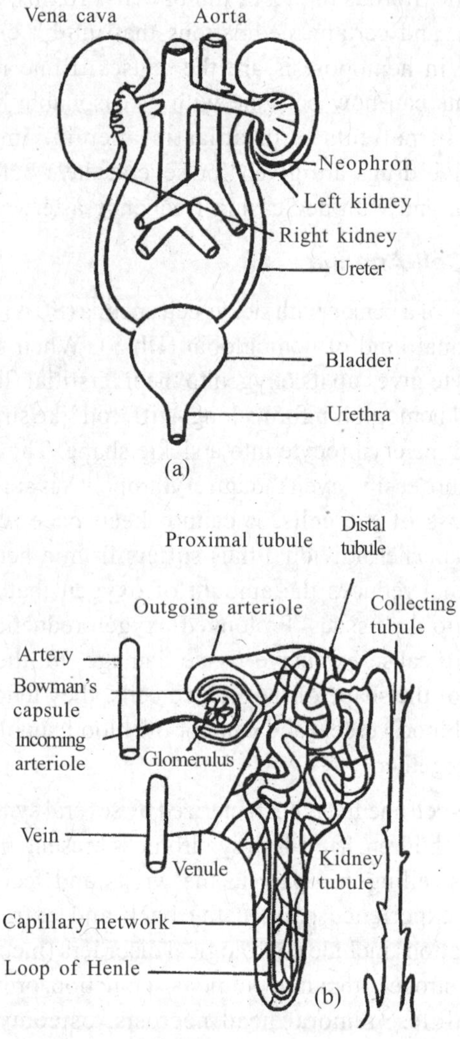

Fig. 7.2: Excretion through the kidneys (a) The human urinary system (b) A kidney nephron and its components, with the surrounding circulatory system

Under certain pathological conditions, other substances can appear in the urine. It is because of this, that urine analysis is such an important part of diagnostic procedure. We have already noted that the presence of glucose and ketone bodies is an indication of diabetes. Among other abnormal constituents may be proteins, which can indicate such kidney diseases as nephritis.

As we have seen that uropoiesis, the urine formation, takes place in kidney tubules or nephrons by a process involving ultrafiltration of blood to yield glomerular filtrate. This filtrate gets transformed into urine after going through tubular reabsorption and active secretion. Functional changes due to disease or damage to various tissues including blood, cause changes in the chemical composition of blood which ultimately gets reflected in the urine composition. That is why urine examination for normal and pathological components yields valuable information regarding diagnosis and prognosis of many diseases. Pathological (abnormal) constituents of the urine are the substances not present in the urine to become detectable by conventional analytical techniques under normal healthy conditions. Their detection in urine is an important diagnostic tool to detect the occurrence of certain pathological conditions or diseases. These substances are reducing sugars (mostly glucose), ketone bodies, proteins, blood and bile constituents–bile pigments and bile salts.

STUDY QUESTIONS

1. Describe briefly the composition and functions of blood.
2. Name the diseases that generally accompany a change in the normal levels of the following blood components:

   (i) Erythrocytes (ii) Leukocytes

   (iii) Platelets (iv) Albumin

   (v) Water
3. Write a detailed note on blood as carrier of oxygen and carbon dioxide.
4. Write a short note on physiology and pathology of urine formation by renal filtration of blood.
5. What is the significance of blood pH regulation in sustaining life how it is brought about?

CHAPTER 8

Food Intake, Digestion and Absorption

Chapter Outlines

- Introduction
- Hunger and appetite
- A road map of digestion and absorption
- Basic processes in digestion and absorption
- Secretions of digestive system
- Saliva
- Gastric juice
- Bile
- Pancreatic juice
- Intestinal juice
- Control of digestive secretions
- Digestion and absorption of carbohydrates
- Digestion and absorption of proteins
- Digestion and absorption of fats
- Intestinal microflora
- Study questions

INTRODUCTION

Utilization of food for nourishing the body involves an array of processes that begin with food intake, followed, in quick succession, by digestion, absorption and transport of nutrients, metabolism and respiration, the latter being action of cellular machinery on the transported nutrients to cause metabolic breakdown, oxidation and energy capture requiring oxygen. The train of processes culminates in excretion of wastes that include food and tissue wastes from the bowl, carbondioxide from the lungs and nitrogenous as well as some mineral wastes and spillage of metabolism through the kidneys. Thus many complex and inter-related processes are in place for affecting the utilization of food by the body of which food intake, digestion and absorption remain most important and involved ones. These three, being discussed here, involve many biochemical reactions and physiological activities.

HUNGER AND APPETITE

Groups of cells in the hypothalamus affect hunger, the primary physiological desire to find and eat food. These cells may sense and monitor blood glucose and other nutrients and read their low levels as a signal to promote feeding.

Hunger (Fig. 8.1) is defined as the physiological need to eat, experienced as a drive for obtaining food, an unpleasant sensation that demands relief. *Appetite* is defined as the psychological desire to eat, a learned motivation and a positive sensation that accompanies the sight, smell, or thought of appealing foods. Hunger is a drive programmed into us by our heredity. Appetite, which is learned, can teach us to ignore hunger or to over-respond to it. Hunger is physiological, while appetite is psychological, and the two do not always coincide. Satiety (feeling full) signals that it is time to stop eating, most likely the result of communication between the stomach and small intestine and the brain's hypothalamus as some overeaters claim they never feel full. Thus a variety of internal/physiological (hunger related) and external/psychological (appetite related) forces affect satiety. Hunger forces like low levels of certain nutrients in the blood combine with appetite forces like easy availability of food to promote feeding.

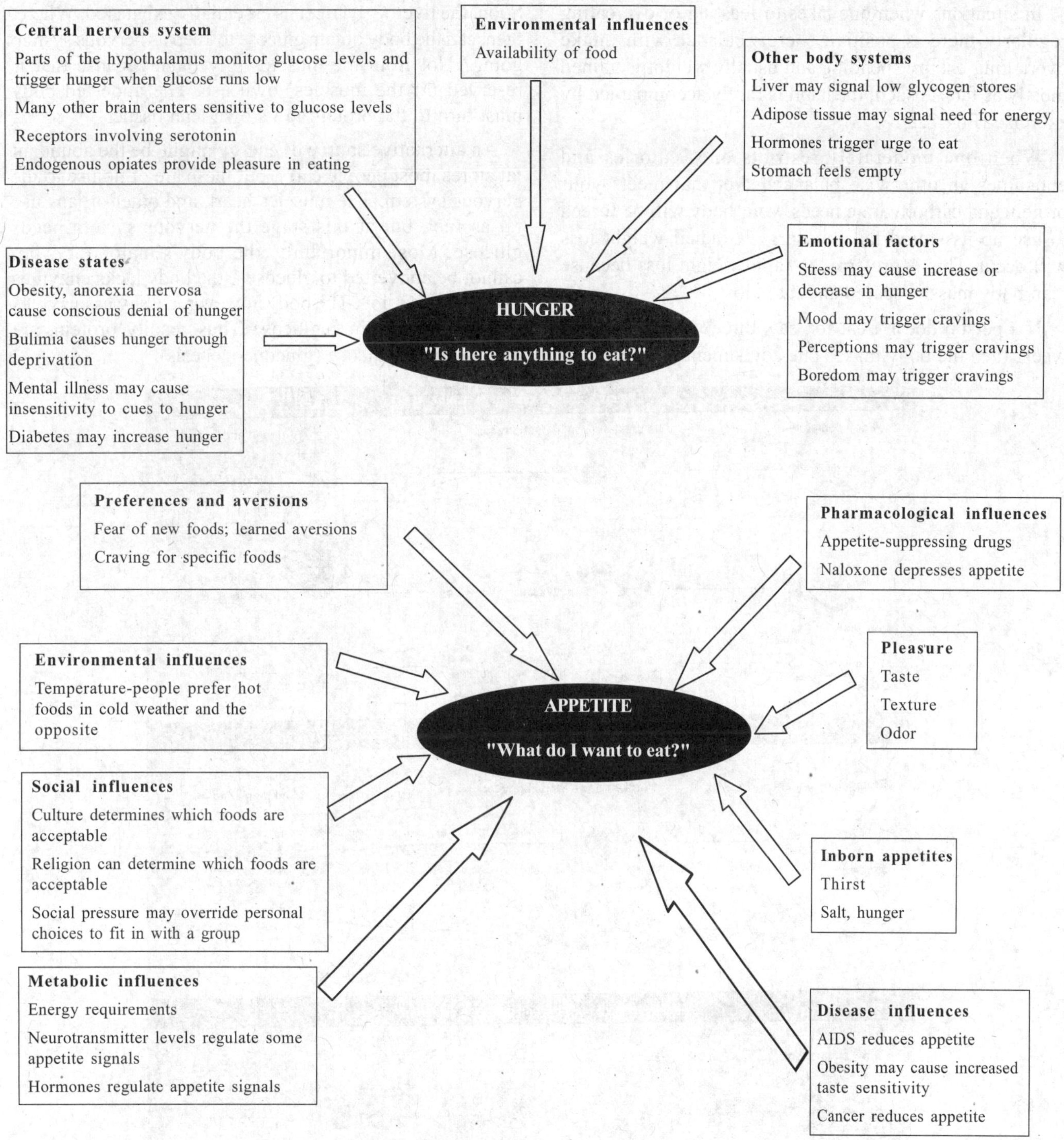

Fig. 8.1: Factors that affect hunger and appetite

Some people argue that the terms hunger and appetite can apply only to human beings as only they can say whether they are hungry or have a specific appetite. However, investigators working with laboratory animals also observe feeding behaviour in animals. Thus hunger and appetite are a set of signals that promote the initiation of feeding and guide the choice of feed items.

In situations when one takes to feasting or overeating regularly there is positive energy balance with intake overtaking energy spending and usually weight is gained mostly as fat. As such, the habit is rarely accompanied by exercise (Fig. 8.2).

When one moderately restricts ones calories and consumes an otherwise balanced diet that meets your protein and carbohydrate needs, your body will be forced to use up its stored fat for energy. Gradual weight loss will occur. This is preferred to rapid weight loss because lean body mass is spared and fat is lost.

If a person doesn't eat for, say, three whole days or a week, then the body makes one adjustment after another. Soon, the liver's glycogen is essentially exhausted. Where, then, can the body obtain glucose to keep its nervous system going? Not from the muscles' glycogen because that is reserved for the muscles' own use. The underfed body must turn to the protein in its own lean tissues.

An alternative source of energy might be the abundant fat stores most people carry, but these are of no use to the nervous system. The muscles heart, and other organs use fat as fuel, but at this stage the nervous system needs glucose. Most importantly, the body's major fuel, fat, cannot be converted to glucose—the body lacks enzymes for this conversion. The body however, possesses enzymes that convert protein to glucose. Thus, readily, proteins are used to make glucose (gluconeogenesis).

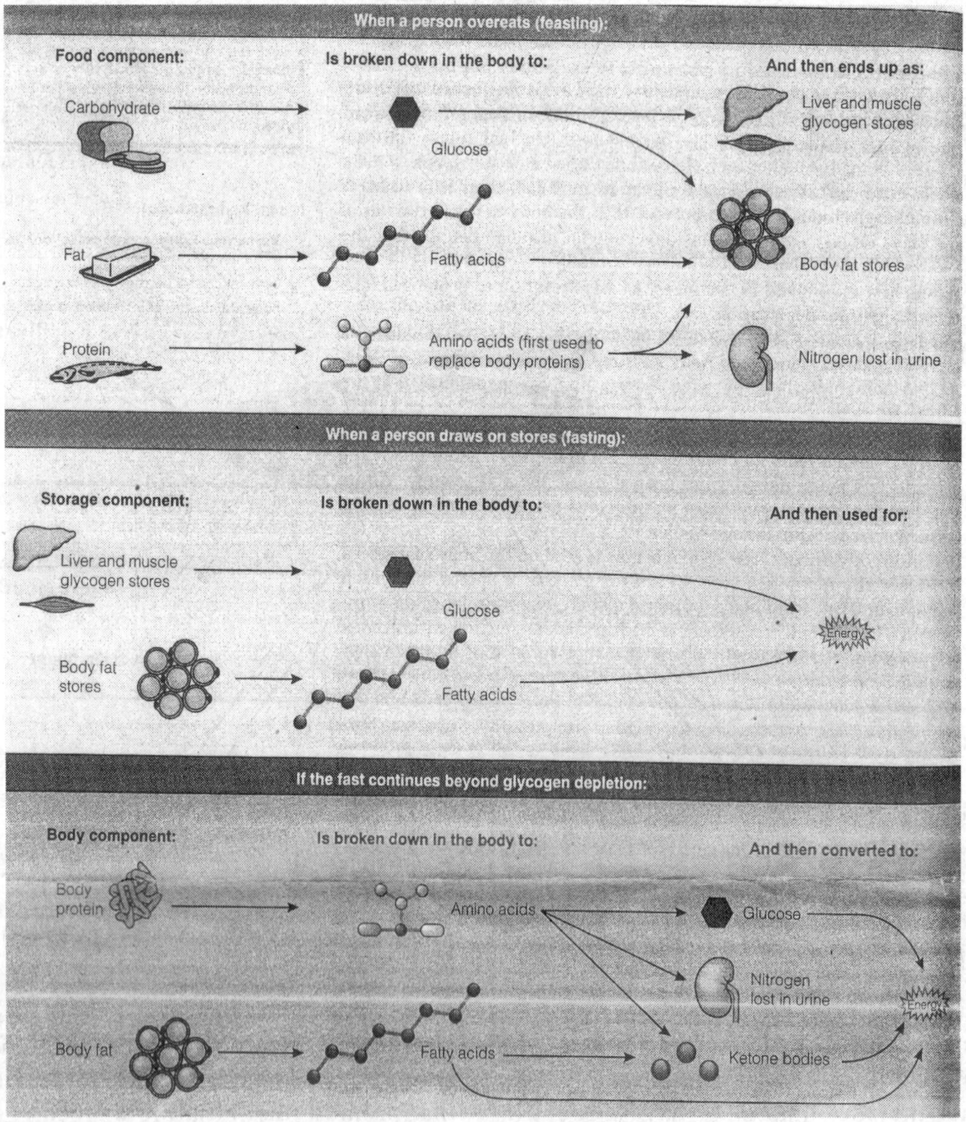

Fig. 8.2: Feasting, fasting and energy balance

A ROAD MAP OF DIGESTION AND ABSORPTION

Because of their complex chemical, often polymeric, structures many components of food cannot as such nourish our bodies. Hence it becomes imperative that there should be an elaborate process which should render complex food materials into simple, diffusible and utilizable forms. This important task is accomplished by digestive system of the body, and the sum total of the chemical and mechanical processes that bring about such transformation are referred to as digestion. It is only after digestion that food components assume molecular sizes and forms that are readily absorbed from the gastrointestinal tract into the blood or lymph circulation.

Large and complex food substances are broken down into smaller ones by chemical reactions that take place in the gastrointestinal tract, also called alimentary canal, of the body. Since most of the chemical reactions taking place in the living systems are catalysed by specific proteins or enzymes, these too, being no exceptions. Therefore, digestion of food components involve occurrence of enzyme catalysed reactions of hydrolytic cleavage of chemical bonds—H and OH groups of water splitting glycosidic, ester and peptide bonds of carbohydrates, proteins fats respectively, resulting in the formation of small, monomeric and diffusible forms of these macronutrients. Digestion, thus is an essential prerequisite for the nourishing action of macronutrients (complex carbohydrates, fats and proteins) because of their polymeric macromolecular nature. Micronutrients (vitamins and minerals), on the other hand, are the food substances that are absorbed by human gastrointestinal tract without affecting much changes in their chemical make up. However, there are some small time exceptions, of certain vitamins (polyglutamate form of folic acid, vitamin A esters and β carotene) undergoing some digestive processing into assimilable forms.

Certain other food substances, of not much nutritional consequence, nucleic acid for instance, also get subjected to digestive hydrolysis.

Digestive enzymes—the kingpins of digestive process—are the indispensable components of digestive secretions of the gastrointestinal tract and associated tissues. Apart from enzymes, digestive secretions also have non enzymic ingredients also participating in digestion and absorption process. Some of them also perform an additional function of protecting the lining of gastrointestinal tract from the hydrolytic action of digestive secretions.

A tube like structure, 5-6 times larger than the height of an adult human, is the site of the activity where digestion and absorption takes place. The tract is aptly named as gastrointestinal tract and extends from mouth to large intestine, spanning oesophagous, stomach and small intestine in between. Further, intestines, both small and large, can be further subdivided into 3-4 portions. Whereas the small intestine comprises duodenum, jejunum and ileum, the larger one has caecum, colon, rectum and anal canal as its four segments. Pancreas and the liver, though not part of gastrointestinal tract, aptly qualify for its associated tissues, for they synthesize and release an array of important digestive secretions.

Given hereunder is the summary of the functioning of different organs of digestive system:

Mouth	:	The lips and cheeks keep food between the teeth during mastication and buccal glands lining the mouth produce saliva.
Tongue	:	Manoeuvres food for mastication, shapes food into a bolus, manoeuvres food for deglutition, detects taste and touch sensations, and initiates digestion of triglycerides.
Salivary glands	:	Produce saliva, which softens, moistens and dissolves foods; cleanses mouth and teeth; and initiates the digestion of starch.
Teeth	:	Cut, tear and pulverize food to reduce solids to smaller particles for swallowing.
Pharynx	:	Receives a bolus from the oral cavity and passes it into the esophagus.
Esophagus	:	Receives a bolus from the pharynx and moves it into the stomach. This requires relaxation of the upper esophageal sphincter and secretion of mucus.
Stomach	:	Mixing waves macerate food, mix it with secretions of gastric glands (gastric juice), and reduce food to chyme. Gastric juice activates pepsin and kills many microbes in food. Intrinsic factor aids absorption of vitamin B_{12}. The stomach serves as a

	:	reservoir for food before releasing it into the small intestine.
Pancreas	:	Pancreatic juice buffers acidic gastric juice in chyme (creating the proper pH for digestion in the small intestine), stops the action of pepsin from the stomach, and contains enzymes that digest carbohydrates, proteins, triglycerides and nucleic acids.
Liver	:	Produces bile, which is needed for the emulsification and absorption of lipids in the small intestine.
Gallbladder	:	Stores and concentrates bile and releases it into the small intestine.
Small intestine	:	Segmentations mix chyme with digestive juices; migrating motility complexes propel chyme toward the ileocecal sphincter; digestive secretions from the small intestine, pancreas, and liver complete the digestion of carbohydrates, proteins, lipids and nucleic acids; circular folds, villi, and microvilli increase surface area for absorption; site where about 90% of nutrients and water are absorbed.
Large intestine	:	Haustral churning, peristalsis and mass peristalsis drive the contents of the colon into the rectum; bacteria produce some B vitamins and vitamin K; absorption of some water, ions and vitamins; defecation.

Thus two groups of organs compose the digestive system, the gastrointestinal (GI) tract, and the accessory digestive organs. The *gastrointestinal (GI) tract*, or *alimentary canal*, is a continuous tube that extends from the mouth to the anus. Organs of the gastrointestinal tract include the mouth, most of the pharynx, esophagus, stomach, small intestine, and large intestine. The length of the GI tract taken from a cadaver is about 9 m (30 ft). In a living person, it is much shorter because the muscles along the walls of GI tract organs are in a state of tonus (sustained contraction). The *accessory digestive organs* include the teeth, tongue, salivary glands, liver, gallbladder and pancreas. Teeth aid in the physical breakdown of food, and the tongue assists in chewing and swallowing. The other accessory digestive organs, however, never come into direct contact with food. They produce or store secretions that flow into GI tract through ducts; the secretions aid in the chemical breakdown of food.

BASIC PROCESSES IN DIGESTION AND ABSORPTION

Overall, the digestive system performs six basic processes:

1. **Partaking:** This process involves taking foods and liquids into the mouth.
2. **Secretion:** Each day, cells within the walls of the GI tract and accessory digestive organs secrete a total of about 7 liters of water, acid, buffers, and enzymes into the lumen of the tract.
3. **Mixing and Propulsion:** Alternating contraction and relaxations of smooth muscle in the walls of the GI tract mix food and secretions and propel them toward the anus. This capability of the GI tract to mix and move material along its length is called *motility*.
4. **Digestion:** Mechanical and chemical processes breakdown ingested food into small molecules. In *mechanical digestion* the teeth cut and grind food before it is swallowed, and then smooth muscles of the stomach and small intestine churn the food. As a result, food molecules become dissolved and thoroughly mixed with digestive enzymes. In *chemical digestion*, the large carbohydrate, lipid, protein, and nucleic acid molecules in food are split into smaller molecules by hydrolysis. Digestive enzymes produced by the salivary glands, tongue, stomach, pancreas and small intestine catalyze these catabolic reactions. A few substances in food can be absorbed without chemical digestion. These include vitamins, ions, cholesterol and water.
5. **Absorption:** The entrance of ingested and secreted fluids, ions and the products of digestion into the epithelial cells lining the lumen of the GI tract is called *absorption*. The absorbed substances pass into blood or lymph and circulate to cells throughout the body.
6. **Defecation:** Wastes, indigestible substances, bacteria, cells sloughed from the lining of the GI tract and digested materials that were not absorbed in their journey through the digestive tract leave the body through anus in a process called *defecation*. The eliminated material is termed *feces*.

SECRETIONS OF DIGESTIVE SYSTEM

Elaborate task of digestion (Fig. 8.3) is accomplished by the coordinated action of a number of secretions, viz., saliva, gastric juice, pancreatic juice, bile and succus entericus or intestinal juice. Whereas saliva, bile and pancreatic juice are secreted through ducts by the tissues that are not integral components of the gastrointestinal tract; the other, namely gastric and intestinal secretions are secreted by the secretory cells of the gastric and intestinal mucosa respectively. Most of these secretions are mixture of enzymes and non-enzyme substances that act on various components of food and render them diffusible and utilizable (Fig. 8.4).

SALIVA

Saliva is colourless viscous mixture of secretions from three pairs of glands, namely parotid (located at the back of mouth below the ear), submaxillary (presents below the lower jaw) and sublingual (situated under the tongue). Saliva solids constitute a mere 1 percent, rest being water making it a very dilute solution of pH ranging between 6.5-7.0, comprising enzymes (α-amylase and lysozyme), glycoprotein-mucin and inorganic constituents thiocynate, chloride, phosphate, sulphate and bicarbonate as anions and sodium, potassium and calcium as cations. Average daily secretion of saliva ranges between 1-2 litres.

The major action of saliva on food is in its lubrication, making its swallowing an easy and effortless affair. With the action of salivary amylase, the enzyme component of saliva, there also begins the digestion in the mouth itself. However, this is of little consequence for food because it doesn't stay for a longer duration in the mouth or oral cavity.

Though saliva is ever present in the mouth; sight, smell or thought of food is said to enhance its flow by reflex stimulation. Mechanical stimulation by a mere presence of food in the mouth and chemical stimulation by its action on the taste buds also augment its flow proportionately and adequately.

GASTRIC JUICE

Normal gastric juice is a clear pale yellow fluid of specific gravity 1.007. Its daily output approximates 2-3.5 litres. It is highly acidic in nature with pH ranging between 1.0-2.0. Secretion of gastric juice, a process mediated through vagus nerve, is elicited by sight, smell, taste and even thought of an appetizing food Gastrin, a hormone secreted by gastric mucosa as a sequel to the food being present in the stomach, also causes the release of gastric secretions.

Chief constituents of gastric juice include hydrochloric acid (0.3-0.4 percent), zymogen-pepsinogen, renin or chymosin (only in infants), mucus, hematopoietic or intrinsic factor for vitamin B_{12} absorption and small, almost symbolic, amounts of enzyme lipase. Natural food substances apart, other known stimulant of gastric secretions are insulin (causes the secretion of acid and pepsin), histamine and alcohol (causes the secretion of acid only). That is why dilute ethyl alcohol (200 ml, 7 percent volume/volume) and histamine (0.04 mg/kg body wt) are used as stimulants of gastric secretion for its collection and subsequent analysis.

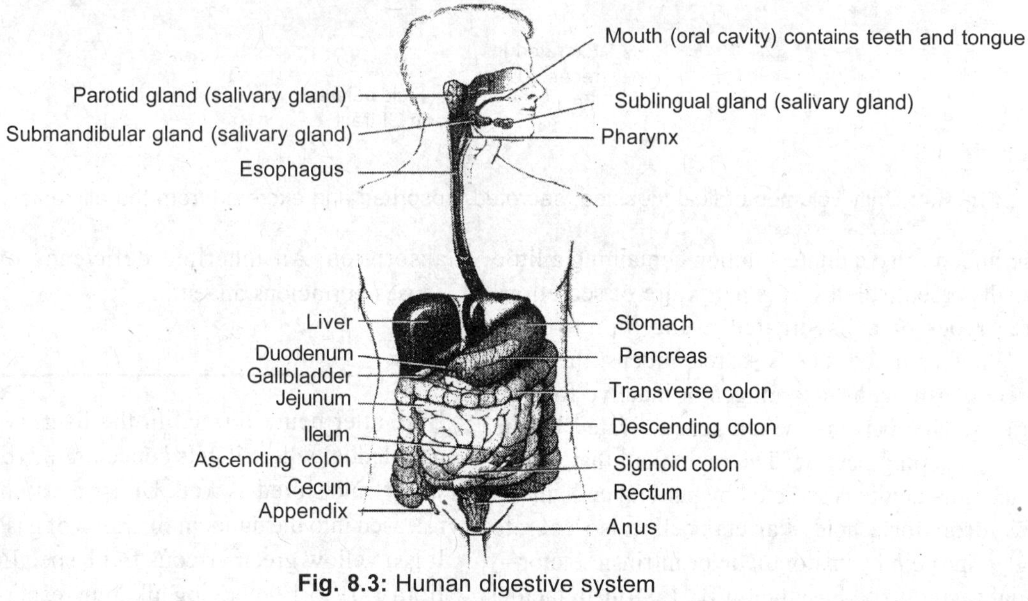

Fig. 8.3: Human digestive system

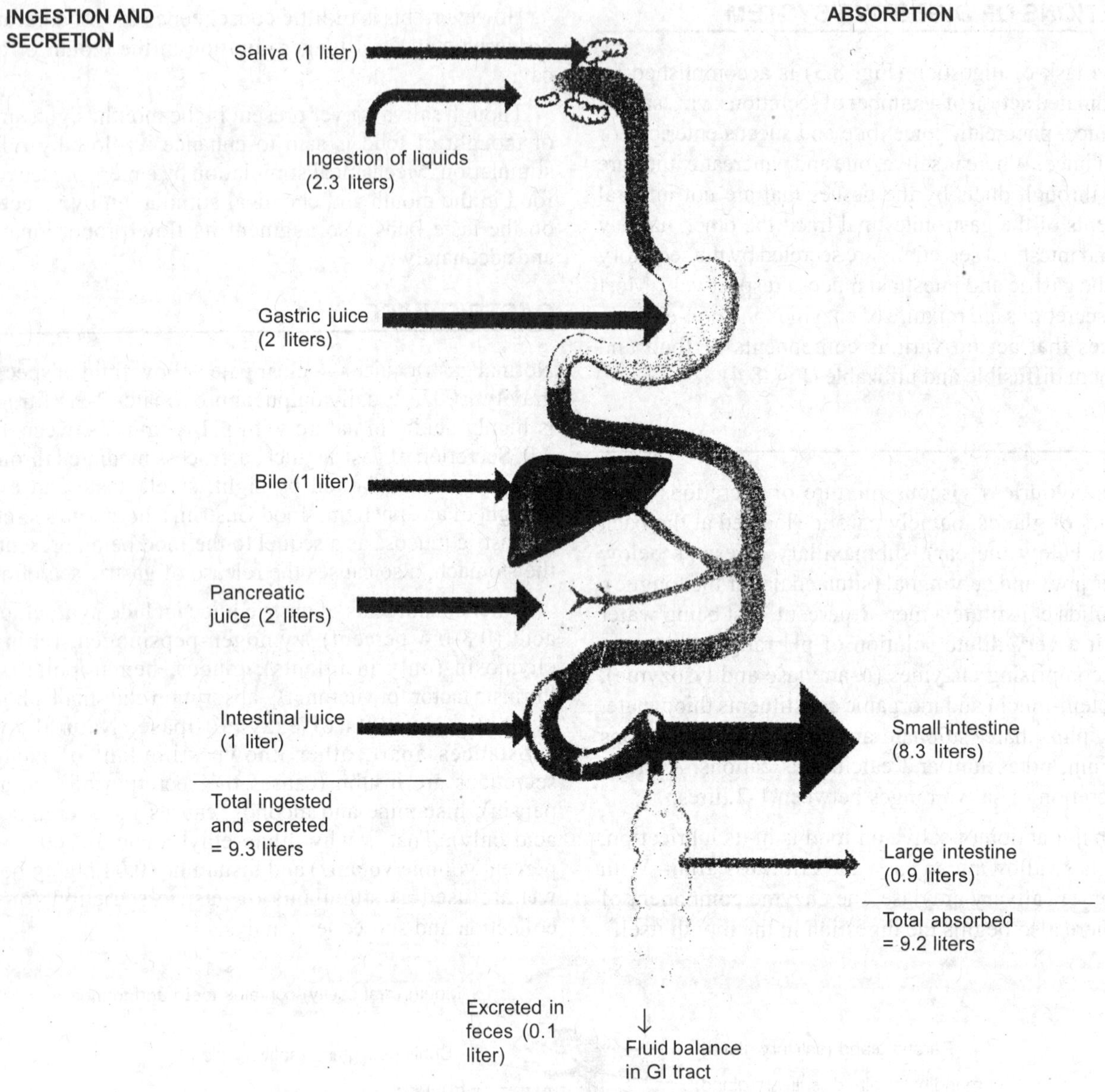

Fig. 8.4: Daily volumes of fluid ingested, secreted, absorbed and excreted from the alimentary canal

Gastric juice is also a dilute solution containing a little more than 1 percent solutes. It is a mixture of secretions from three types of cells situated in the lining of the stomach. Whereas mucous cells secrete mucus, the chief cells secrete pepsinogen—a zymogen or inactive form of proteolytic enzyme pepsin—which gets activated by the cleavage of a capping peptide. The ingredient that makes gastric juice rank acidic is secreted by parietal cells in the form of hydrochloric acid. Parietal cells also secrete another glycoprotein haematopoietic or intrinsic factor—an essential prerequisite for vitamin B_{12} (extrinsic factor) absorption. An inherited deficiency of intrinsic factor causes pernicious anaemia.

BILE

Bile, after being formed in the liver, is passed on to the gallbladder where it gets concentrated (by reabsorption of water) and stored as well. Under the stimulus of food, it is released into the duodenum region of gastrointestinal tract. It is a yellow green viscous fluid, specific gravity ranging from 1.01 to 1.04 having alkaline reaction (pH 7.2-8.5), a characteristic odour and bitter taste. The normal volume secreted daily into the duodenum ranges between 500 ml to 1100 ml. Its principal constituents are bile salts, bile pigments, lipids (including fats, lecithin and other phosphatides and cholesterol), proteins (mucin and nucleoproteins) and inorganic ions such as bicarbonate, chloride, sodium, potassium, iron, copper, calcium, magnesium and zinc. Bile salts, sodium glycocholate and sodium taurocholate are the main functionally digestive ingredients of bile. Others, namely lecithin (phosphatidyl choline), sodium and potassium salts of fatty acids (soaps), bicarbonates and chlorides of sodium and potassium and protein mucin also play roles in the digestion and absorption of foods. Bilirubin and its oxidation products, biliverdin, are the pigments of bile. Bile owes its colour to these pigments. Bile pigments along with cholesterol comprise the main endogenous excretory materials present in bile. Other endogenous substances that may also find their way into bile for excretion albeit at a far smaller quantitative levels are thyroid hormones (thyroxine) and steroid hormones. Apart from these, liver uses bile as a vehicle for eliminating compounds of foreign origin (chemical and toxic substances, such as metals, toxins and drug metabolites for instance). Most of the excretory substances, both of exogenous and endogenous origin, are present as conjugates of glucuronic acid as glucuronide to tone down their toxicity and enhance solubility.

Unlike most of other reactions of gastrointestinal tract, bile doesn't contain any enzyme. This, however, doesn't undermine its contribution to digestion in the intestinal tract. Bile salts, owing to their being surfaceactants (having surface tension lowering property) cause emulsification of fats and fat soluble vitamins and by doing so they increase their surface area, facilitating the action of lipolytic enzymes on fats.

PANCREATIC JUICE

Pancreatic juice is an alkaline secretion of exocrine pancreatic cells reaching gastrointestinal tract through pancreatic duct. It is also a dilute 1 percent solution, its 99 percent being constituted by water. Among solid constituents, enzymes, glycoprotein, mucin and inorganic ions (bicarbonate, chloride, sodium and potassium) are the principle ones. Of enzymes, there is an array of proteases (Trypsinogen, chymotrypsinogen, procarboxylase A and B and proelastase) all secreted in zymogen forms. Lipase along with small amount of phospholipase (zymogen prophospolipase form) and cholesterol esterase and α-amylase are the lipid and carbohydrate digesting enzymes. Small amounts of ribonuclease (RNAse) and deoxyribonuclease (DNAse) are nevertheless sufficient for the digestion of small proportion of nucleic acids in food.

Presence of almost a complete range of nutrient hydrolyzing enzymes in pancreatic juice makes it the dominant contributor of intestinal dietary digestion. Further, the proportion of different enzymes vary in keeping with the composition of the blood ingested.

A high fat diet, for instance, induce the secretion of a pancreatic juice containing higher proportion of lipolytic enzymes.

INTESTINAL JUICE

Intestinal juice or succus entericus is secreted by crypts of Liberkuhn and glands of Brunner present in the intestinal mucosa. Whereas glands of Brunner are located in the duodenum, only the crypts of Liberkuhn are present all though the mucosa of small intestine. The composite secretion of these two glands contains mucin, serotonin and the some electrolytes that are present in the pancreatic juice, bicarbonate being an exception for its lower content in intestinal juice. These components create a favorable atmosphere for the digestion and absorption of partially digested food products. Apart from intestinal mucosa, includes intracellular enzymes, i.e., disaccharides (maltose, sucrose, lactose, isomaltose), dipeptidases, aminopeptidases, nucleosidases, nucleotidases and phosphatases.

CONTROL OF DIGESTIVE SECRETIONS

Nervous and mechanical stimulation apart, the digestive secretions are also regulated by hormonal interplay. These hormones are synthesized in the gastrointestinal mucosa where the hormone synthesizing cells lie interspersed between other mucosal cells. They secrete their respective hormonal secretion into the blood circulation as a sequel to the arrival of food in the gut from where they reach respective target organs. Although several substances with such activities have been encountered in the alimentary canal; four of them, namely gastrin, secretin, cholecystokinin and somatostatin; have been found to act through hormonal target tissue interactions on the gastrointestinal secretary tissues. Table 8.1 sums up the role of these gastrointestinal hormones in the regulation of digestive secretions.

Table 8.1: Hormones that regulate digestion

Hormone	*Stimulus and site of secretion*	*Actions*
Gastrin	Distension of stomach, partially digested proteins and caffeine in stomach, and high pH of stomach chyme stimulate gastrin secretion by enteroendocrine G cells, located mainly in the mucosa of pyloric antrum of stomach.	*Major effects:* Promote secretion of gastric juice, increases gastric motility, and promotes growth of gastric mucosa. *Minor effects:* Constricts lower esophageal sphincter, relaxes pyloric sphincter.
Secretin	Acidic (high H+ level) chyme that enters the small intestine stimulates secretion of secretin by enteroendocrine S cells in the mucosa of the duodenum.	*Major effects:* Stimulates secretion of pancreatic juice and bile that are rich in HCO_3^- (bicarbonate ions). *Minor effects:* Inhibits secretion of gastric juice, promotes normal growth and maintenance of the pancreas, and enhances effects of CCK.
Cholecystokinin (CCK)	Partially digested proteins (amino acids), triglycerides, and fatty acids that enter the small intestine stimulate secretion of CCK by enteroendocrine CCK cells in the mucosa of the small intestine; CCK is also released in the brain.	*Major effects:* Stimulates secretion of pancreatic juice rich in digestive enzymes, causes ejection of bile from the gallbladder and opening of the sphincter of the hepatopancreatic ampulla (sphincter of Oddi), and induces satiety (feeling full to satisfaction). *Minor effects:* Inhibits gastric emptying, promotes normal growth and maintenance of the pancreas, and enhances effects of secretin.
Somatostatin	This gastrointestinal secretion acts on gastric mucosa.	Causes inhibition of HCl and pepsin secretion by gastric mucosa.

Self shielding of the gastrointestinal tract from the onslaught of digestive enzymes:

Since cells of the gastrointestinal mucosa and those of digestive glands are constituted by proteins, lipids, and to a much smaller extent, by carbohydrates, it becomes necessary to explain the puzzling fact that these cells remain unharmed in the presence of highly hydrolytic enzymes (proteolytic, lipolytic and amylolytic). The following points reveal the reality behind this puzzle:

i. In the cells that store and secrete the digestive enzymes, they (the digestive enzymes) are well segregated from other cellular contents by being encased in membrane surrounded vacuoles.

ii. The hydrolytic enzymes, the proteolytic and lipolytic ones especially, are stored and secreted in inactive zymogen or proenzyme forms that get activated only on exposure to specific substances in gut lumen.

iii. While in action in gut lumen, they are of no threat to the mucosal cells because they are very effectively sheathed—both mechanically (gut mucus creates a physical barrier) and chemically (gastric mucus has antitrypsin factors and an enormous buffering capacity) by a coating of mucus.

DIGESTION AND ABSORPTION OF CARBOHYDRATES

Carbohydrates: Ingested food on entering the mouth gets chopped down and chewed into fine particles by the action of teeth. During the course of this action, it also gets mixed up with saliva. Saliva, apart from lubricating food also initiates enzymatic action on starch through its salivary amylase, or ptyalin. However, the action, that involves conversion of starch to maltose, is of minor consequence as the presence of food in the mouth is too short to allow any worthwhile action by salivary amylase. The optimum pH for the action of salivary amylase is slightly acidic to neutral (6.8 to 7.0).

The food mixed with saliva digestion descends down the stomach, where it gets mixed up with gastric juice. The extremely low pH of the gastric juice (1.0-2.0) inactivates salivary amylase making salivary digestion a mercurial and symbolic affair. The human gastric juice doesn't contain any carbohydrate splicing enzyme. In a sharp contrast, first stomach (rumen) of all cattle (ruminants) inhabits microorganisms that produce a special cellulose splitting enzyme, cellulase or 1-4 glycosidase) that hydrolyzes cellulose to glucose.

But no such enzyme activity is present in the stomach or any other part of the alimentary canal. That explains the gross inefficiency of human beings in utilizing cellulose material (grass, fodder etc) as energy yielding food material.

The semi digested food materials leaving stomach is called chyme, which on entering the small intestine, has most of its carbohydrate content in an undigested state. However, the carbohydrate hydrolyzing enzymes of pancreatic juice and intestinal mucosa convert complex carbohydrates into simple monosaccharides in a systematic and coordinated manner. First of all, pancreatic amylase enzyme (pH optima 6.5 to 7.1) acts on 1-4 glycosidic linkages of starch, both soluble (amylose) and insoluble (amylopectin). However, 1-6 glycosidic linkage of amylopectin remain intact.

Digestion products of amylose by the action of pancreatic amylase are maltotriose and maltose. But action of this enzyme on amylopection also produces isomaltose and branched dextrins of small chain lengths. Since amylase enzyme doesn't act on the outermost 1-4 linkages, free glucose is not formed by the action of -amylase.

Finally, the carbohydrate digestion products (disaccharides and oligosaccharides) and dietary disaccharides (Lactose and Sucrose) are hydrolyzed by oligosaccharidase (α-dextrinase) and disaccharidases (sucrose, maltase, lactase and isomaltase) enzymes on the brush border membrane of the small intestine. This phase of carbohydrate digestion that occurs at the permeability barriers (cell membranes) of the small intestine is referred to as intracellular phase. Hence, the net effect of enzymatic digestion of carbohydrates produces mainly monosaccharide glucose along with small amounts of fructose and galactose.

Monosaccharides, the end products of carbohydrate digestion are absorbed by active transport (glucose and galactose) and facilitated diffusion (fructose).

Whereas absorption of glucose and galactose is carrier mediated, energy (ATP) dependent sodium linked symport (A molecule of glucose or galactose is absorbed concomitantly with a Na+) that works against a concentration gradient, the absorption of fructose in contrast is carrier mediated but energy independent and in accordance with concentration gradient (facilitated diffusion).

DIGESTION AND ABSORPTION OF PROTEINS

Protein digestion begins in the stomach as saliva contains no known proteolytic enzyme. However, enzymes present in gastric and pancreatic secretion (mostly endopeptidases) and intestinal mucosal cells (mostly exopeptidases) bring about the hydrolysis of proteins into their component amino acids.

Broadly speaking, the enzymes carrying out protein digestion can be studied under two heads, the endopeptidases and the exopeptidases. Whereas the former hydrolyze specific peptide bonds of protein chains that are positioned in the middle of the molecules. Pepsin of the gastric juice and trypsin and chymotrypsin of the pancreatic juice (all secreted in their respective zymogen form) are all endopeptidases. Exopeptidases, on the other hand, act on the terminal peptide bonds removing amino acids either from the carboxy (carboxy peptidases) or the aminoterminals (amino peptidases) of the proteins (Table 8.2).

Pepsin, the enzyme first to act on proteins in the stomach, mostly attack those peptide bonds that are formed between acidic amino acids (L-glutamic acid and aspartic acid) and aromatic amino acids (L-phenylalanine, L-tyrosine and L-tryptophan). However, this enzyme has not been found to be highly specific and hydrolyzes, albeit much slowly, the other peptide bonds as well.

Pepsin, as had been mentioned earlier, is secreted as zymogen 'pepsinogen' and is converted to pepsin by hydrochloride acid of gastric juice at the beginning of digestion and by pepsin itself (autocatalytically). The digestive action of this proteolytic enzyme involves converting proteins to a mixture of polypeptides of different chain lengths (proteoses and peptones). A sizable part (about 10 percent) of the protein digestion is credited to the action of pepsin. The optimum pH for its action is between 1.5 to 2.2.

Table 8.2: Enzymes of protein digestion			
Active enzymes	*Zymogen*	*Activator*	*Specificity*
Pepsin	Pepsinogen	HCl Autoactivation by pepsin	R ↓ | R ↓ | —CO—NH—CHCO—NH—CH—CO— R' = Tyr, Phe R = Asp Glnl
Trypsin	Trypsinogen	Enteropeptidase trypsin	R | ↓ R | —CO—NH—CH—CO—NH—CHCO— R = Arg, Lys
Chymotrypsin	Chymotrypsinogen	Trypsin	R | ↓ R | —CO—NH—CHCO—NHCHCO— R = Tyr, Tyr, phe
Elastase	Proelastase	Trypsin	↓ R | ↓ R | —CO—NHCHCO—NHCHCO— R = Ala, Gly, Ser
Carboxy- peptidase A	Procarboxy- peptidase A	Trypsin	↓ R | —CO—NH—CH—COO R = All amino acids except basic and imino acids
Carboxy- peptidase B	Procarboxy- peptidase B	Trypsin	↓ R | —CO—NHCH—COO⁻ R = Arg, Lys

Renin, another enzyme, a component of infants' gastric juice, converts the milk protein casein into paracasein which, by combining with Ca++, coagulates and stays in the stomach for a longer period and accomplishes its digestion.

In the duodenum, as many as four proteolytic enzymes of the pancreatic secretion, transform the partially digested protein products into a mixture of amino acids and small peptides. All the four peptidases have different peptide bond digestion specification. Trypsin, an all powerful endopeptidase, is also secreted in zymogen (trypsinogen) form. The enzyme is activated initially by another intestinal enzyme, the enteropeptidase and auto catalytically by trypsin later on during the progress of digestive process. Again, the activation involves the removal of a hexapeptide, known as masking peptide. Trypsin specifically hydrolyzes those peptide bonds where the carboxyl group is contributed by basic amino acids; arginine and lysine.

Chymotrypsin, another endopeptidase of pancreatic juice has to be converted from inactive chymotrypsinogen form to active chymotrypsin prior to its action. It hydrolyzes those peptide bonds whose carboxyl groups are contributed by aromatic amino acids; tryptophan, tyrosine and phenylalanine. Whereas pH optima for both the enzymes (trypsin and chymotrypsin) is near 8.0 the trypsin additionally requires Ca++ for its activity. Carboxypeptidase, both A and B, hydrolyze carboxyterminal peptide bonds, the former hydrolyzing carboxy terminal peptide bonds involving all but basic (arginine and lysine) and imino (proline) amino acids, and the latter attacking those carboxy terminal peptide bonds that have arginine and lysine as the end amino acids. Carboxy peptidase A, therefore, is more versatile of the two. Elastase, in keeping with its name, hydrolyzes elastic (fibrins) proteins at peptide bonds involving glycine, leucine, isoleucine and valine amino acids.

The final mopping up operation in protein digestion is performed by the amino peptidases and dipeptidases present in the intestinal mucosal cells. An aminopeptidase, as the name points out acts on peptide bonds involving amino terminal amino acids of an oligopeptide. Dipeptidase also do not lag behind in justifying their names and hydrolyze the lone peptide bond that exists between the two amino acids of a dipeptide. Several aminopeptidases and dipeptidases with separate amino acid specifications have been identified.

The net effect of this enzymatic action is the conversion of all the proteins present in the food into their constituent amino acids, the forms in which they are absorbed and utilized for the synthesis of body proteins.

Dietary proteins, on being hydrolyzed to their constituent amino acids in the gastrointestinal tract, are absorbed by the small intestine and finally get into the portal blood. The mode of amino acid absorption seems to be through energy dependent active transport process, much like that of sugar monosaccharides (glucose and galactose) absorption.

The carrier system is also similar (if not the same), requiring the presence of Na^+. Thus amino acids are also transported with sodium. Further, vitamin B_6 is also required for the passage of amino acids through the serosal side of intestinal mucosa. The neutral and hydrophilic amino acids are absorbed more readily as compared to basic and hydrophobic amino acids. There operates at least four transport systems, one each for neutral, basic, acidic and imino (proline and hydroxyproline) groups of amino acids.

Besides, small intestine may also absorb some small peptides that get hydrolyzed into amino acids through intracellular digestion by aminopeptidases and dipeptidases. However, when larger segments are absorbed and transferred into the blood circulation, owing to a defect in the intestinal mucosa (as happens in the disease like non-tropical sprue) they may cause immunological sensitivity as proteins and polypeptides are antigenic in nature. In this disease the affected individuals become allergic to gluten, the wheat protein because of its incomplete digestion and entry into blood to cause immunogenicity and the resultant symptoms of allergy or hypersensitivity.

DIGESTION AND ABSORPTION OF FATS

Effective digestion of fats takes place only in small intestine, for saliva contains no fat digesting enzyme (lipase) and gastric lipase is handicapped functionally owing to highly acidic environment (pH 1-2) of gastric juice, not at all conducive to the action of lipase (optimum pH 7.0). However, stomach contributes towards fat digestion by its churning action on food which emulsifies fats. In the small intestine (duodenum), the food fats are further acted upon by bile. Bile salts present in this secretion further intensify the emulsification of fats by their surface tension lowering action and convert fat droplets into still finer particles. Phosphatidyl choline, another surfaceactant present in the bile, further augments this (emulsification) process transforming emulsified fats into micelles that are supramolecular aggregates in which the hydrophobic components are localized in the interior and hydrophilic portions lie on the exterior to facilitate the action of pancreatic lipase by greatly increasing the surface area of the fat particles. The enzyme (lipase) being hydrophilic in nature acts only at the interface of fat particles and aqueous phase. Further, pancreatic lipase is an α-lipase and thus it acts specifically at 1st and 3rd ester linkages of a fat (triacylglycerol) molecule thereby converting it to 2-monoacylglycerol. The 2-monoacylglycerol in turn is isomerized to 1-monoacylglycerol by an isomerase and a part of it is further hydrolyzed by the α-lipase to glycerol and free fatty acid. However, it becomes pertinent to note that some fat absorption from luminal side also take place at the monoacylglycerol stage. Pancreatic juice also contains small amounts of phospholiapse and cholesterolesterase that act on phospholipids and cholesterylesters present in foods and the products of such action are also absorbed through the cells of small intestinal mucosa. But quantitatively, they constitute a small and insignificant proportion of total dietary fat.

Thus the process of fat digestion results in the formation of glycerol, free fatty acids and monoacylglycerol, all rolled into miscelles along with bile salts. It is at this stage that micelles get transported through the microvilli of the intestinal mucosal cell membranes by passive diffusion. Once within the mucosal epithelial cells, the long chain (C12 to C18) fatty acids get reesterified with monoacyl and diacylglycerols so as to resynthesize triacylglycerol. These triacylglycerols become part of lipoprotein complexes, the chylomicrons that pass through lacteals and thoracic duct (lymphatic system) into the blood. That precisely is the reason why lymph or blood plasma presents a milky appearance shortly after a fat-rich meal. In contrast, short to medium chain (C4 to C10) fatty acids and glycerol pass from mucosal cells to liver by portal circulation. Bile salts, as part of mixed micelles with glyceride products, are not absorbed along with them. The bile salts after making the products of fat digestion absorbed in the proximal part of the small intestine are themselves absorbed in the distal part and pass from mucosal cells to liver and recycle again and again between intestine and liver or in enterohepatic circulation (Fig. 8.5).

Once in blood, the lipids are transported to various tissues as chylomicrons, lipoproteins and non-esterified fatty acids.

Long-chain fatty acids and monoglycerides are absorbed into lacteals; other products of digestion are absorbed into blood capillaries (Fig. 8.6).

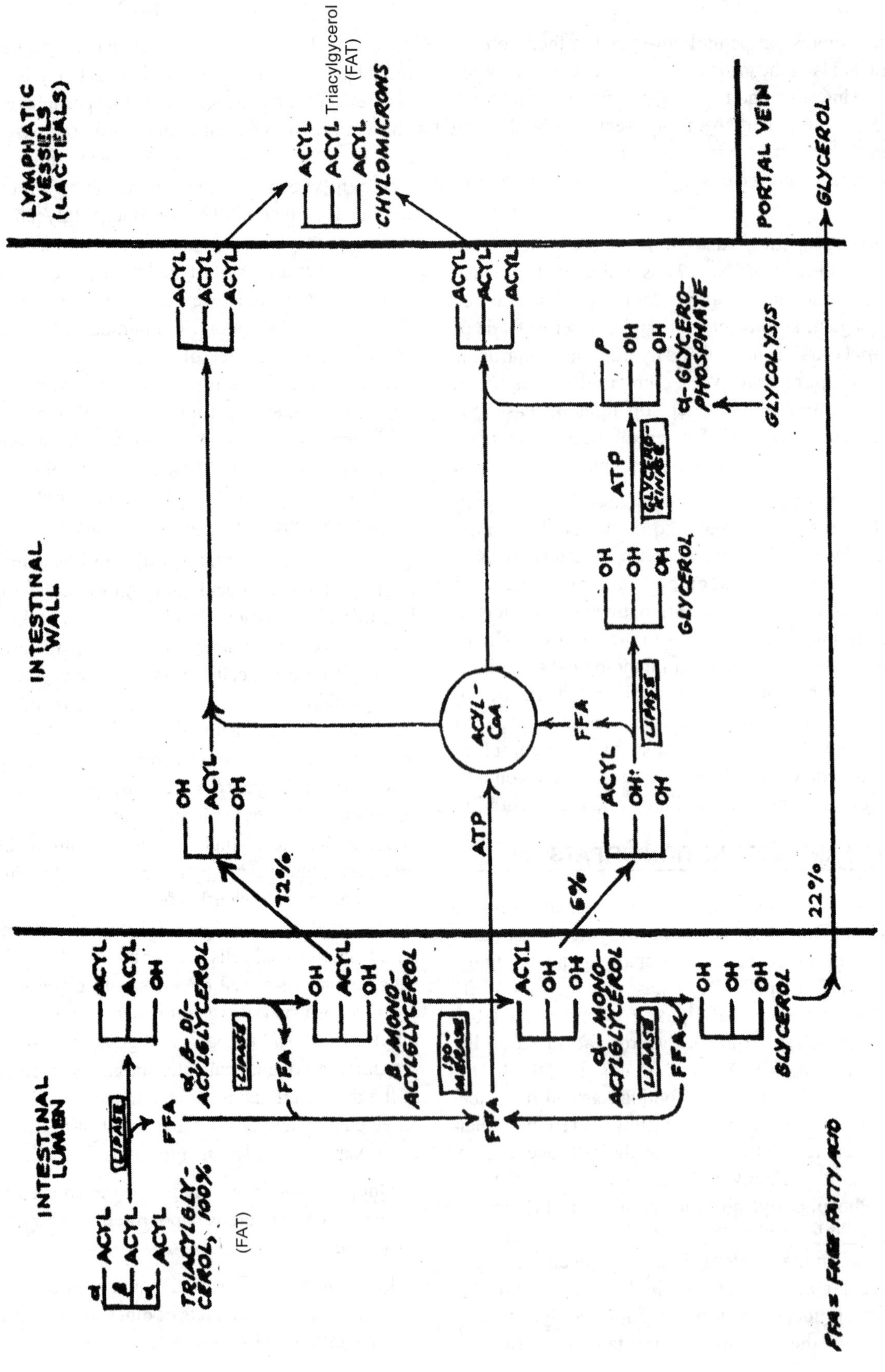

Fig 8.5: Digestion and absorption of fats in small intestine (A schematic diagram)

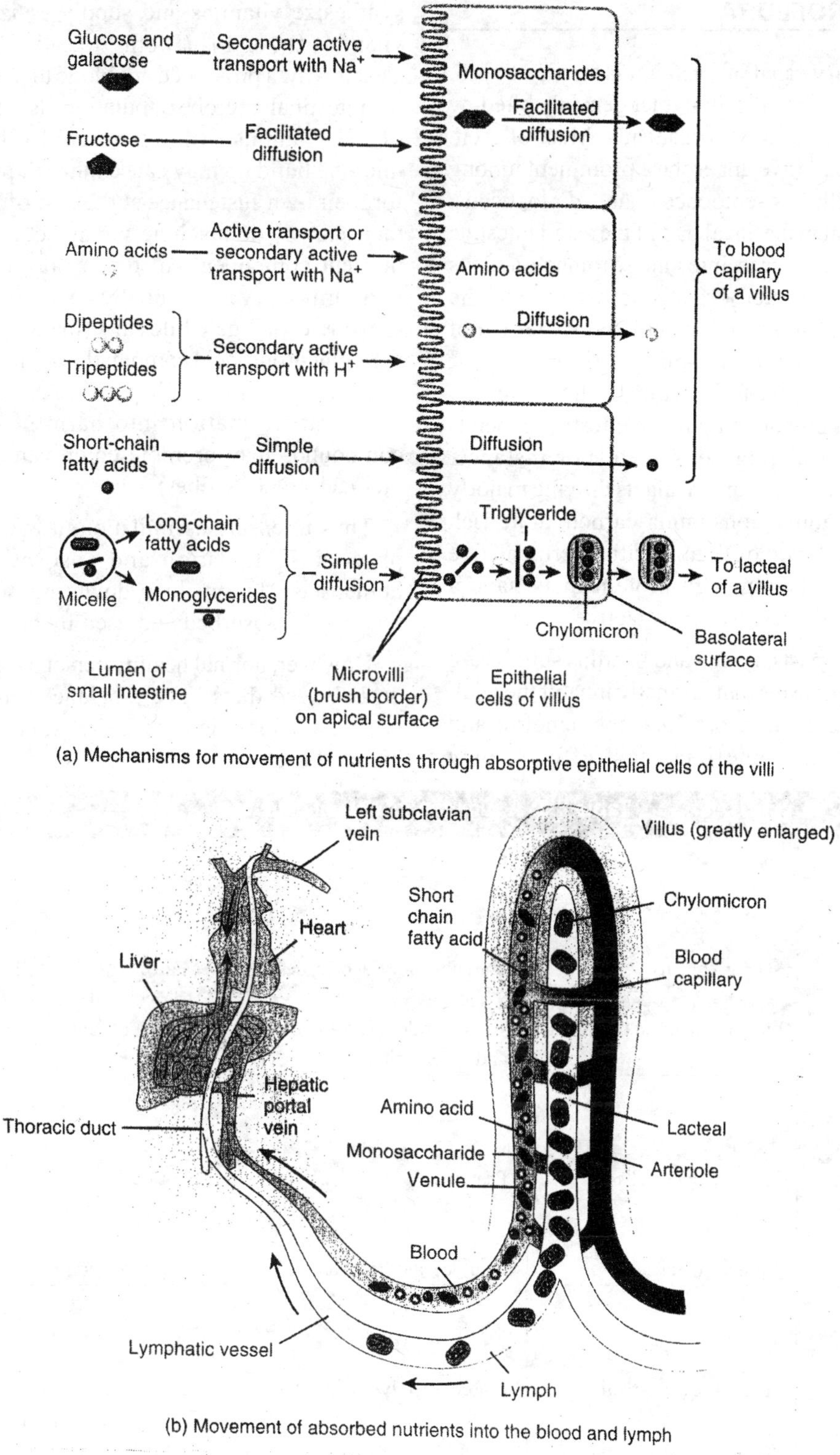

Fig. 8.6: Absorption of digested nutrients in the small intestine (A simplified view). For simplicity, all digested foods are shown in the lumen of the small intestine, even though some nutrients are digested by brush-border enzymes

INTESTINAL MICROFLORA

Though the alimentary canal of an infant is sterile at birth, as the age progresses, the intestinal tract gets inhabited by more than 100 species of microorganisms. Most of them are obligatory or facultative anaerobes, prominent among which are lactobacillus, streptococcus and diplococcus, species mostly present in the distal part of the small intestine or proximal part of the large intestine. Stomach and its vicinity does not have microorganisms because of the highly acidic environment prevalent over there, not conducive to the survival and proliferation of microorganisms. Most of the times, the types of microorganisms that predominate in the intestine depends upon the type of diet being consumed. For instance, lactobacillus species are abundant in infants thriving majorly on milk. Likewise, adults consuming carbohydrate rich diets has a high population of gram positive fermentative organisms and those taking high protein diets have a preponderance of gram negative putrefactive bacteria.

Escherichia coli, yeasts, molds and bacillus subtilis are some of the microorganisms that normally inhabit the adult intestinal tract. Intestinal microflora has benefits and shortcomings. Among beneficial host effects, they synthesize vitamins and supply a sizable proportion of vitamins B_{12} and H (Biotin) to satisfy host requirements. That is why, a prolonged antibiotic therapy that extinguishes the intestinal microbe population also induces a deficiency of the vitamins. Among harmful effects, an excessive microbe build up may cause nutrient pilferage using them for their own sustenance at the cost of human health. Also their enzymatic machinery may act on nutrient and non-nutrient components of dietary origin, converting them into harmful, even potentially toxic, compounds. They may as well deconjugate bile salts (making bile salts free from their glucuronic acid combinations) and hamper their cyclic participation in enterohepatic circulation and promoting their transformation into harmful compounds (such compounds may promote colon cancer especially when diet lacks dietary fiber).

Thus to ensure assimilation, it is underscored that the process of digestion and absorption contributes to homeostasis by breaking down ingested food into forms that can be absorbed and used by body cells (Table 8.3).

However, normal healthy persons sustaining themselves on balanced diets have a balanced intestinal microflora having a symbiotic humane relationship with its humble human host.

Table 8.3: A summary of acts of digestion

Enzymes	*Source*	*Substrates*	*Products*
Saliva			
Salivary amylase	Salivary glands	Starches (polysaccharides)	Maltose (disaccharide), maltotriose (trisaccharide), and α-dextrins.
Lingual lipase	Lingual glands in the tongue	Triglycerides (fats and oils) and other lipids	Fatty acids and diglycerides.
Gastric Juice			
Pepsin (activated from pepsinogen by pepsin and hydrochloric acid	Stomach chief cells	Proteins	Peptides.
Gastric lipase	Stomach chief cells	Triglycerides (fats and oils)	Fatty acids and monoglycerides.
Pancreatic Juice			
Pancreatic amylase	Pancreatic acinar cells	Starches (polysaccharides)	Maltose (disaccharide), maltotriose (trisaccharide), and α-dextrins.
Trypsin (activated from trypsinogen by ente-kinase)	Pancreatic acinar cells	Proteins	Peptides.

Contd.

Contd.

Chymotrypsin (activated from chymotrypsinogen by trypsin)	Pancreatic acinar cells	Proteins	Peptides.
Elastase (activated from proelastase by trypsin)	Pancreatic acinar cells	Proteins	Peptides.
Carboxypeptidase (activated from procarboxypeptidase by trypsin)	Pancreatic acinar cells	Amino acid at carboxyl end of peptides	Amino acids and peptides.
Pancreatic lipase	Pancreatic acinar cells	Triglycerides (fats and oils) that have been emulsified by bile salts.	Fatty acids and monoglycerides.
Nucleases			
Ribonuclease	Pancreatic acinar cells	Ribonucleic acid	Nucleotides.
Deoxyribonuclease	Pancreatic acinar cells	Deoxyribonucleic acid	Nucleotides.
Brush Border			
α-Dextrinase	Small intestine	α-Dextrins	Glucose.
Maltase	Small intestine	Maltose	Glucose.
Sucrase	Small intestine	Sucrose	Glucose and fructose.
Lactase	Small intestine	Lactose	Glucose and galactose.
Enterokinase	Small intestine	Trypsinogen	Trypsin.
Peptidases			
Aminopeptidase	Small intestine	Amino acid at amino end of peptides	Amino acids and peptides.
Dipeptidase	Small intestine	Dipeptides	Amino acids.
Nucleosidases and phosphatases	Small intestine	Nucleotides	Nitrogenous bases, pentoses and phosphates.

STUDY QUESTIONS

1. Write a brief note on gastrointestinal secretions that are instrumental in the process of digestion.
2. What roles do different enzymes play in the digestion of carbohydrates?
3. Explain precisely the role of exo and endopeptidases in protein digestion.
4. Pin-pointing the similarities and differences, explain the absorption of the products of carbohydrate and protein digestion.
5. Why digestion and absorption of fats is a process more complex than that of other macronutrients? Explain giving a brief account of the digestion and absorption of fats.
6. Explain the following:

   i. Incomplete protein digestion.

   ii. Fat malabsorption.

CHAPTER 9

Food-Energy Transformations

Chapter Outlines

- Underpinnings of energy transformation
- Direct calorimetry
- Units of energy measurement
- Specific fuel factors
- Basal metabolic rate (BMR)
- Specific dynamic action (SDA)
- Respiratory quotient
- Factors affecting total energy requirements
- Estimation of daily energy requirements
- Study questions

UNDERPINNINGS OF ENERGY TRANSFORMATION

Understanding the essence of energy metabolism offers us an insight into mother nature's benevolence in bestowing bounties on plants, animals and human beings. Organisms ranging from tiny microbes to animals and humans capture and transform potential energy from macronutrients of food into utilizable chemical energy. Carbondioxide, a byproduct of animal energy metabolism, is cycled through the plant kingdom while oxygen, a byproduct of plant energy metabolism, is cycled through the animal kingdom; both using the byproducts of each other in their acts of transferring energy to useful forms. The most interesting is the way in which human beings interconnect energy through ATP-ADP cycle, ATP being the carrier and currency of energy.

As a matter of fact, energy, an all important ingredient for human survival and sustenance, comes from the oxidation of carbohydrates, fat and to some extent, proteins. A part of this energy liberated from nutrient oxidation is converted into chemical energy of ATP (energy currency) and the rest dissipates as heat; the efficiency of this conversion being about 40-50 percent. Energy demand for internal (heart and lung and other vital organ functioning, nutrient and metabolic transport, osmotic and biosynthetic activity etc.) as well as external work, locomotion and other activity of skeletal muscles is met out of this chemical energy or energy currency. The end outcome of internal work is also heat, as energy input used for heart and lung functioning, for instance, is also transformed into heat by the friction of blood with blood vessels and that of air with respiratory air passages. Likewise, energy expended on biosynthetic work, e.g., on protein or any other macromolecular synthesis is sure to be released as heat during their catabolism and the resultant energy utilization. Similarly, energy used up on external work done on the environment, by carrying an object of certain weight to a specific height, is stored as potential energy, and is released as heat when the same object descends down through that height. Also energy utilized in peddling a tricycle is transformed, into heat produced by the friction of wheels and the road. Thus one arrives at the generalization that energy upheavals taking place in human body are summed up as heat dissipated from the body and the work done by it on environment. As a corollary to this, one can also state that in a resting healthy adult (with no activity or external work), all energy transformations occurring within the body appear as heat.

The following two equations narrate the energy balance positions in an adult (growth completed) and an adolescent (growth underway) respectively.

For Adults:

Total energy transformed = Total heat dissipated + External work done on environment

For Adolescents:

Total energy transformed = Total energy dissipated + External work done on environment + Energy stored in biosynthesis

DIRECT CALORIMETRY

If in a room sized calorimeter, the subject is performing all its activities, and the amount of heat generated is also measured accurately, it would be equal to that subject's actual energy expenditure. However, this direct measurement of heat loss-direct calorimetry is complicated and expensive exercise and very difficult to perform practically. The technique of direct calorimetry was first used in the end of 18th century with the construction of first human calorimeter by Atwater with the help of physicist Rosa in U.S.A. Further large calorimeter was built again in U.S.A. by Armsby in Pennsylvania state university in the beginning of 20th century. The technique involves putting the individual in a specially constructed chamber (calorimeter) which has specially been constructed with insulated walls from where no heat can either enter or escape through the calorimeter body.

The heat lost by the experimental subject goes fully to increase the temperature of water flowing through the water ducts in the calorimeter walls. By accurate measurement of the temperature increase at different intervals of time during the progress of the experiment and the volume of water flowing through the coils, it is possible to calculate the energy expenditure of the subject during a given period of time. The energy expended by the subject, as measured by direct calorimeter, is related to net energy intake (total energy of food-energy lost in faeces and urine). Atwater measured the energy intake and energy expenditure of humans using this technique and proved that there is a considerable degree of agreement between energy input and output. His work conclusively proved that human body runs like an efficient combustion engine and theory of vitalism has no role, whatsoever, in explaining the working of human machine.

However, it became abundantly clear to Atwater and many of his contemporaries working on energy metabolism that the assessment of energy expenditure by directly measuring heat loss is cumbersome, complicated and exorbitantly expensive, and needed replacement by another, practically viable and scientifically precise technique. Taking a cue from the observation of 18th century scientist 'Antoine Lavosier', better known as the father of nutrition, that oxygen consumption and heat production were closely related, Atwater and Rosa also proved beyond doubt the validity of direct quantitative relationship of energy production and oxygen consumption. This generalization laid down the foundation of indirect calorimetry or the technique of calculating energy expenditure in kilocalories (k cal), i.e., in nutritional calories (Cal) from oxygen consumption (Fig. 9.1).

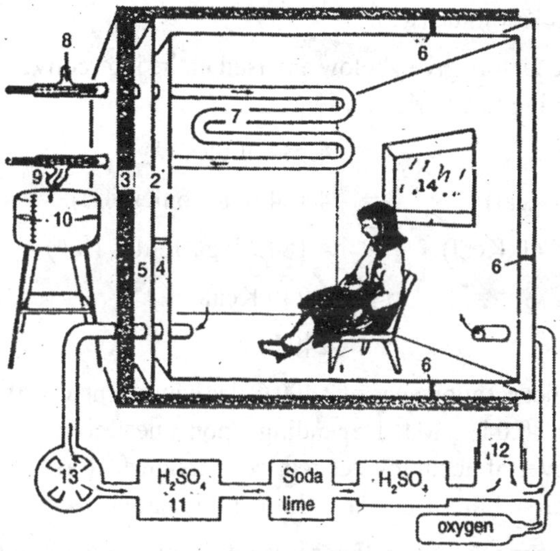

Fig. 9.1: Schematic diagram of Atwater-Benedict Human Calorimeter. The water flows in the tubes at (7) and its temperature is measured at the inlet (8) and the outlet (9). The air leaves the calorimeter aided by a fan, water is removed from it by sulphuric acid and CO_2 by soda lime, and then goes back to the chamber with O_2 added at a measured rate (12). The calorimeter possesses an efficient thermal insulation. The heat gained by flowing water is a fairly accurate indication of the external heat produced by the subject. Activities of the subject can be observed through the double glass in the windows in 14

The technique is simple, comparatively less expensive and has the potential of measuring energy expenditure in both resting state and state of activity. Due to these characteristics, indirect calorimetry has been practised as the technique of choice in energy expenditure determinations.

UNITS OF ENERGY MEASUREMENT

As the preceding discussion, at the very outset of the chapter, makes it amply clear that all forms of energy in living bodies ultimately appear as heat, it becomes natural to use units of heat for expressing all sorts of energy exchanges in caloric unit of heat, which is defined as the amount of heat needed to raise the temperature of 1g of water from 14.5°C to 15.5°C.

Likewise, one nutritional calorie (Cal.) equivalent to a kilo calorie (Kcal) is the amount of heat required to raise the temperature of a kilogram of water from 14.5 to 15.5°C.

Though calorie is the popular and the most prevalent unit of heat measurement, the units devised by S.F. (International system for such measurements) are Joule (J) and Kilojoule (KJ).

The factors given below are used in the interconversion pertaining to calorie and Joule.

1 calorie	=	4.184 Joules (J)
1 Cal (Kcal)	=	4.184 Kilo Joules (KJ)
1000 Cal (Kcal)	=	4.184 Mega Joules (MJ)
1 KJ	=	0.240 Kcal
1 MJ	=	240 Kcal.

A dietary allowance of 2,400 Cal is equivalent to 10041.6 KJ or 10.0416 MJ. Depending upon one's convenience and level of accuracy desired, conversion factors of 4.18 or even 4.2 are used for Calorie-Joule conversion.

Energy inherent in foods is used up by living organisms for survival, sustenance and activity. Human beings being no exceptions, also conform to this cardinal principle. The energy yielding nutrients of food are carbohydrates, proteins and fats, releasing energy as a consequence of systematic, stepwise, enzyme catalyzed catabolic oxidation.

The byproducts of oxidation are carbondioxide and water. The gross energy contents of foodstuffs are readily determined by means of an instrument known as bomb calorimeter (Fig. 9.2).

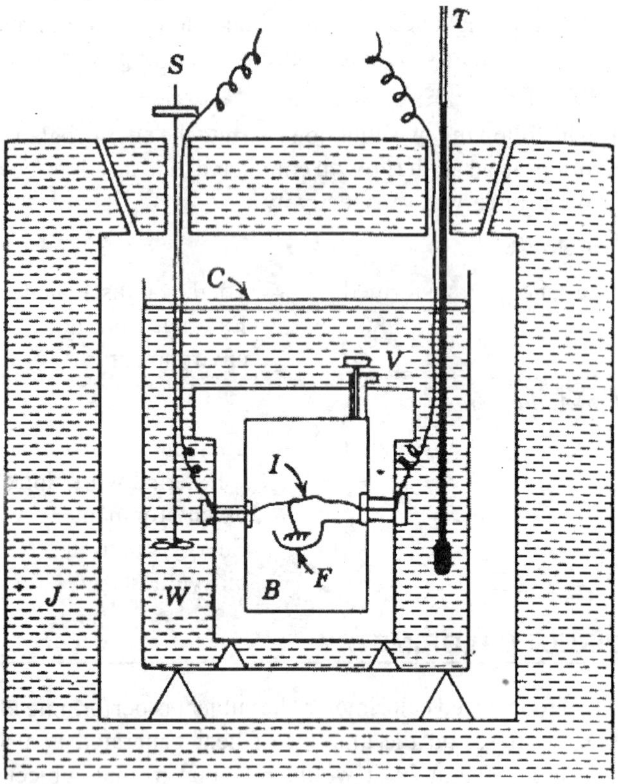

Fig. 9.2: Cross-section of bomb calorimeter, J = water jacket; W = weighed amount of water; S = stirrer; T = thermometer; F = platinum sample dish; B = bomb chamber; I = ignition wire

The most important part of the apparatus is a bomb, a sturdy steel container with a platinum plated copper lining, covered by a tightly fitting strong screw cap or cover. A dried food sample, weighed accurately and pressed into a pellet, is put in the bomb. Since oxygen aids in combustion, a strong stream of oxygen (290-310 lbs/inch) is let in by opening the oxygen valve before the onset of sample ignition. Since the bomb lies immersed in another well insulated container having a known volume of water. The heat evolved by the combustion of the food sample is taken up by water, change in temperature of water is noted down by a sensitive differential temperature thermometer which can sense temperature accurately upto 0.01 degree Celsius by measuring temperatures in the beginning (before ignition of sample) and end of the experiment. Since the heat evolved by sample combustion is taken up by water and calorimeter, the caloric value of the food sample is obtained in the following manner:

Weight of oil sample	=	2.7 g
Water weight (M_1)	=	5000 g
Water equivalent of the calorimeter (M_2S_2)	=	1000 g
Specific heat of water (S_1)	=	1
Initial temperature of water (T_1)	=	28°C
Final temperature of water (T_2)	=	32°C
Rise in temperature (T_2 - T_1) (32°C - 28°C)	=	4°C
Heat gained by water	=	$M_1 \times S_1 \times (T_2 - T_1)$
	=	$5000 \times 1 \times (32 - 28)$
	=	$5000 \times 1 \times 4$
	=	20000 calories
Heat gained by calorimeter	=	$M_2 \times S_2 \times (T_2 - T_1)$
	=	$1000 \times 4 = 4000$
Total heat gained in calories	=	20,000 + 4,000 = 24,000
Since, heat gained by water and calorimeter	=	Heat lost by sample combustion
	=	24,000 calories
Fuel value of 2.7 g of sample	=	24000 calories
Fuel value of 1 g of sample	=	$\frac{24000}{2.7}$
	=	8.9 kcal.
Hence fuel value of 1 g of oil	=	8.9 cal.

(Heat of combustion)

Gross energy values, obtained by ignition of foodstuffs in the bomb calorimeter are equivalent to their heat of combustion. However, the energy extracted from the same foodstuffs by the body (physiological energy values) is generally less than that obtained by bomb colorimeter combustion, the reason being nutrient digestion, absorption and oxidation is never a complete affair.

In the case of proteins, the fact of nitrogen containing groups being incompletely oxidized in the body, further contributes towards lowering down their (proteins) physiological fuel values. On an average, in a healthy human adult, approximately 1.25 Cal energy of every gram of absorbed protein is lost as urinary nitrogen in the form of urea. By applying these corrections Atwater and Bryant arrived at energy values derived by the bodily oxidation of 1 gram of carbohydrates, proteins fats and alcohol and termed them as physiological fuel values or energy conversion factors. After the names of these great nutritionists they are also known as Atwater Bryant energy factors (Table 9.1 and Fig. 9.3).

Finally, one can sum up this discussion by writing the following equation:

Physiological energy value = Gross energy value–Energy lost in digestion/absorption/metabolism.

Applications: In order to compute the energy value of a diet, first its macronutrient contents are estimated by chemical analysis and thereafter the energy value is calculated using following equation:

Energy value (Cal) = (Pm × P) + (Fm × F) + (Cm × C)

Where Pm, Fm and Cm are the protein, fat and carbohydrate contents in grams respectively as determined by proximate analyses and P, F and C are their respective energy conversion factors. In this way extractable energy content of a mixed diet can be calculated with a fair degree of accuracy.

SPECIFIC FUEL FACTORS

Every food item has specific co-efficient of digestibility. In the case of foods of animal origin, milk, meat and eggs, for instance, the co-efficient of protein digestibility is around 97 percent as compared to 98 and 90 percent for those from refined and whole wheat flours respectively. Hence, many a time specific fuel values (factors), and not the physiologic fuel values, are listed in the food composition tables. That precisely explains the discrepancy between

Table 9.1: Energy contents (gross energy values) and physiological fuel values of proximate principles and alcohol

Name of the substance	*Gross energy value (Heat of combustion) (Cal/g)*	*Digestibility co-efficient*	*Urinary/ respiratory loss (Cal/g)*	*Physiological energy value (Cal/g)*
Carbohydrate	4.15	0.99		4.0
Fat	9.45	0.95		9.0
Protein	5.65	0.92	1.25 (Urinary)	4.0
Alcohol	07.1	1.00	0.1 (Respiratory)	7.0

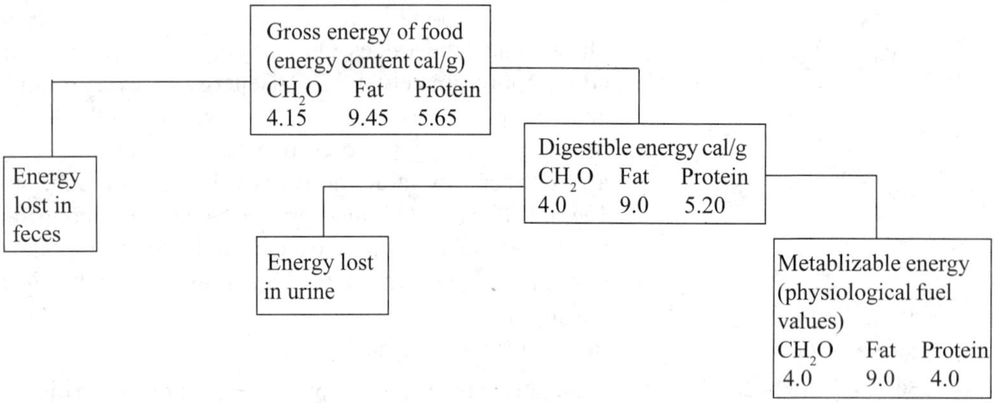

Fig. 9.3: Gross energy values and available energy values of macronutrient substances

the values calculated on the basis of proximate composition and physiological fuel values on one hand and the tabulated values on the other (tabulated values are mostly lower than the calculated values). A decrease in the digestibility of the given macronutrient occurring in a foodstuff is due to its interaction with other nutritional and non-nutritional factors present in the same foodstuff, that may hamper the absorption or utilization to varying extents.

BASAL METABOLIC RATE (BMR)

The term 'basal metabolism' refers to the minimum energy required to maintain life sustaining vital activities such as the functional activities of organs like brain, kidney, liver, heart, lungs; the secretary activities of glands, the peristaltic movements of the gastrointestinal tract, maintenance of body temperature etc. The rate of basal metabolism (basal metabolic rate or BMR) is determined by either measuring the energy output or the state of oxygen consumption of the subject in post absorptive state (10-12 hours after last meal) in a state of complete physical and mental rest, reclining but not asleep, in a room with comfortable temperature and humidity. The BMR of an average adult male (reference Indian man age 20-39 years, wt 60 kg) is 1515 Cal and that of an adult female (reference Indian woman age 20-39 years, wt 50 kg) is 1170 Cal.

It has been found that brain and nervous tissue account for more energy expenditure in basal conditions as compared to other vital organs like heart, kidneys, lungs and liver. The fact that heat loss of an individual is proportional to its skin surface makes it logical to relate BMR with surface area. A thin and tall individual has a greater surface area than a dwarf and fat person of the same weight, and therefore the former has a higher BMR than the latter. BMR values can be predicted by equations.

In nutritional and clinical practice, BMR is calculated in calories per square metre of body surface per hour, or alternatively, in kilo Joule per square metre of body surface per hour. To calculate body surface area, the following equation by Dubois and Dubois is made use of:

$$S = 0.007184 \times W0.425 \times H\ 0.725$$

Where,

S = Surface area in square metres

W = Body weight in kilograms

H = Height in centimetres

Solving the equation further by taking logs.

$$\log_{10} S = \log 100.007184 + 0.425 \log_{10} W + 0.725 \log_{10} H$$

or

$$\log_{10} S = 3.8564 + 0.425 \log_{10} W + 0.725 \log_{10} H$$

The surface area is calculated by taking the anti log of the whole sum of the right hand side. Alternatively, surface area can also be calculated from nomograms (Fig. 9.4).

Measurement of BMR

BMR values of the subjects are measured in the laboratory making use of the technique of indirect calorimetry. Earlier on, the oxygen consumptions were measured by the Benedict's Roth closed circuit breathing apparatus. However, due to cumbersome nature of the measurement,

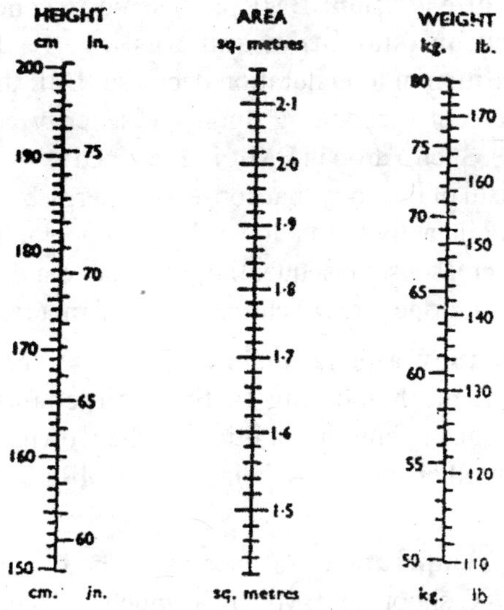

Fig. 9.4: Nomograms for the calculation of body surface area

it has been replaced by more precise and convenient Douglas bag and Maxplank's respirometer apparatus (Fig. 9.5).

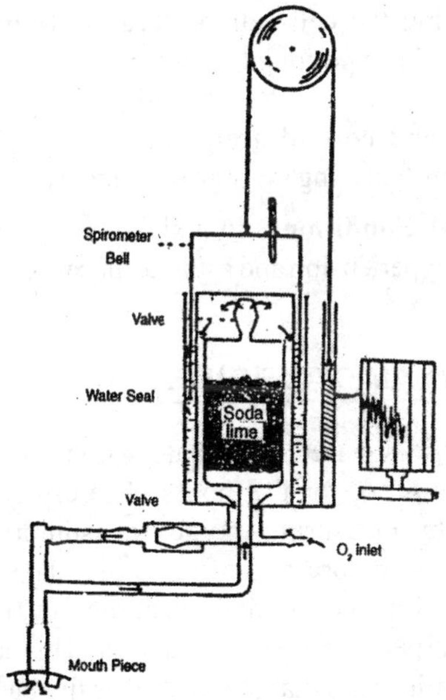

Fig. 9.5: Schematic diagram of the Benedict-Roth Spirometer used for measuring oxygen consumption

Douglas Bag Method

The air tight bag, as name indicates, has a capacity of 100 or 200 liters. The subject breaths through a mouthpiece (nose is clipped) which has separate valves for inspiration and expiration. Whereas room air is inspired, breathing out is made into the Douglas bag. The breathing out into the bag is continued for 5-6 minutes (time exactly noted) and the air composition of the expired air (CO_2 and O_2 contents) is ascertained by a gas meter. With the help of these values, oxygen consumption, carbondioxide production and respiratory quotients are determined and finally the heat expenditure is calculated. The method is useful in determining energy expenditure not only in basal state but also in various stages of human activities (Fig. 9.6).

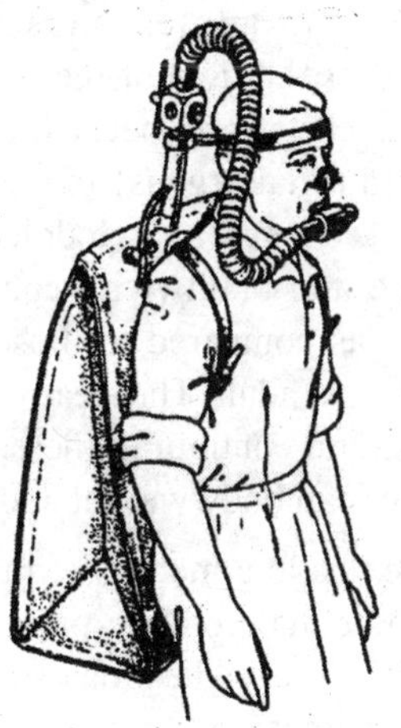

Fig. 9.6: Person breathing out into the Douglas bag

Max Plank's Respirometer Method

The working is similar to that of Douglas bag, the only difference is in its being portable and more convenient for in field conditions.

Calculation of BMR

An adult male weighing 55 kg, inspire 1200 ml of oxygen and breathes out 984 ml. of carbondioxide in 6 minutes. Calculate his BMR:

$$\text{Respiratory Quotent} = \frac{\text{Volume of } CO_2}{\text{Volume of } O_2}$$

$$= \frac{984}{1200} = 0.82$$

At R.Q. value 0.82, 1 litre of oxygen consumption releases 4.825 (approx 4.8) Kcal m^2 from nutrient oxidation. Therefore heat produced = 4.8 × 1.2 = 5.76 Cal. in 6 minutes for 1.2 sq meter surfsce area

Heat produced in 24 hours = 5.76 × 10 × 24

= 1382.4 Cal

Hence BMR of the adult human subject is 1382.4 Cal/day.

Factors Affecting Basal Metabolic Rate (BMR)

Since BMR is the rate at which body oxidizes its own stored fuels in the fasting, resting and reclining state (also known as the basal state) in a comfortably warm room, it is equivalent to the energy required to maintain the life sustaining metabolic activity. There are a number of factors that affect this basal metabolism.

Age: BMR is high in infancy peaking at the age of 5 years. Then it declines gradually throughout childhood, accelerating a little in adolescence and declining continuously thereafter throughout the rest of life. BMR increases intensely in early years because of rapid increase in the size of viscera (vital organs) in relation to surface area or body weight. Therefore, a toddler has relatively larger liver intestine and brain (with comparatively less developed muscles) as compared to those of a muscular (with well built muscles) adult. The steady decline in BMR starting in twenties, and continuing thereafter is due to a gradual reduction in lean body weight and increase in fat.

Gender: Females have a metabolic rate 5-10 percent less than that of their male counterparts. The influence partly at least, is due to a higher mass of comparatively inert (metabolically) adipose tissue in women. Adipose (fat) cells of the body are metabolically active but contain a substantial amount of metabolically inert fat, so that the larger fat mass of a woman has a lower BMR per unit body weight than a man. However, the oxygen uptake is calculated in terms of lean body weight, a woman's BMR value also tends to be near to that of a man of comparable surface area.

Surface Area: Since much of the basal metabolism is meant to maintain vital activities, including body temperature and the energy expended on this is lost to the surroundings as heat through skin surface; the BMR is directly proportional to the surface area. That is why it is customary to express BMR as calories/square meter/hour.

Climate: Although, the effect of environmental temperature is uncertain, some sporadic data do indicate that BMR is higher in temperate or cold climates as compared to tropical environs, like in our country. Low environmental temperature, somehow or the other, seems to increase the energy expenditure in basal state.

Race: BMR is higher in occidental (western) races vis-à-vis orientals. Indians, for instance, have been found to have a lower BMR than the Europeans. The difference has been found to be due to racial diversity.

State of Nutrition: BMR is lowered in conditions of malnutrition, starvation and wasting. Fasting and undernutrition of long duration decrease BMR to as much as 20 percent (depending upon the severity and/or the duration). Such a drop in BMR is explained as the adaptive mechanism of the body that conserves energy by adjusting its metabolic activity to a lower level of operation. A part of the decrease is consequential, i.e., due to a decrease in weight and surface area of chronically undernourished body.

Pregnancy and lactation: BMR is increased in expectant mother owing to the maintenance of the metabolism of fetus in addition to their own. Likewise nursing mothers also have heightened BMRs, for obvious reasons.

Body Temperature: An increase in body temperature above 37°C shoots up BMR by as much as 14 percent for every degree Celsius increase in temperature.

Sleep: During sleep, BMR is lower than that in woken-up state. This may be due to a slight decrease in body temperature during sleep.

Endocrine Secretions: Thyroid hormones (thyroxine, T4, and triiodothyronine T3) stimulate oxidation and heat production within the cells, thyroidectomy (removal of thyroid glands) in experimental animals brings about a marked decrease in the BMR. Similarly, hypothyroidism (myxoedema) and colloid goiter decrease BMR, and hyperthyroidism (Cushing's syndrome) increases it.

Pathological Conditions: Pyrexia (fever), leukemia, polycythemia, hypertension and asthma; all cause elevation in BMR.

SPECIFIC DYNAMIC ACTION (SDA)

Metabolic rate is increased immediately after ingestion of food and remains so, for 6-8 hours. The effect can be demonstrated by measuring oxygen consumption of a resting individual before and after eating. The oxygen consumption and the concomitant heat out put rise upon eating even if the person remains in resting and immobilized state. The elevation in metabolic rate over the basal state upon ingesting food, has been termed as specific dynamic action (SDA) or calorigenic effect of foods. It has also been well established that the SDA is something over and above the result of the exertions of mastication, swallowing and increased mobility of gastrointestinal tract.

Further, the effect varies with the type of food that actually supplies the calories. If the calories are, exclusively derived from proteins, SDA is 20 to 30 percent of the total caloric equivalent of the ingested protein. The SDA is intermediate with carbohydrates, resulting in 5-10 percent of the total caloric value. The SDA is minimum with fats, a mere 0-4 percent of the caloric value of the ingested fats. On a mixed diet, SDA is 10-12 percent. The effect, first of all recognized by Rubner (1902), is only too important, to be measured in working out the energy requirements of an individual.

The reason why food is withheld from a person, when subjected to the determination of BMR, is that heat output would be higher than that in the resting state.

The extra energy expenditure is not solely because of requirements of digestion and absorption of ingested food. No doubt, synthesis of the constituents of digestive juice is an energy expending process in itself, this accounts for a very small fraction of the effect. Intravenous injections of amino acids, for instance, produce an SDA only a little lower than that of their oral ingestion. Surprisingly the SDA effect is not observed in hepatectomized (with liver removed) animals (rats).

The most plausible explanation to-date, proposed by Hans Krebs is that this effect (SDA) of foods is due to the energy requirements for ATP synthesis needed for the processing and storage of nutrients. The minimum effect observed in fat intake may be due to the reason that storage of fat (TG) in the adipose tissue require minimum expenditure in terms of ATP utilization, only 1-2 percent of their potential ATP yield. The intermediate effect, the case of carbohydrate feeding may be due to energy expenditure for storing carbohydrates in the form of glycogen and amounts to 5 percent of its potential ATP output. The ATP requirement accordingly stimulate oxidative phosphorylation or ATP synthesis.

The highest SDA of protein foods is thought to be due to the deamination of amino acids, which occurs in the liver after absorption and ultimately results in the formation of urea. Other products formed from amino acids, e.g., creatine, porphyrin and purine, needing glycine for their formation, or pantothenic acid, needing cysteine for its formation; also contribute towards SDA.

Whatever be the subtle causes of SDA, it is for sure that the amount of energy available on food ingestion is less than its actual caloric value. Therefore, while computing the food requirement of a given individual, it becomes imperative to add up to its caloric requirements an extra 10 percent of the BMR to compensate for SDA because the usual mixed Indian diet has a caloriginic effect of this order.

Oxygen Consumption and Heat Output

Since there is a direct quantitative relationship between oxygen consumption, carbondioxide production and macronutrient oxidation, it has been inferred by experiments that the amount (in grams) of carbohydrate, protein and fat oxidized by one litre of oxygen are 1.25, 0.83 and 0.49 and energy values produced (in calories) are 5.0, 4.6, 4.5 respectively. To generalize, a litre of oxygen consumed in macronutrient oxidation by an adult on Indian diet, produces 4.5-5.0 Cal. of heat.

RESPIRATORY QUOTIENT

The total rate of body metabolism is assessed by monitoring the rate of oxygen uptake by the lungs. As the macronutrients and alcohol (dietary fuels) are oxidized in the tissues, oxygen is inhaled by the lungs and the end product of oxidation; carbondioxide water and urea, excreted by the lungs, skin and kidneys respectively. If we measure the value of respiratory gases in inspired and expired airs and calculate the ratio of moles of CO_2 produced to those of O_2 consumed, the resultant quotient is known as respiratory quotient or (R.Q.).

$$RQ = \frac{\text{Moles of } CO_2 \text{ in expired air}}{\text{Moles of } O_2 \text{ inspired air}}$$

The R.Q. varies when either carbohydrates or proteins are oxidized solely because equal amounts of each type of macronutrient depending upon its specific molecular structure, consume and produce specific amounts of oxygen and carbondioxide respectively. For instance, R.Q. is I for carbohydrate oxidation because the amount of oxygen needed is exactly equivalent to that of carbondioxide produced as evident by the following reaction. Depicting glucose oxidation:

$$C_6H_{12}O_6 + 6O_2 \quad 6CO_2 + 6H_2O$$

$$\frac{6CO_2}{6O_2} = 1.0$$

For fat, R.Q. value is 0.7 as they require more oxygen to produce less carbondioxide as evident from following reaction of fat (Tristearin) oxidation.

$$2C_{57}H_{110}O_6 + 163O_2 + 100H_2O$$

$$\frac{114\ CO_2}{163O_2} = 0.70$$

Calculation of R.Q. for protein is difficult as they are incompletely oxidized to urea. However if we take into account this factor the ratio of CO_2 produced to O_2 consumed turns out to be 1:1.2 equal to R.Q. of 0.82. In the case of a mixed diet comprising carbohydrate, fat and protein, it also becomes possible to estimate the quantitative proportion of the three fuel sources by determining the R.Q. of the mixed diet. Further, when we determine BMR in post absorptive state (when the body fulfills energy need by oxidizing carbohydrate, fat and protein in 5:4:1, is convenient to compute the heat equivalent of respiratory exchange by taking an R.Q. of 0.82 and caloric equivalent of 4.825 per litre of oxygen consumed for this R.Q. Furthermore an average Indian meal (carbohydrate: protein: fat; 70:20:10) also corresponds to an R.Q. of 0.85 and a caloric equivalent of 4.84 per litre of oxygen (at standard, temperature and pressure). R.Q. decreases in prolonged fasting or diabetes mellitus when fats become the virtual energy source.

As different foodstuffs have specific proximate composition, their oxidation by cellular respiratory processes in body tissues could require different volumes of O_2 and also liberate different volumes of CO_2. Hence different dietary intakes would have separate R.Q. values as well as caloric equivalents per litre of oxygen used. Table 9.2 lists the non-protein R.Q. values.

Table 9.2: R.Q. (Non-protein) and heat produced per litre of oxygen consumed

R.Q. (Non-protein)	*Heat produced (Cal/litre)*
1.00	5.047
0.95	4.998
0.90	4.924
0.85	4.862
0.80	4.801
0.75	4.739
0.70	4.686

Besides, nutritionists have also calculated the caloric equivalents of oxygen and the quantities of carbohydrate and fat oxidized on a mixed diet.

FACTORS AFFECTING TOTAL ENERGY REQUIREMENTS

Total energy expenditure in a healthy individual is, in effect a sum of total internal and external works performed by the body. On the cellular and subcellular level, these works are performed by countless metabolic reactions that occur in different subcellular organelles of the cells of tissues making human body. Prominent among such, cellular structures are mitochondria. External work is performed when the person is active mechanically, e.g., a person walking a mile or a farmer ploughing his field. Hence the energy used up in performing external work is referred to as energy spent on activity. Muscles, both skeletal and smooth, have a built in mechanism of intermittent functioning and resting between two contractions. Skeletal muscles are primarily involved in the performance of external work. Internal work, in contrast, is performed by parenchyma (heart, brain, liver, kidney, diaphragm and endocrine glands). Cells of the parenchymal tissues are abundantly involved in the metabolic (oxidative and biosynthetic) processes essential to the tissue sustenance and survival. Thus it is also apt and logical to hold parenchyma and muscles responsible for energy expenditure on basal metabolism and activity respectively (Tables 9.3, 9.4 and 9.5).

Table 9.3: Resting oxygen consumption by the chief organs of healthy man

Organ	*Oxygen consumption ml/min*	*% of resting metabolism*
Liver (including splanchnic area)	65	26.0
Brain	48	19.2
Heart	17	6.8
Kidney	27	10.8
Skeletal muscle	45	18.0
Rest of the tissues	48	19.2
Total	250	100.0

Table 9.4: Age and gender difference in B.M.R.

Age in Years	*B.M.R. in Kcal/sq m/hour*	
	Male	*Female*
2	57.0	52.5
6	53.0	50.6
10	48.5	45.9
16	45.7	38.8
20	41.4	36.1
30	39.3	35.7
40	38.0	35.7
50	36.7	34.0
60	35.5	32.6

Table 9.5: Classification of physical activity in term of energy expenditure		
Grade of work	*Men Kcal/min/60 kg*	*Women Kcal/min/50 kg*
Light	2.0-4.9	1.5-3.4
Moderate	5.0-7.4	3.5-5.4
Heavy	7.5-9.9	5.5-7.5
Very heavy	10.0-13.0 or above	7.6-10.0 or above

In different tissues too, the respiratory rates differ widely. Kidney, for instance, respire at a far higher rate than heart and liver. The heart and liver, in turn, respire at a higher rate than the adipose tissue, skin skeleton, ligaments and blood, for metabolic activity and energy expenditure. Hence the term "body cell mass" used to refer to parenchyma and muscle tissue combine, encompassing almost all those components of the body that are majorly responsible for energy expenditure. This precisely is the reason, why body cell mass, and not body weight (which includes adipose tissue too) has a direct relationship with energy expenditure. Thus the process of determining the energy requirements of a person entails separation of the composite total energy expenditure into the following definable and measurable physiological factors:

1. Basal metabolism (BMR).
2. Calorigenic or specific dynamic action of foods (SDA of foods).
3. Activity.

Whereas the comparatively less variable ones (the first two) have already been discussed in this chapter, the most variable factor (the activity), affects energy requirements the most. As the level of activity increases, it also heightens up the cellular metabolic processes to furnish more and more energy to make body cope with increased energy demand. Whereas, on an average, a person expends about 50-60 Cal./hour in basal state, an intense activity may involve an energy expenditure six times this value.

ESTIMATION OF DAILY ENERGY REQUIREMENTS

Daily energy requirement of a person is defined as—the level of energy intake from food that can balance energy expenditure when the individual has a body size, composition and level of physical activity, consistent with long term good health and that will allow for maintenance of economically necessary and socially desirable activity. In children, expectant and nursing mothers, energy intake needs to cover the requirement of energy for tissue growth and deposition or milk secretion. In fact, the daily energy requirement is the sum total of these factors, namely, basal metabolism, activity and thermic effect of food also known as specific dynamic action on SDA.

By doing repeated experiments using the technique of indirect calorimetry, nutritionists have worked out prediction equation for BMR or basal metabolism and computed the 24 hours energy requirement by activity break up method is terms of BMR limits. For Indian population, the daily energy requirement estimates are worked out as per Indian Council for Medical Research (ICMR) guidelines as given under: (Table 9.6).

Table 9.6: BMR prediction for adults in Kcal/hour		
Sex	*Age (in years)*	*ICMR expert group prediction equation*
Male	18-30	14.5 × BW (kg) + 645
	30-60	11.6 × BW (kg) + 833
	>60	13.5 × BW (kg) + 463
Female	18-30	14.0 × BW (kg) + 471
	30-60	8.3 × BW (kg) + 788
	> 60	10.0 × BW (kg) + 561

Using BMR values, 24 hours energy requirements can be estimated through computation by activity break up method in terms of BMR units (Table 9.7).

Table 9.7: Estimates of energy requirements of adults (Kcal/24 hours)				
Daily activity	*Duration in hours*	*Rate of energy expenditure in BMR units*		
		Sedentary	*Moderate*	*Heavy*
Sleep	8	1.0	1.0	1.0
Occupational	8	1.7	2.8	4.5
Non-occupational activity	8	2.2	2.0	2.0
Average for 24 hours		1.6	1.9	2.5
Total energy expenditure during 24 hours in Kcal				
Reference man, 60 kg		2424	2882	3788
Reference woman, 50 kg		1872	2223	2995

Energy Requirements for Maintenance

Energy requirements per 24 hours for maintenance is the energy needed for minimal activity, rest and sleep and for diet induced thermogenesis. Any intake below this level over a long period of time would lead to tissue depletion and loss of body weight.

Dietary Composition As Energy and Well Being Source

In a balanced diet, fats should provide 20-30% of the total calories intake, protein; 10-12% and rest carbohydrates. Besides, adequate micronutrient and dietary fiber need to be provided through vegetables, fruits and whole cereals and pulses. Clean potable water becomes the other important ingredient of daily diet.

STUDY QUESTIONS

1. Explain what is meant by the following terms:
   i. Calorie.
   ii. Joule.
   iii. Bomb calorimeter.
   iv. Respiration calorimetry.
   v. Respiratory quotient.
2. What do you understand by the terms 'Indirect Calorimetry'? How, with the help of this technique, can you calculate the energy value of food consumed by a person over 24 hours?
3. What are the physiological fuel values of carbohydrate, fat and protein? Why do they differ from the energy values obtained from 'Bomb calorimeter combustion', of these macronutrients.
4. Explain the terms 'Basal metabolism' and 'Calorigenic effect of foods'. How do you estimate basal metabolism of a person and how it is modified by different factors.
5. Discuss briefly the factors that affect the total caloric needs of healthy person.
6. Explain in brief the method to estimate the daily energy requirements of adults.

CHAPTER 10

Metabolic Transformations of Food

Chapter Outlines

- Introduction
- Anaerobic metabolism of carbohydrates
- Aerobic metabolism
- Respiration: Electron transport chain and oxidative phosphorylation
- Metabolism of lipids
- Metabolism of proteins
- Protein synthesis
- Inborn errors of protein metabolism
- Study questions

INTRODUCTION

Metabolism is the sum of all the chemical processes carried out by living organisms. It includes anabolism, reactions that require energy to synthesize complex molecules from simpler ones, and catabolism, reactions that release energy by breaking complex, molecules into simpler ones. Anabolism is needed for growth, reproduction, and repair of cellular structures. Catabolism provides the organism with energy for its life processes, including movement, transport, and the synthesis of complex molecules-that is, anabolism.

All catabolic reactions involve electron transfer, which allows energy to be captured in high-energy bonds in ATP and similar molecules. Electron transfer is directly related to oxidation and reduction. Oxidation can be defined as the loss of electrons. Though many substances combine with oxygen and transfer electrons to oxygen, oxygen need not be present if another electron acceptor is available. Reduction can be defined as the gain of electrons. When a substance loses electrons, or is oxidized, energy is released, but another substance must gain electrons, or be reduced, at the same time. For example, during the oxidation of organic molecules, hydrogen atoms are removed and used to reduce oxygen to form water.

$2H_2$	+	O_2	$\rightarrow$	$2H_2O$
Hydrogen		Oxygen		Water

In this reaction hydrogen is an electron donor, or reducing agent, and oxygen is an electron acceptor, or oxidizing agent. Because oxidation and reduction must occur simultaneously, the reactions in which they occur are also called redox reactions.

Among all living beings, human beings are termed 'heterotrophs' in the ways in which they obtain energy. The various ways different organisms capture energy can be classified in which as autotrophy, self-feeding, or heterotrophy other-feeding. Autotrophs use carbon dioxide to synthesize organic molecules. They include photoautotrophs, which obtain energy from light (plants and certain microbes), and chemoautotrophs, which obtain energy from oxidizing simple inorganic substances such as sulfides and nitrites (some microbes). Heterotrophs use readymade organic molecules obtained from plants.

Autotrophic metabolism, especially photosynthesis, is important as a means of energy capture in plants and many free-living microorganisms. However, autotrophic, microorganisms do not usually cause disease. On the other hand disease causing organisms are those that thrive on other living forms for life sustenance. That is the reason why almost all infectious microorganisms are chemoheterotrophs and depend on their hosts (Fig. 10.1).

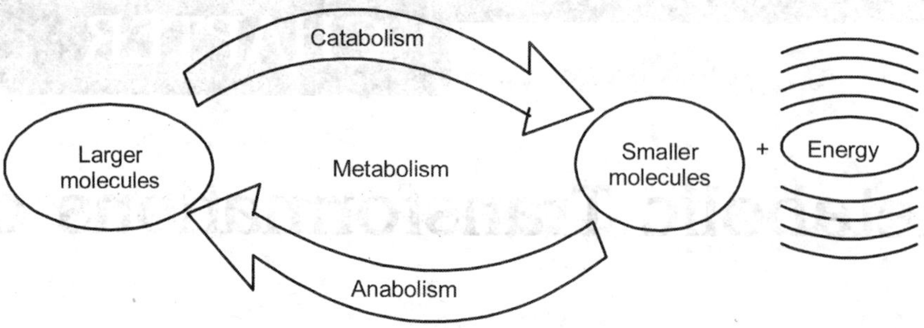

Fig. 10.1: Catabolic reactions break down large molecules into smaller ones, releasing energy. Organisms capture some of this energy for their life processes. Anabolic reactions use energy to build large molecules from smaller components. The molecules synthesized in this way are used to growth, reproduction and repair

The basic energy yielding metabolic processes (Figs. 10.2, 10.3, 10.4) include glycolysis (oxidation of glucose to pyruvate), fermentation (conversion or pyruvate to ethyl alcohol, lactic acid, or other organic compounds), and aerobic respiration (oxidation of pyruvate to carbon dioxide and water). Glycolysis and fermentation do not require oxygen and transfer only a small amount of the energy in a glucose molecule to ATP. Aerobic respiration does require oxygen as an electron acceptor and captures a relatively large amount of the energy in a glucose molecule to ATP. Complete oxidation of glucose by glycolysis and aerobic respiration can be summarized as follows:

$$\underset{\text{Glucose}}{C_6H_{12}O_6} + \underset{\text{Oxygen}}{O_2} \rightarrow \underset{\text{Carbon dioxide}}{CO_2} + \underset{\text{Water}}{H_2O} + \text{Energy}$$

Plants obtain energy by photosynthesis, the use of light energy and hydrogen from water or other compounds to reduce carbon dioxide to an organic substance containing more energy. The synthesis of glucose by photosynthesis in green plants, cyanobacteria and algae is summarized as follows:

$$\underset{\text{Carbon dioxide}}{CO_2} + \underset{\text{water}}{H_2O} \xrightarrow[\text{Chlorophyll}]{\text{Light energy}} \underset{\text{Glucose}}{C_6H_{12}O_6} \text{ and other carbohydrates} + \underset{\text{Oxygen}}{O_2}$$

Plants and some photosynthetic microorganisms then use of the glucose or other carbohydrates made in this way for energy. Respiration and photosynthesis are related in Figure 10.5.

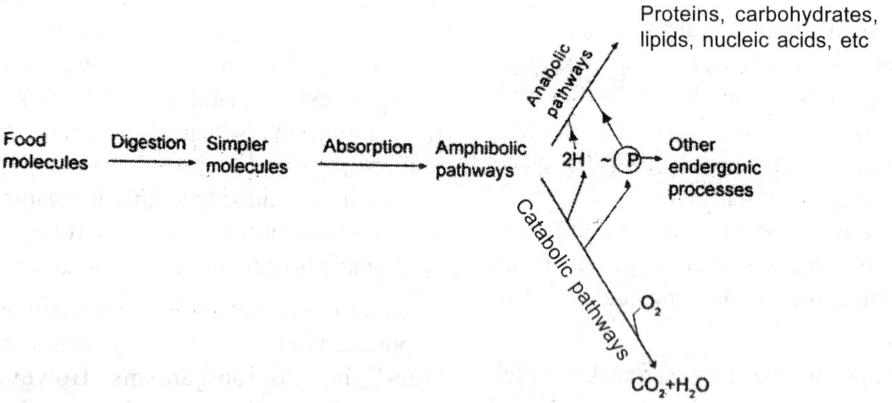

Fig. 10.2: Overview of metabolism: The 3 major categories of metabolic pathways. Catabolic pathways release free energy in the form of high-energy phosphate (-P) to power the anabolic pathways. Amphibolic pathways serve as the bridges between the other two

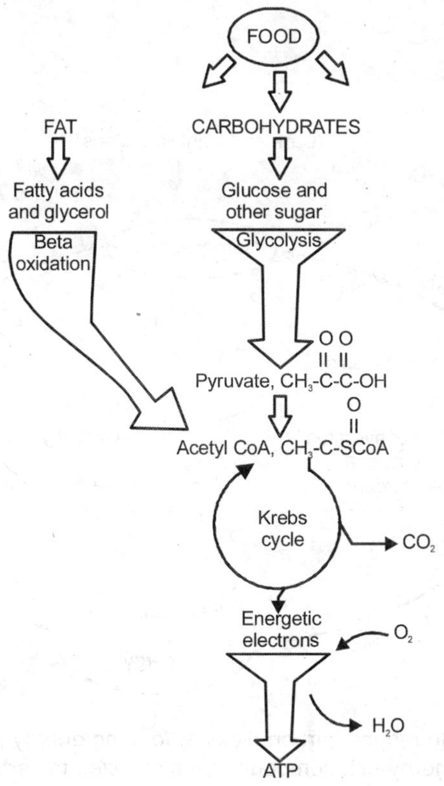

Fig. 10.3: Metabolism of three major classes of nutrients (macronutrients)

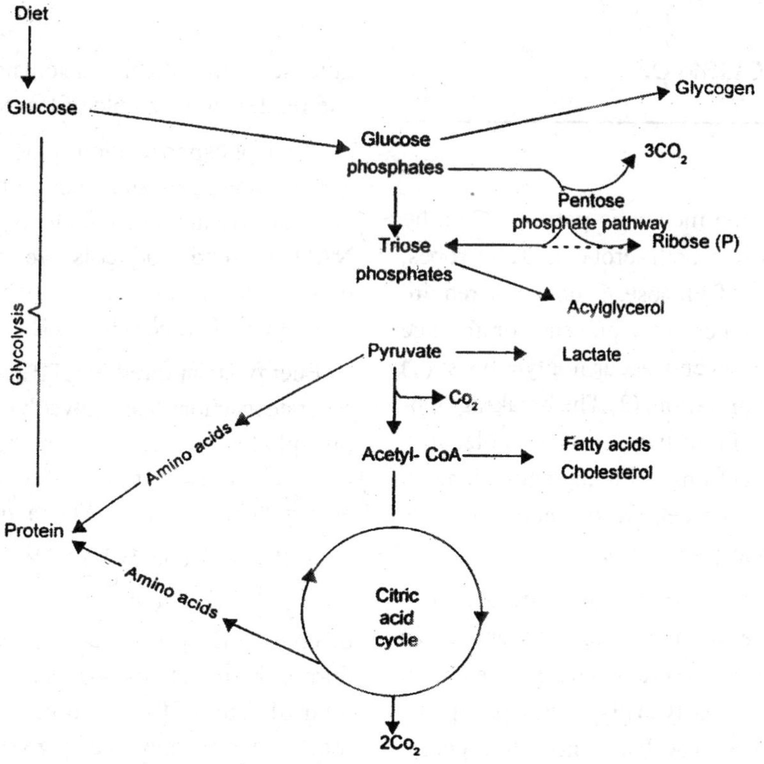

Fig. 10.4: A bird's eyeview of carbohydrate metabolism showing the major routes

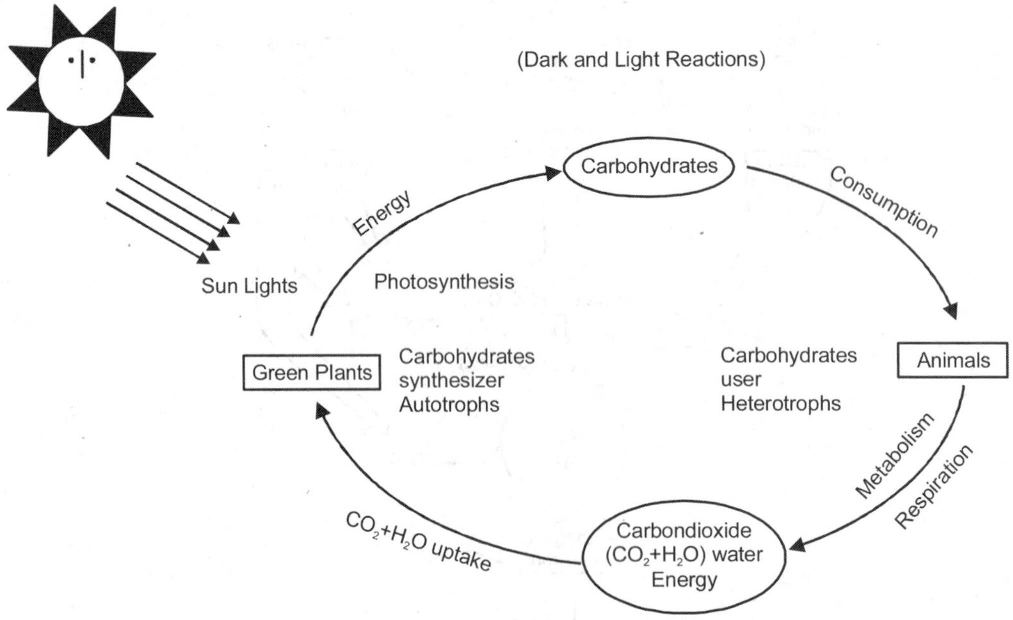

Fig. 10.5: In photosynthesis, light energy is used to reduce carbon dioxide, forming energy-rich compounds such as glucose and other carbohydrates. In aerobic respiration, energy-rich compounds are oxidized to carbon dioxide and water, and some of the energy released is captured for use in life processes. (The form of photosynthesis shown here is carried out by higher plants, cyanobacteria and algae. Thus this is photoautotrophy or getting energy for sustenance from light)

ANAEROBIC METABOLISM OF CARBOHYDRATES

Glycolysis

Glycolysis (Fig. 10.6) is the metabolic pathway used by most heterotrophic organisms, both aerobes and anaerobes, for the initial breakdown of glucose. It does not require oxygen, but it can occur either in the presence or absence of oxygen. Four important events occur in glycolysis: (1) Initial priming by phosphorylation, (2) The breaking of 6-carbon molecule (glucose) into two 3-carbon molecules, (3) The transfer of two electrons (reducing equivalents in the coenzyme NAD, (4) The capture of energy as ATP, and (5) Substrate level phosphorylation.

Initial priming or addition of a phosphate group to glucose, from ATP, increases the molecule's energy as phosphate groups commonly serve as energy carriers in biochemical reactions. Thus early in glycolysis, phosphate groups from two molecules of ATP are added to glucose. This expenditure of two ATPs raises the energy level of glucose so that it can participate in subsequent reactions and renders it incapable of leaving the cell.

After phosphorylation, glucose in broken into two 3-carbon molecules and each molecule is oxidized as two electrons (reducing equivalents) are transferred from it to NAD. The end product is two molecules of pyruvic acid, or pyruvate (the ionized form) and two molecules of reduced NAD (2NADH + $2H^+$).

Energy is captured in ATP at the substrate level in two separate reactions late in glycolysis. With ADP and inorganic phosphate (P_i) available in the cytoplasm, the energy released from substrate molecules in used to form high-energy bonds between ADP and P_i

$$ADP + P_i + energy \rightarrow ATP$$

Glycolysis provides cells with a relatively small amount of energy. Energy is captured in two molecules of ATP during the metabolism of each 3-carbon molecule, and a total of four ATPs are formed as one 6-carbon glucose molecule is metabolized by glycolysis to two molecules of pyruvate. Because energy from two ATPs was used in the initial phosphorylations, glycolysis results in a net energy capture of only two ATPs per glucose molecule. When atmospheric oxygen is present and the organism has the enzymes to carry out aerobic metabolism, electrons from reduced NAD are transferred to oxygen during biological oxidation, as is explained later, and two reduced NAD furnish 6 ATPs, taking the number of ATP to 8 aerobic condition (Fig. 10.6).

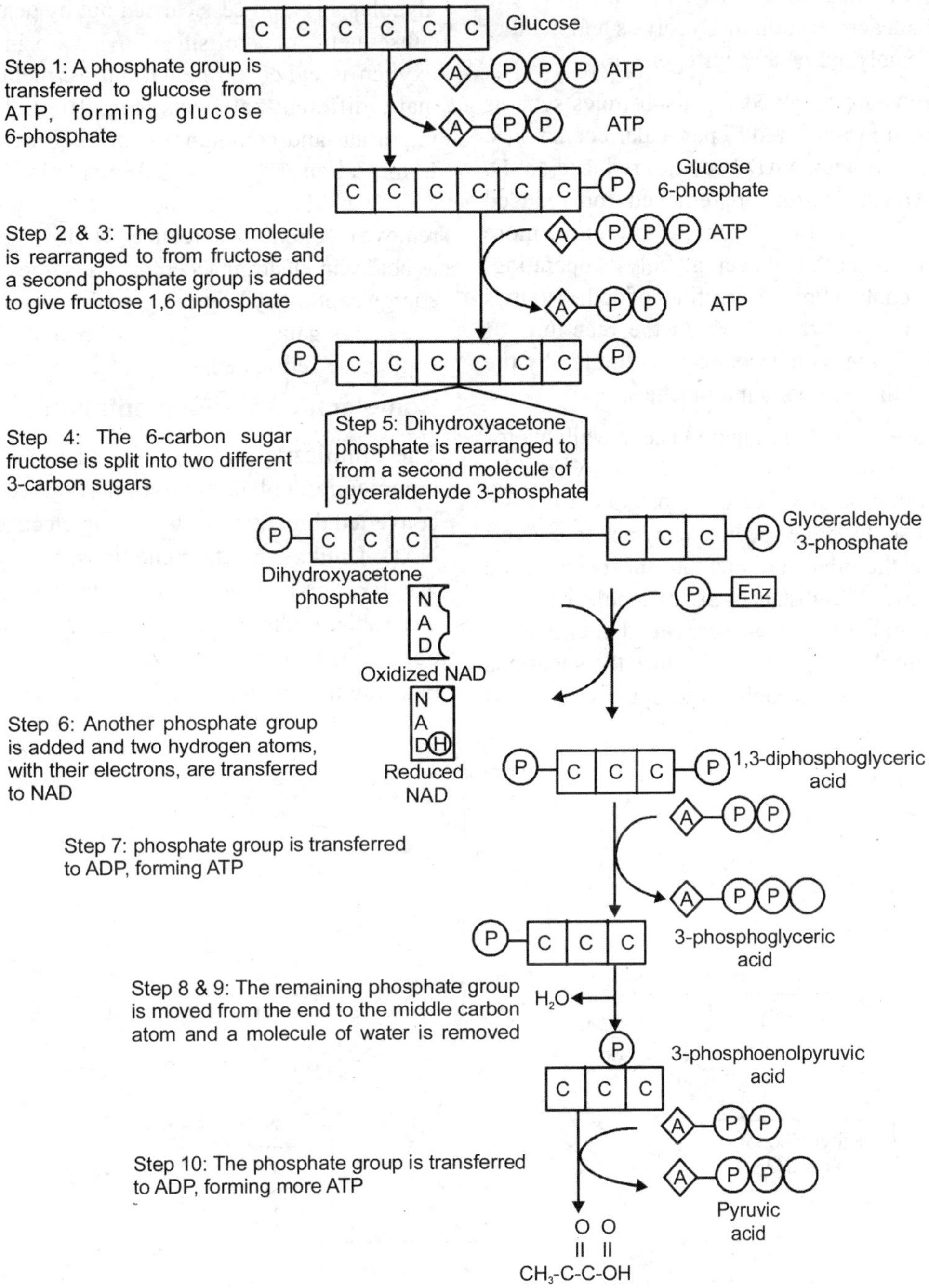

Fig. 10.6: The reactions of glycolysis. In steps 1 and 3, two molecules of ATP are used. In steps 7 and 10, two molecules of ATP are formed. Since each glucose molecule yields two and the 3-carbon sugars that undergo reactions 7 and 10, four molecules of ATP are actually formed, giving a net yield to two ATP per glucose

Two additional features of glycolysis illustrate principles that apply to metabolic pathways in general:

1. Each reaction is catalyzed by a specific enzyme. Though enzyme names have been omitted in this chapter for the sake of avoiding complexity, it is important to remember that each reaction in glycolysis and in other pathways is catalyzed by a specific enzyme.
2. When electrons are removed from substrates such as glucose, they are transferred to particular coenzymes. In glycolysis, oxidized NAD becomes reduced NAD. As explained next, electrons are removed from reduced NAD during fermentation, freeing it to remove more electrons from glucose and keep glycolysis operating. Because cells contain limited quantities of both enzymes and coenzymes, the rate at which the reactions of glycolysis and other pathways occur is limited by the availability of these important molecules.

Though glucose is the main sugar nutrient available for metabolism to most organisms, some energy can be obtained from other sugars like galactose and fructose. The organisms usually have specific enzymes to convert a sugar to one or the other intermediate substance in the glycolytic pathway. (All substances in a metabolic pathway between the first and last substance are called intermediate substances, or simply, intermediates). Once the sugar has entered glycolysis, it is metabolized to pyruvic acid and then fermented or metabolized aerobically by processes that are described here.

Fermentation

Anaerobic metabolism of glucose or another sugar by glycolysis is a process carried out by nearly all cells. The subsequent metabolism of pyruvate in the absence of oxygen is called fermentation. Fermentation occurs by many different pathways (Fig. 10.7). Two of the most important and commonly occurring are homolactic-acid fermentation and alcoholic fermentation. Neither captures energy in ATP from the metabolism of pyruvate, but both remove electrons from reduced NAD so that it can continue to act as an electron acceptor. Thus, they indirectly foster energy capture by keeping glycolysis going. However, the net energy gain is a molecule or two of ATP per molecule of glucose fermented.

Homolactic Acid Fermentation

The simplest pathway for pyruvate metabolism is homolactic acid fermentation (Fig. 10.8). Pyruvate is converted directly to lactate using electrons from reduced NAD. Unlike other fermentations, this type produces no gas. It occurs in mammalian cells like muscle cells under anaerobic conditions of strenuous muscular activity. It also occurs in lactobacilli and streptococci bacteria. This pathway in lactobacilli is used in making some cheeses.

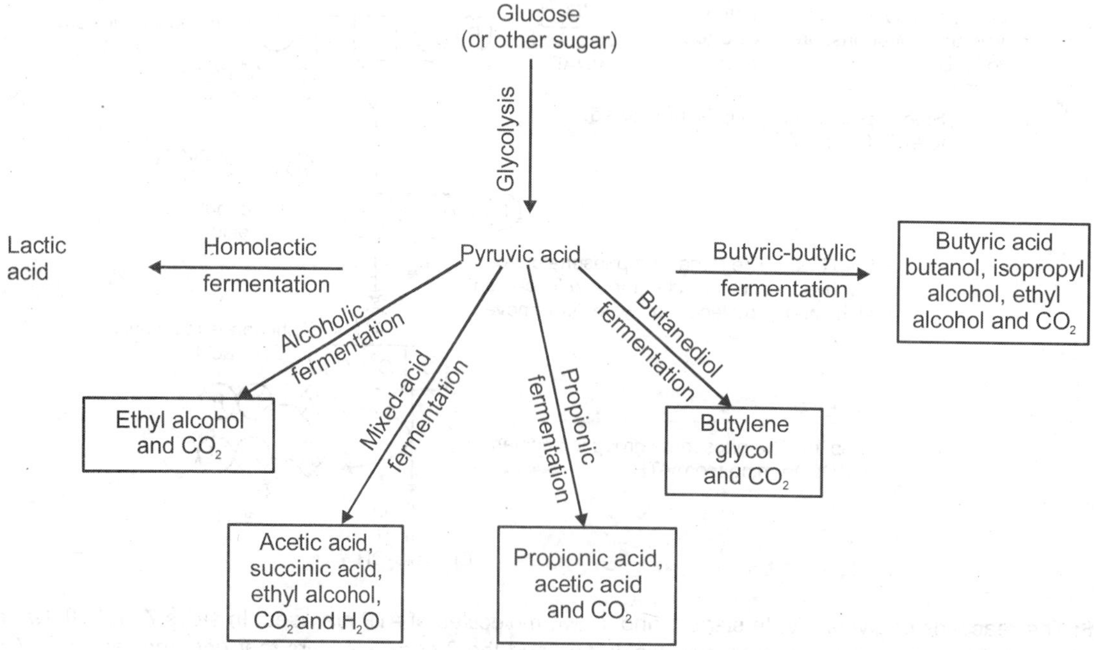

Fig. 10.7: Some of the fermentation pathway

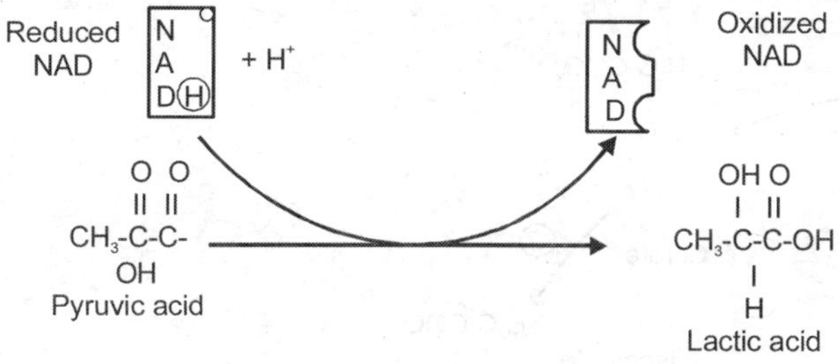

Fig. 10.8: In homolactic acid fermentation, pyruvic acid is reduced to lactic acid by the reduced NAD from step 6 of glycolysis

Alcoholic Fermentation

In alcoholic fermentation (Fig. 10.9), carbon dioxide is released from pyruvate to form the intermediate acetaldehyde, which is quickly reduced to ethyl alcohol by electrons from reduced NAD. Alcoholic fermentation, while rare in bacteria, is common in yeasts and is used in making bread and wine. This, however, doesn't occur in human beings.

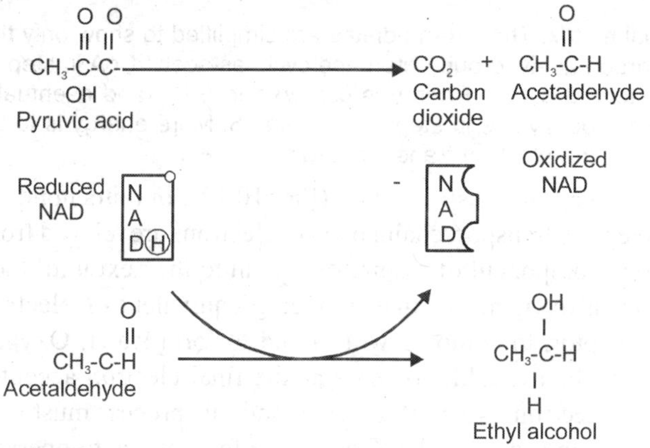

Fig. 10.9: Alcoholic fermentation is a two-step process. A molecule of carbon dioxide is first removed from pyruvic acid to form acetaldehyde. Acetaldehyde is then reduced to ethyl alcohol by reduced NAD

AEROBIC METABOLISM

As we have noted, most organisms obtain some energy by metabolizing glucose to pyruvate by glycolysis. Among these metabolizing organisms, both anaerobes and aerobes carry out these reactions ubiquitously. Anaerobes are organisms that do not use oxygen; they include some that are killed by exposure to oxygen. Aerobes are organisms that do use oxygen; they include some that must have oxygen. In addition, a significant number of species of microorganisms are facultative anaerobes, which use oxygen if it is available but can function without it. Though aerobic organisms, such as higher organisms including human beings obtain some of their energy from glycolysis, they use glycolysis chiefly as a prelude to a much more productive process, one that allows them to obtain far more of the energy potentially available in glucose. This process is aerobic respiration via the Krebs cycle and oxidative phosphorylation.

The Krebs Cycle

The Krebs cycle, named after Hans Krebs, who identified its steps in the late 1930s, metabolizes 2-carbon units called acetyl groups to CO_2 and H_2O. Its also called the tricarboxylic acid (TCA) cycle because some molecules in the cycle have three carboxyl (COOH) groups or the citric acid cycle because citric acid is its important intermediate.

Before pyruvate, the product of glycolysis, can enter the Krebs cycle, it must first be converted to acetyl-CoA. This complex reaction involves the transfer of electrons to NAD, removal of one molecule of CO_2, and addition of coenzyme A (Fig. 10.10).

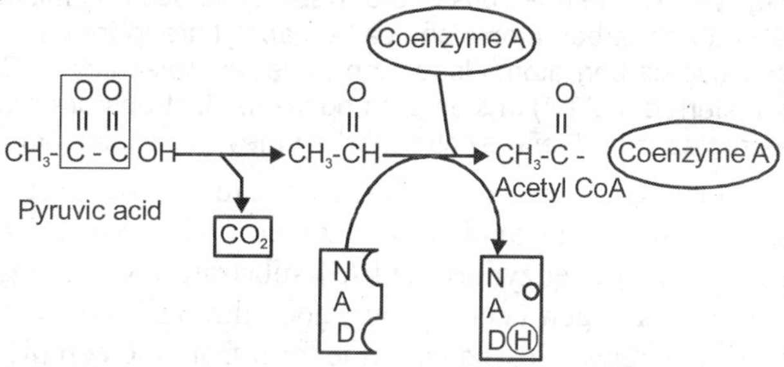

Fig. 10.10: The entry into the Krebs cycle. Pyruvic acid loses a molecule of CO_2 and is oxidized by NAD. The resulting 2-carbon acetyl group is attached to co-enzyme A forming acetyl-CoA

The Krebs cycle is a sequence of reaction in which acetyl groups are oxidized to carbon dioxide. Hydrogen atoms are also removed and their electrons transferred to coenzymes that serve as electron carriers (Fig. 10.11).

(The hydrogens, as we will see, are eventually combined with oxygen to form water). Each reaction in the Krebs cycle is controlled by a specific enzyme, and the molecules are passed from one enzyme to the next as they go through the cycle. The reactions constitute a cycle because oxaloacetic acid (oxaloacetate), a first reactant, is regenerated at the end of the cycle. As one acetyl group is metabolized, oxaloacetate combines with another and goes through the cycle again.

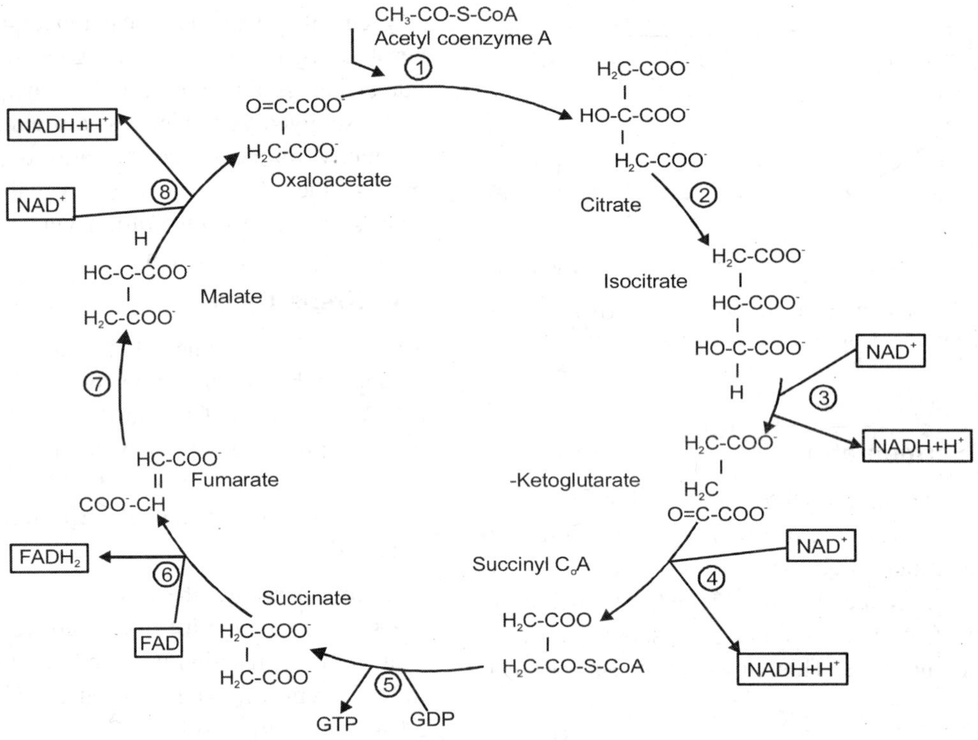

Fig. 10.11: The reactions of the Krebs cycle occur in mitochondrial matrix. The intermediates are simplified to show only the number of carbon atoms and carbon acetyl group for each. A 2-carbon acetyl group enters the cycle as acetyl-CoA in step 1, and two carbon atoms leave the cycle as molecules of CO_2 in steps 3 and 4. Energy is captured in GTP (and eventually transferred to ATP) in step 5. In addition, electrons are removed by coenzymes in steps 3, 4, 6 and 8. More energy is to be extracted from these electrons when they are subsequently fed into the electron transport chain

Certain events in the Krebs cycle are of special significance: (1) oxidation of carbon, (2) removal of electrons to coenzymes, and (3) substrate-level energy capture. As each acetyl group goes through the cycle, two molecules of carbon dioxide form from the complete oxidation of its two carbons. Four pairs of electrons are transferred to coenzymes: Three pairs to NAD and one pair to FAD. Much energy is derived from these electrons in the next phase of respiration, as we will soon see. Finally, some energy is captured in a high-energy bond in guanosine triphosphate (GTP). This reaction takes place at the substrate level. That is, it occurs directly in the course of a reaction of the Krebs cycle. Energy in GTP is easily transferred to ATP. Note that because each glucose molecule produces two molecules of acetyl-CoA, the quantities of the products just given must be doubled to represent the metabolism of a single glucose molecule.

RESPIRATION: ELECTRON TRANSPORT CHAIN AND OXIDATIVE PHOSPHORYLATION

Reduced NAD and reduced FAD from the Krebs cycle and some other metabolic pathways feed their electrons or reducing equivalents into a series of coenzymes called an electron transport chain (Fig. 10.12). In mitochondrial electron transport chain, pairs of electrons are relayed from one component of respiratory chain to the next until they reach oxygen, the final reducing equivalent or electron acceptor, to combine with it and to form water. Oxygen must be available to serve as the final electron acceptor for electron transport to occur, and this process must take place in order for the Krebs cycle to continue to operate. Unless electrons are continuously transferred from reduced NAD and FAD to oxygen via the electron transport chain, these enzymes cannot accept more electrons from the Krebs cycle, and the entire process will come to a grinding halt. From the metabolism of a single glucose molecule 12 pairs of electrons are transported by NAD and FAD to other electron carriers in the biological oxidation pathway. Eight pairs come from the Krebs cycle, 2 pairs from glycolysis, and 2 pairs from the conversion of pyruvate to acetyl-CoA.

At three sites in the electron transport chain, some of the energy of the electrons is captured in high-energy bonds as inorganic phosphate combines with ADP to form ATP in the process of oxidative phosphorylation. Electron

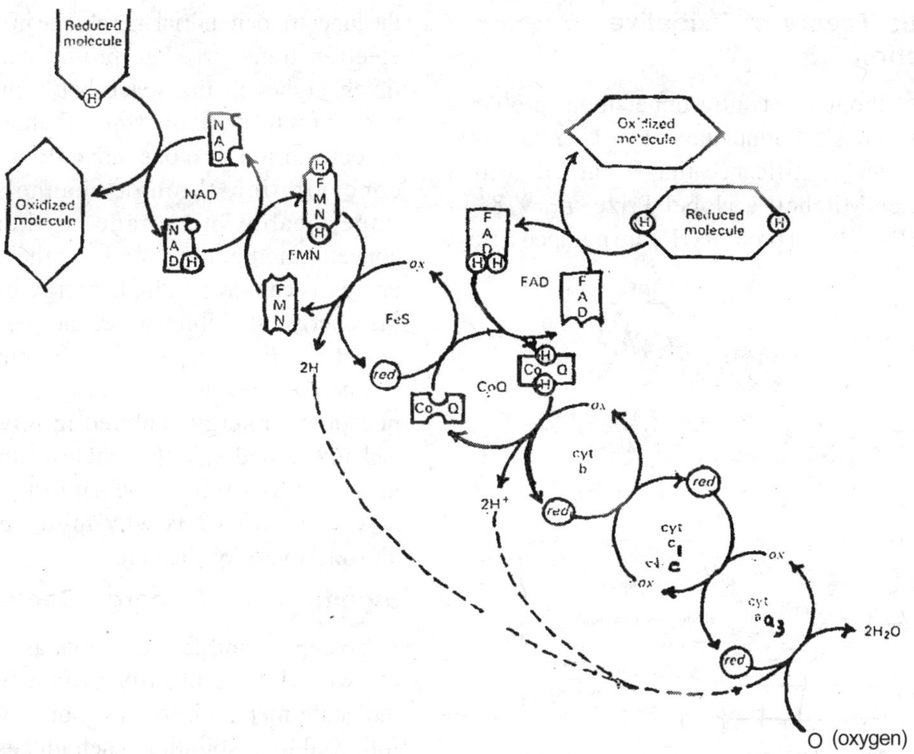

Fig. 10.12: Respiratory chain or the electron transport chain. Each carrier is reduced as it picks up electrons and is oxidized as it passes them on to the next carrier in the chain. Eventually, the electrons combine with the final electron acceptor, oxygen, to form water. Note that FAD feeds its electrons into the chain at a lower point than does NAD. Because of the arrangement of those carriers in the inner mitochondrial membrane, and because some carriers accept hydrogen atoms while others can carry only electrons, protons (H+ ions) are picked up inside the matrix and dropped off outside it during electron transport. The proton gradient created in this way is used to make ATP, the energy currency

transport and oxidative phosphorylation can be likened to a series of waterfalls where the water makes many small drops and three larger ones (Fig. 10.13). In most electron transfer (the small drops) only small amount of energy are released. At three points (the larger drops) more energy is released, and thus is captured in high-energy bonds.

In our waterfall analogy, we can think of water entering the falls at two sites, one higher up the mountain than the other. Water from the higher site falls farther than water entering a little lower down the mountain. Electrons entering the electron transport chain at NAD start at the top, and their descent released enough energy to make three ATPs. Electron entering at FAD start some way down the chain and contribute only enough energy to make two ATPs. Thus, during aerobic metabolism of a glucose molecule, the 10 pairs of electrons from NAD produce 30 ATPs and 2 pairs from FAD produce 4 ATPs, for a total of 34 ATPs. Four substrate-level ATPs, make a total yield of 38 ATPs per glucose molecule.

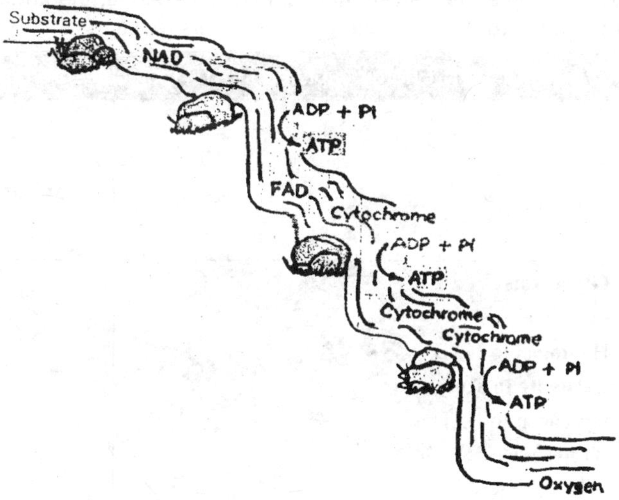

Fig. 10.13: The respiratory chain is seen as a waterfall. As the electrons are passed from coenzyme to coenzyme in the chain, they fall in energy, and some of the energy they lose is harnessed to make ATP

Chemiosmotic Theory of Oxidative Phosphorylation

Energy capture, though not fully understood, probably occurs by chemiosmosis. Formulation of the chemiosmotic theory was of such significance that it earned British biochemist Peter Mitchell a Nobel Prize in 1978. In chemiosmosis (Fig. 10.14) protons (H^+) are pumped across the inner mitochondrial membrane in eukaryotic cells during electron transport. The proton concentration becomes much higher in the space between the inner and outer mitochondrial membranes than in the matrix of the mitochondrion. Protons move from their region of higher concentration through channels in the otherwise impermeable membrane to their region of lower concentration in the matrix. As they cross the membrane, energy is captured in high-energy bonds in ATP, much as the energy of falling water can be captured by a water wheel or turbine by driving the membrane located ATP synthetase enzyme into synthesizing ATP from ADP and phosphate. Energy captured in prokaryotic cells, which lack mitochondria, is thought to occur in the cell membrane in a process similar to chemiosmosis in mitochondrial membranes. That is why mitochondria are known as 'Power House' of the cell.

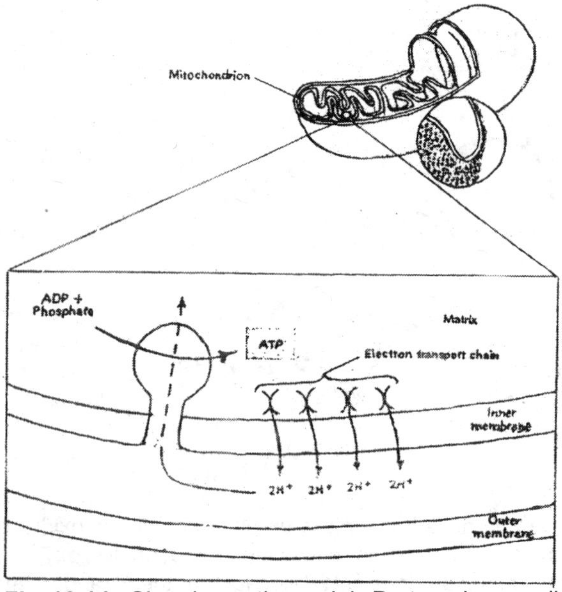

Fig 10.14: Chemiosmotic model. Protons 'pumped' out of the matrix during electron transport pass back in through channels in the inner membrane. The channels are associated with enzymes that phosphorylate ADP to make ATP. By some mechanism not yet fully understood, the flow of protons provides the energy to drive this reaction

Significance of Energy Capture

In glycolysis and fermentation, as we noted earlier, a net of two ATPs is usually produced for every glucose molecule metabolized anaerobically. When glycolysis is followed by respiration, each glucose molecule produces 2 ATPs in the Krebs cycle at the substrate level and 34 ATPs by oxidative phosphorylation. Thus, a glucose molecule metabolized aerobically yields 38 ATPs, but when metabolized anaerobically yields only 2 ATPs (Table 10.1). Hence, 19 times as much energy is captured in aerobic metabolism as in anaerobic metabolism. Thus, aerobic organisms in environments with ample oxygen generally grow rapidly but they would die if oxygen is depleted.

Table 10.1: Energy captured in ATP molecules from a glucose molecule by anaerobic and aerobic metabolism

Metabolic process	*Number of ATP Molecules*	
	Anaerobic conditions	*Aerobic conditions*
Glycolysis		
Substrate level	4	4
Hydrogen to NAD	0	6
Pyruvate to acetyl-CoA		
Hydrogen to NAD	0	6
Krebs cycle		
Substrate level	0	2
Hydrogen to NAD	0	18
Hydrogen to FAD	0	4
Less energy for initial phosphorylation	-2	-2
Total	2	38

However, mother nature maintains its atmosphere oxygen abundant to keep all aerobes alive and respiring.

METABOLISM OF LIPIDS

For most organisms, including microorganisms, glucose is a major source of energy. However, organisms cal also metabolize, albeit sparingly, lipids and protein for energy.

Lipids As a Source of Energy

Most animals including human beings, can obtain energy from lipids. The following examples give a general idea of how such a process occurs. Fats are hydrolyzed to glycerol and three fatty acids. The glycerol is metabolized by glycolysis. The fatty acids, which usually have an even number of carbons (16, 18 or 20), are broken down into 2 carbon pieces by a metabolic pathway called beta oxidation. In this process the beta carbon, the second carbon from the carboxyl group of a fatty acid, is oxidized, and the carbon chain is broken. Coenzyme A is attached to each piece to form acetyl-CoA, which is then metabolized through the Kreb cycle to obtain additional energy. Whereas Figure 10.15 sums up the fatty acid metabolism, Figure 10.16 provides an overall picture of catabolic breakdown of fats.

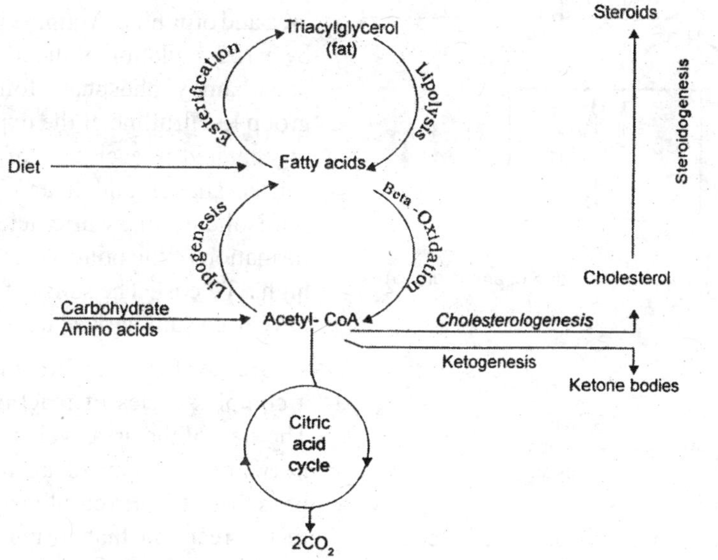

Fig. 10.15: Overview of fatty acid metabolism showing the major end products. Ketone bodies comprise the substances acetoacetate, D-hydroxybutyrate and acetone

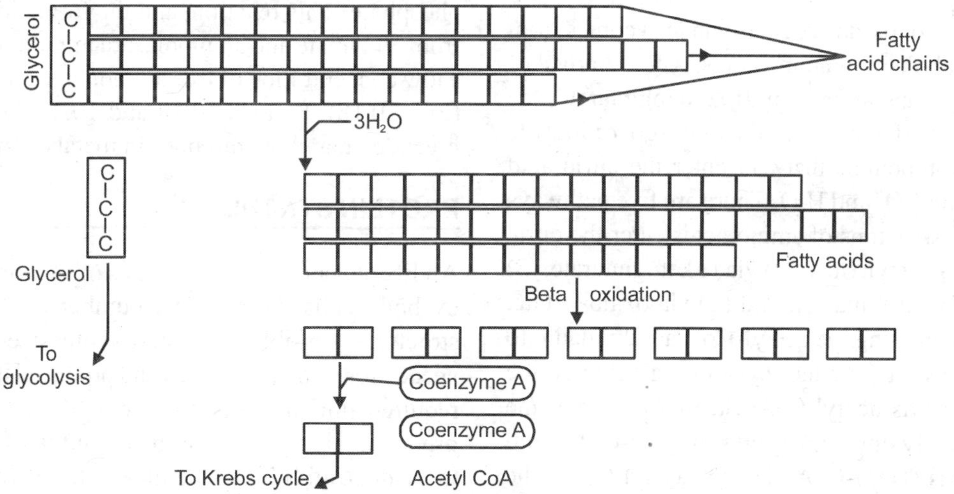

Fig. 10.16: The catabolism of fats. Triglycerides are hydrolyzed into glycerol and fatty acids. The glycerol is broken down via glycolysis. The fatty acids are broken down into 2 carbon units and fed into the Krebs cycle, where they are metabolized to produce additional energy

METABOLISM OF PROTEINS

Proteins also can be metabolized for energy. They are first hydrolyzed into individual amino acids by proteolytic (protein-digesting) enzymes. Then the amino acids are deaminated, that is, their amino groups are removed. The resulting deaminated molecules enter glycolysis, fermentation, or the Krebs cycle (Fig. 10.17).

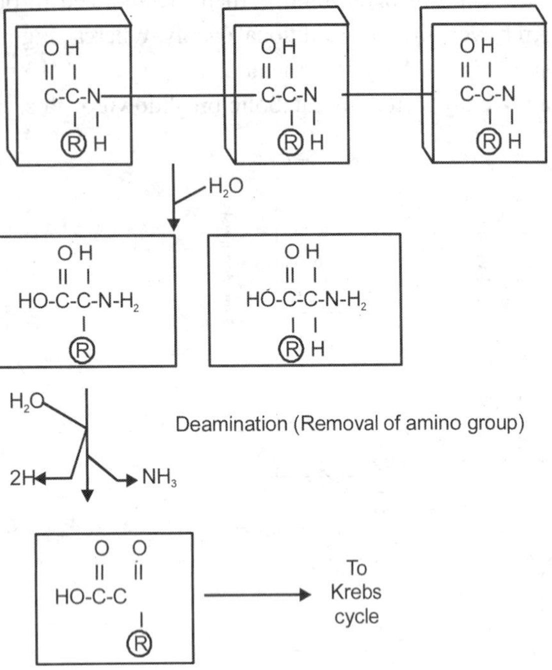

Fig. 10.17: The catabolism of proteins. Polypeptides are hydrolyzed to amino acids. The amino acids are deaminated, and the resulting molecules enter pathways leadings to the Krebs cycle

A small fraction of oxidative energy in man comes from the oxidative catabolism of amino acids. After removal of amino groups by trans-amination of α-ketoglutarate, the carbon skeletons of amino acids undergo oxidative degradation to compounds that can enter the citric acid cycle for oxidation CO_2 and H_2O. There are five pathways by which carbon skeletons of amino acids enter the citric acid cycle: (1) via acetyl-CoA, (2) via α-ketoglutarate, (3) via succinate, (4) via fumarate, and (5) via oxaloacetate. The amino acids entering via acetyl-CoA are divided into two groups. The first (alanine, cysteine, glycine serine and threonine) yields acetyl-CoA via pyruvate, and the second (leucine, lysine, phenylalanine, tyrosine and tryptophan) yields acetyl-CoA via acetoacetyl-CoA. The amino acids proline, histidine, arginine, glutamine and glutamic acid enter via α-ketoglutarate; methionine, isoleucine, and valine enter via succinate; four carbon atoms of phenylalanine and tyrosine enter via fumarate; and asparagines and aspartic acid via oxaloacetate. A number of human genetic defects in amino acid catabolic pathways occur. Phenylketonuria is a particularly serious and relatively common defect.

Ammonotelic animals (bony fishes, tadpoles) excrete amino nitrogen from their gills as ammonia, which derives from the hydrolysis of glutamine. Ureotelic animals (most terrestrial animals) excrete amino nitrogen as urea. Urea is formed in the liver by the urea cycle, discovered by Hand Krebs and Kurt Henseleit in 1932. Arginine is the immediate precursor of urea by the action of arginase, which yields urea and ornithine. Arginine is resynthesized from ornithine by carbamoylation of the latter to citrulline at the expense of carbamoyl phosphate, followed by addition of an amino group to citrulline at the expense of aspartate. Orithine is regenerated in each turn of the cycle. Uricotelic animals (birds, snakes and lizards) excrete amino nitrogen in semisolid form as uric acid a derivative of purine. The formation of the nontoxic urea and of solid uric acid has a high ATP cost. The salient features of protein metabolism have been summarized here through brief text and figures.

Urea cycle for the formation of urea takes place through a complex series of reactions known as the urea cycle. The start of the urea cycle may be regarded as the reaction between the amino acid ornithine and carbamoyl phosphate, to form citrulline, ornithine is finally regenerated in the reaction that forms urea, thus giving rise to the cyclic form of the overall reaction.

Free ammonia is needed for the synthesis of carbamoyl phosphate. This reaction, and the formation of glutamine, from glutamate and ammonia, are important in maintaining a low concentration of free ammonia, which is highly toxic (Fig. 10.18). Figures 10.19 and 10.20 depict amino acid breakdown and overall protein metabolism respectively.

PROTEIN SYNTHESIS

All life depends on the synthesis of new protein molecules by body cells. Of the vast number of different protein structures possible, each cell synthesized only the ones needed for its own purposes and produced them in precisely required amounts; this is true of every cell of every living organism, be it bacterium, or human being. In every individual, all cellular chemical activities are programmed by a genetic code unique to that individual. The genetic code itself is contained within the chromosomes inside every cell nucleus.

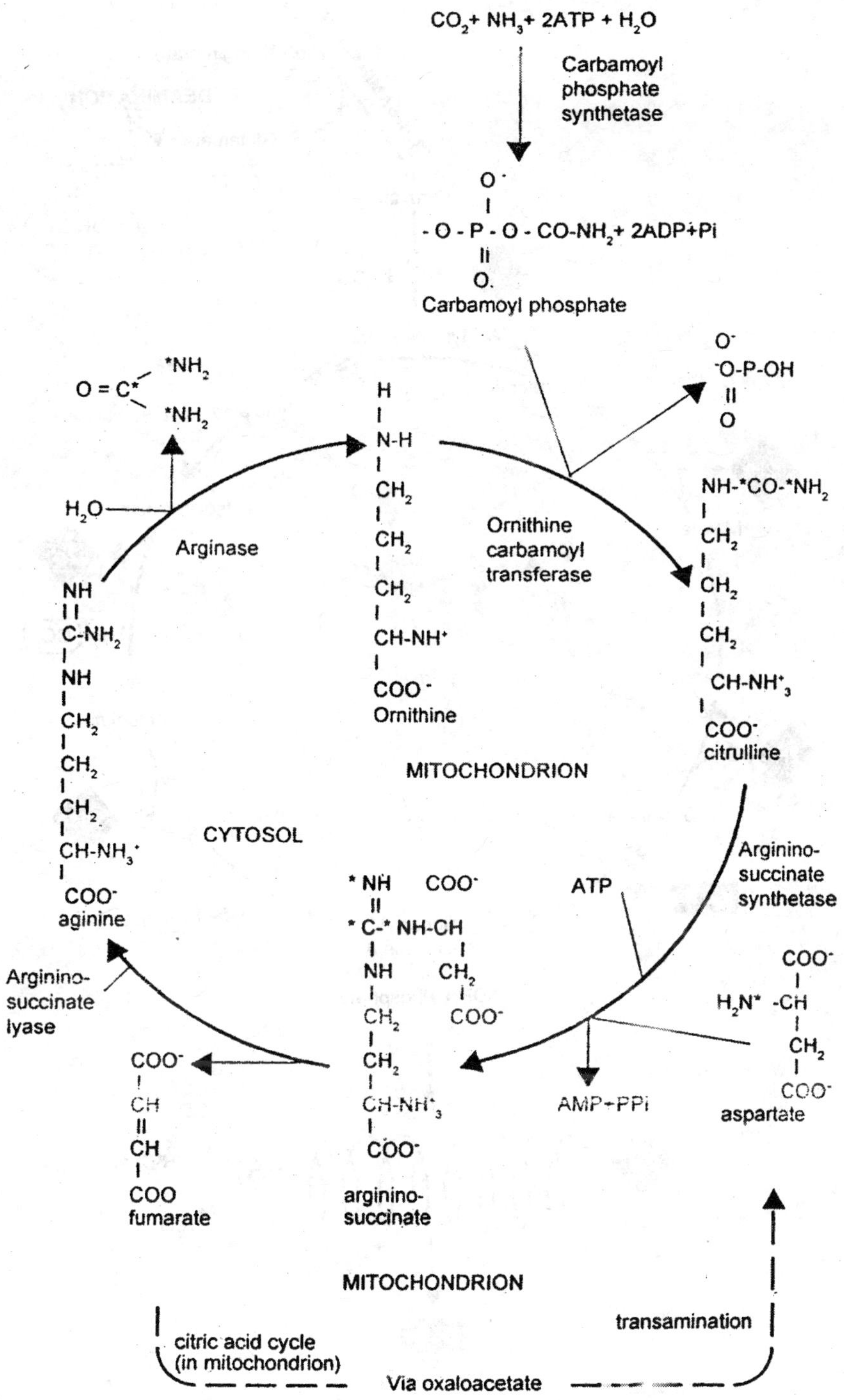

Fig. 10.18: Urea (Krebs Henseleit): Cycle one of the nitrogens of urea comes from aspartate as a result of aspartate transaminase (GOT) reaction

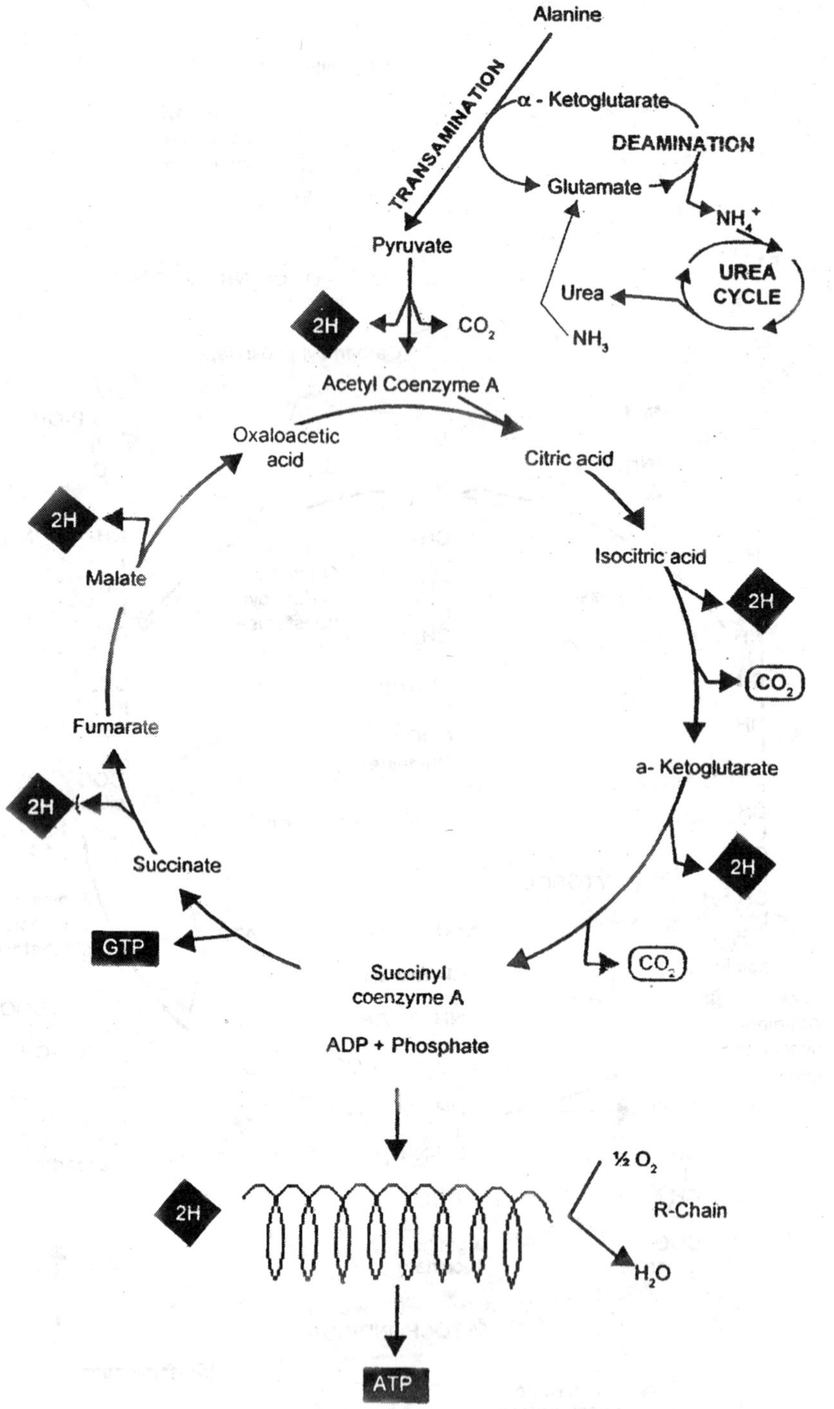

Fig. 10.19: Amino acid catabolism in a nutshell

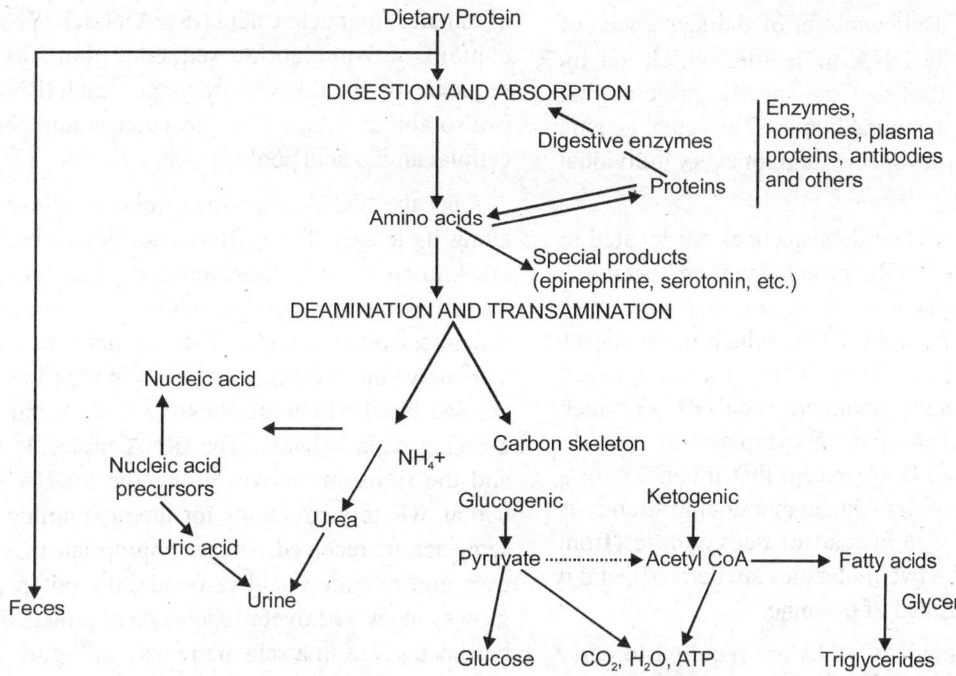

Fig. 10.20: Overall protein metabolism

'Deciphering' The Genetic Code

Chromosomes have long been recognized as being responsible for duplicating and transmitting the genetic message, and that the actual units heredity were a component of the chromosomes known as deoxyribonucleic acid (DNA). But the actual molecular structure and behaviour of DNA remained a mystery until 1953, when Watson and Crick unravelled its chemical organization and proposed a model for its biochemical action. These scientists determined that the DNA molecule was an elongated double helix, whose two twisting and intertwined strands were composed of linked subunits called nucleotides.

Watson and Crick proposed that the two strands of a DNA molecule were held together by hydrogen bonds between specific nucleotide bases. The specificity of nucleotide bonding means that a new DNA molecule can be constructed from a single strand of the old DNA molecule. The single strand serves as a pattern (template) to define a complementary strand. Thus, the information contained in a given pair of nucleotide chains is duplicated precisely, and hereditary information is transmitted from generation to generation. The cell-duplicating mechanism is so perfect that every cell in an individual contains identical nucleotide sequences in its DNA (Fig. 10.21).

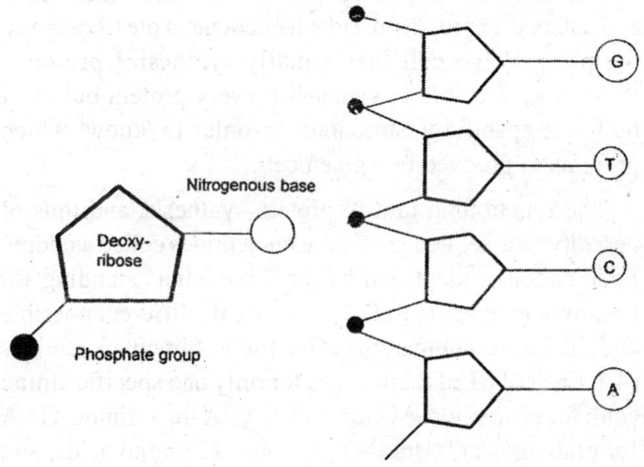

Fig. 10.21: Part of nucleotide (DNA) chain

Each nucleotide consists of deoxyribose (a 5 carbon sugar), phosphate, and a nitrogen containing base. There are four different bases (adenine, guanine, cytosine and thymine), and therefore four different kinds of nucleotides, usually expressed as A, G, C and T. The sugar of one nucleotide is always attached to the phosphate group of the next, forming the 'backbone' of the DNA molecule, with the different bases branching off as side chains

The genetic code itself consists of the sequences of nucleotides within the DNA molecule, which act by programming the synthesis of the specific proteins that make up each species including human. The actual genetic code is different for every species and for every individual within a species.

The DNA and its nucleotide sequences are located in the nucleus of the cell, but the protein synthesis occurs in the cytoplasm. The genetic information, therefore, must somehow be carried from the DNA, which never leaves the cell nucleus, to the site of action. This is accomplished by another macromolecule, ribonucleic acid (RNA), which exists in both the nucleus and the cytoplasm of the cell. RNA is very similar to DNA except that it consists of a single strand of nucleotides instead of a double strand, its 5 carbon sugar is ribose instead of deoxyribose (from which the names of the two molecules are derived), and it contains uracil (U) instead of thymine.

Actually, several kinds of RNA are required to carry out the instructions of the DNA. Messenger ribonucleic acid (mRNA) is produced in the nucleus of the cell modeled by a single strand of DNA which partially separates from its complementry strand for this purpose. The completed mRNA molecule then moves through the nuclear membrane and enters the cytoplasm. Here it encounters the ribosomes, the parts of the cell that actually synthesize proteins. Ribosomes are able to synthesize every protein but must be given specific 'instructions' in order to 'know' which proteins to produce in a given cell.

The functioning unit of protein synthesis, and thus of heredity, is a sequence of three nucleotides celled a codon. Each codon is identified by the three letters standing for its component nucleotides. There are 64 different possible codons from combinations of the four different nucleotides (4^3). Each of 61 of them codes for only one specific amino acid; for example, AAG for lysine, AGA for arginine, GAA for glutamic acid. But there are only 22 amino acids, and so some may be called for by more than one codon L Lysine, for example, is coded by either AAG or AAA, and serine by UCU, UCC, UCA or UCG. The remaining three codons are chain-terminating (or 'nonsense') codons, which signal the end of a particular message sequence.

The Making of a Polypeptide

In the bloodstream, ready to enter the cell cytoplasm at an instant's notice, is a supply of amino acids that have resulted both from digestion of dietary protein and from breakdown of cellular protein. Waiting in the cytoplasm are molecules of transfer ribonucleic acid (tRNA). Each tRNA molecule contains a 3-nucleotide sequence that 'fits' a similar sequence on the mRNA strand, and each tRNA molecule is also able to attach to a particular amino acid from the cellular amino acid pool.

Once the mRNA enters the cytoplasm, ribosomes cluster along its length. The mRNA and its attached ribosomes are known as polyribosome complex. Each ribosome moved along the strand of mRNA, touching two codons at a time. Codon by codon, a tRNA molecule and its amino acid arrive on the scene. Enzymes in the ribosome form a peptide bond which attaches the new amino acid to the growing peptide chain. The tRNA molecule is released, and the ribosome moves along the mRNA to the next codon, where instructions for the next amino acid in the sequence are received. As each appropriate tRNA molecule carrying its amino acid responds, the polypeptide chain grows longer. The overall sequence of protein biosynthesis has been given in a schematic way in Figure 10.22.

INBORN ERRORS OF PROTEIN METABOLISM

Despite its amazing complexity, the protein synthesizing process functions to perfection in virtually every individual. But in some conditions, a key component of the mechanism fails to work. These inborn errors of metabolism are due to inherited defects that result in biochemical abnormalities, often with serious clinical symptoms. We consider here one of the most familiar of such diseases, phenylketonuria or PKU.

Usually, defects are the result of damage to a single gene, the unit by which hereditary traits are transmitted. Genes can be described as the set of nucleotide codons on a DNA molecule that direct the formation of a particular protein from its component amino acids. However, it is convenient to refer to genes in terms of their net effect, as has been traditional since Gregor Mendal first suggested their existence a century ago.

A damaged gene is known as a mutant. Mutations result from factors, such as exposure to radiation, that interfere with the replication of the DNA molecule. If even a single nucleotide were missing, or if an incorrect nucleotide were to replace a correct one, the mRNA strand would be transmitting the 'wrong' information and keying the addition of an incorrect amino acid. If the resulting protein were a metabolic enzyme, the metabolic process for which it was necessary could not take place.

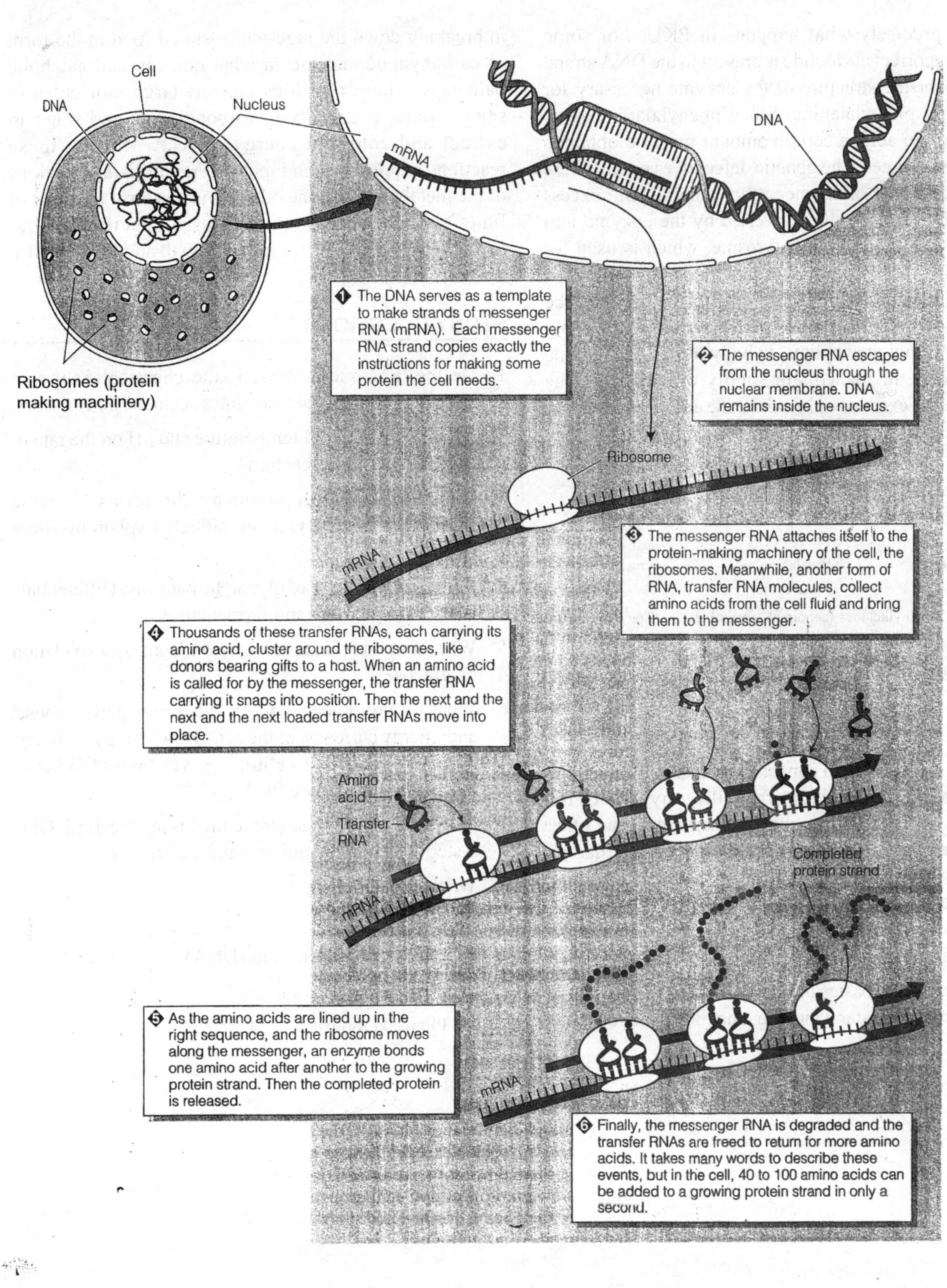

Fig. 10.22: A schematic sketch of protein biosynthesis

This is precisely what happens in PKU. For some reason, an incorrect nucleotide is present in the DNA strand that codes for the structure of the enzyme necessary for metabolizing phenylalanine. Since phenylalanine is an essential amino acid, a certain amount must be obtained from dietary sources. The genetic defect does not interfere with the utilization of this necessary amount. But excess phenylalanine is normally converted by the enzyme into the non-essential amino acid tyrosine, which is used for growth and other functions. If this pathway is blocked because the enzyme is missing, phenylalanine must be metabolized by alternate pathways and accumulates, along with its abnormal metabolites, in body fluids. At the same time, there is an inadequate supply of tyrosine. The combination of excessive phenylalanine and its byproducts, and inadequate tyrosine, results in the symptoms found in untreated phenylketonuric patients. The condition of PKU can be diagrammed as follows:

Normal individual: phenylalanine ⟶ tyrosine (Low)
↓ (minor route)
phenylketones (abnormal metabolites) (Trace amounts)

(minor route)
PKU: phenylalanine ⟶ tyrosine
↓ (main pathway)
phenylketones (abnormal metabolites) (Large amounts)

The symptoms, which appear in infants between 6 and 18 months of age, include irritability, hyperactivity, convulsive seizures, lighter skin and hair color than other family members, moderate to severe mental retardation, and a general slowdown of physical growth and development. Untreated individuals have a short life expectancy, with only a 25 percent chance of surviving past the third decade.

By studying the basics of metabolic transformations of food, one can understand the role, chemical reactions play in breaking down the ingested or stored food in the form of carbohydrate and fat, in what one can call catabolic pathways. These reactions convert large molecules to smaller ones, eventually to carbondioxide and water to extract and conserve energy as ATP. Most of these reactions require oxygen input. Energy utilizing reactions of the metabolism, on the other hand, perform a variety of functions most of which are tissue specific cellular including biosynthesis for tissue growth and maintenance and nutrient storage.

STUDY QUESTIONS

1. Define 'Enzymes'. What is the chemical nature of enzymes? Explain how enzymes act in the body tissues.
2. What is the effect of temperature and pH on the rate of enzyme catalyzed reaction?
3. What do you understand by the terms 'enzyme specificity' and 'enzyme inhibition'? Explain by citing examples.
4. Give a brief account of glycolytic pathway. Differentiate between glycolysis and fermentation.
5. Write a comprehensive essay on 'complete oxidation of glucose'.
6. What do you understand by the terms 'power house' and 'energy currency' of the cell? How 'energy currency' is generated in the cellular power house? What is oxidative phosphorylation?
7. Name the body tissue where urea is synthesized. Give a step-wise description of urea cycle.
8. Write short notes on:
   i. Photosynthesis.
   ii. Deoxyribonucleic acid (DNA).
   iii. Fatty acid oxidation.
   iv. Phenylketonuria.

CHAPTER 11

Appraisal of Nutritional Status

Chapter Outlines

- Nutritional assessment
- Anthropometry
- Clinical signs of deficiency
- Dietary assessments
- Role of vital and health statistics in nutritional assessment
- Ecological and family factors that determine nutritional status
- Biochemical evaluation
- Study questions

NUTRITIONAL ASSESSMENT

Nutrition has become an increasing concern to professionals involved with preventive as well as curative health care, as evidence mounts to implicate dietary factors in the incidence of coronary heart disease, cancer, diabetes, and other illnesses. Poor nutritional status is sometimes associated with prolonged recovery periods following illness or injury, adding to the duration and cost of hospitalization.

We are all food consumers. As economic consumers, we select and purchase food. As biological consumers, we ingest, absorb, and metabolize it. Both processes have become centers of attention. Books, magazines, newspaper articles, and radio and television programmes provide a constant flow of information about food budgeting, 'healthful eating', 'wise marketing', menu planning and 'gourmet cookery'. But despite our preoccupation with food and demand for information about it, and despite the fact that we have an abundance of food in this country, many people, either through ignorance or neglect, choose foods that do not provide adequate or balanced supplies of key nutrients.

Since good nutrition is consonant with good health, nutritional shortcomings and disorders and nutrient-related problems must be identified, not only in patients populations but in the presumably healthy general public as well. Four major methods—anthropometric, clinical, biochemical and dietary—are used to assess nutritional status. The particular measurements used in the assessment depend on whether it is a minimal or screening assessment of an essentially healthy individual; whether it is a detailed and specific assessment of a patient who is unhealthy and may need complex support systems; or whether it is an examination of a population to determine the incidence of malnutrition. Because a particular finding may be due to any of several causes, no one of these methods is sufficient to diagnose a nutritional deficiency state. A child's failure to achieve an adequate rate of growth, for example, could be documented by anthropometric measurements but might be caused by heredity, disease, nutrition, or other factors. Only biochemical, clinical and dietary data could confirm that the growth failure was caused by inadequate nutrient intake or some other factors.

These assessment tools are also used to identify individuals or populations who are "at risk" of developing nutritional deficiencies, as well as to evaluate the effectiveness of nutrition education or supplementary feeding programes. They can also determine relationships between nutrient intake and the onset or prevention of chronic nutrition-related disease, such as coronary heart disease, diabetes, and some forms of cancer. No association between a disease condition and nutritional factors can be determined if food intake patterns are not known. These methods can also help to identify nutrients that may be inadequately provided by the available food supply and necessary dietary changes can be instituted.

Further, in a particular individual, clinical symptoms of nutrient deficiency and abnormalities of growth, development, or physiological functions are the ultimate results of long-standing deprivations. Visible signs of nutritional deficiency do not appear until the body's stores of nutrients have been depleted. For most nutrients, this will happen only after daily intake has fallen far short of need for a prolonged period of time. Examination of an individual's food behavior may suggest the existence of a nutritional deficiency, and laboratory tests may confirm the tentative diagnosis. On the other hand, biochemical data can indicate tissue depletion of nutrients before clinical signs become apparent, and a study of food intake patterns may then strengthen the argument. A variety of standardized anthropometric, clinical, biochemical, and dietary assessment techniques are, therefore, necessary to determine nutritional status of individuals and groups. Each of these methods has advantages and disadvantages, but taken together they can confirm suspicions and provide the factual basis for corrective measures.

The process undertaken to determine the state of nutrition of a person, or a group of persons or a population is termed as nutritional assessment. It is an index of the impact of nutrition on the survival, health and performances status, and is estimated by determining and describing the nutritional status of persons or population in relation to those physiological and economical variables that affect and explain the nutrition of that population. The aim of making nutritional assessment is to identify the vulnerable groups and the causative factors for such vulnerability.

Nutritional status of an individual is defined as the state of his health as affected by the intake and utilization of nutrients and is a reflection of the balance between their dietary intake and expenditure. As a matter of fact, nutritional well being of a person can be described at several levels. Normal nutrition refers to a state of sufficiency of nutrients and energy intake—neither excess nor deficiency—and is the ideal situation that tends to bring the highest level of wellness. However, deficient nutrition triggers a sequence of events commencing with tissue depletion of nutrients, followed in succession by biochemical changes and clinical signs and symptoms. Expectedly, excessive intake or overnutrition of one or more nutrients induce tissue (including blood) excess of nutrients resulting in biochemical and clinical changes.

Nutritional assessment is of value in identifying individuals or groups with one or more of the following conditions:

i. Overt or manifest malnutrition.

ii. Covert or latent nutrient deficiency.

iii. Risk of developing malnutrition.

iv. Risk of developing nutrient related diseases.

v. Available resources to assist affected people in overcoming nutritional problems.

Apart from these, an individual's nutritional requirements for growth, maintenance, tissue repletion during health, illness and stress are also estimated by undertaking his nutritional assessment. As a sequel to such an estimation, suitable nutritional care and appropriate dietary counseling are also initiated, in a follow up action. Above all, conclusions drawn through nutritional assessment also become the guiding principles for evolving specific intervention programmes for the targeted community and population groups. Further, quantitative data obtained from nutritional assessment studies is made use of in convincing ministers, legislators and officials to initiate, encourage, support and sustain direct action programmes for the benefit of public health and nutrition.

Nutritional status of an individual can be assessed by a variety of techniques which can be grouped under four heads; namely anthropometric, dietary, biochemical and clinical. Techniques falling under each group measure different states of nutrition, and many a time, do not correlate well with each other. Whereas dietary surveys evaluate current food intake and biochemical determinations the nearly current nutritional standing, the clinical and anthropometric examinations evaluate a nutritional status of comparatively longer term. However, a thoughtful combination of different techniques can generate useful data that grossly determine and describe the nutritional status of individual or population groups.

Since nutritional status of an individual is a reflection of the balance between dietary intake and expenditure of the nutrients; it is positive when the intake is more than the expenditure and leads to the accumulation of the surplus nutrients or fuels in certain tissues. In the other situation, when expenditure exceeds the intake, nutrient reserves get depleted in the tissues, as a result of body's bid to make up for the shortfall.

Efforts to obtain reliable information regarding nutritional status, meet with many difficulties, arising mostly due to body's ability to adapt to adverse conditions of both deficiency and excess in such a way that changes in biochemical and functional characteristics become evident only after the occurrence of substantial impairment in the nutritional status.

Methods of assessment, therefore, should be highly specific and sensitive. The complex and intertwined relationships between dietary deficiency, disease, and personal environment variables also make it particularly difficult to determine whether or not health impairment can be linked specifically to diet, and whether or not any nutritional deficiency is secondary to some other defects. These and related aspects can only be taken care of by a systematic study of the patterns of biochemical, physiological, pathological and biochemical responses to deficiency and excess of nutrients and applying this knowledge in practical situations.

Despite all these limitations, nutritional assessment has an immense significance in nutritional monitoring and surveillance of the population. Whereas nutritional monitoring is the determination of nutritional status of the population either continuously or periodically in order to explore the possibility of a nutritional intervention or to see the effectiveness of some intervention programmes already in force; nutritional surveillance refers to the early detection of the nutritional problems of the community so as to initiate early attempts aimed at their correction and rectification.

ANTHROPOMETRY

Beginning with anthropometric methods, we set out to acquire familiarity with the techniques of nutritional assessment. The term anthropometry has a Greek origin meaning human (anthropos) measurements (metery). The technique involves the measurements of whole body (body weight) and part thereof (physique, e.g., height, thickness of skin folds, arm muscle head and chest circumferences). These apart, the technique (anthropometry) also involves the assessment of age and energy exchange. Anthropometric data, in essence, is a measure of all those indices that reflect the long-term energy balance and protein status of individual. Intake and balance positions of other nutrients affect anthropometric indices not directly but indirectly by affecting the energy and protein metabolism. Secondly, there may be a wide variation in the methods and measurements employed in anthropometry, both in terms of number and level of complexity and it is desirable to select the given method and indices keeping in view the aims and objectives of the study and nature of the target group. Given hereunder is a brief discussion on various anthropometric measurements (Fig. 11.1).

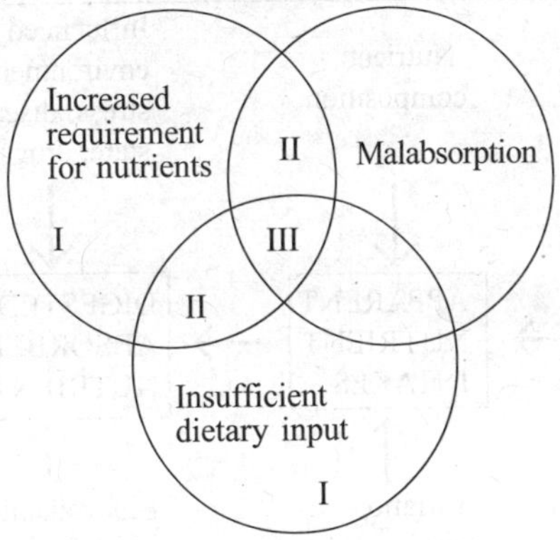

Fig. 11.1: Important causative factors of low individual nutritional status. Schematic diagram showing three important determinants of nutritional status. Individuals in the area I are least vulnerable, in the area II comparatively more vulnerable and in the area III; most vulnerable

Age

Age is ascertained from authenticated records like municipal corporation, birth register, certificates and horoscopes. Exact age estimation is of great significance when one's targeted population involves young children where the incidence of malnutrition is found to be very high.

Weight

If weight measurements are of value in charting out the growth patterns during infancy and childhood, they are equally useful in the detection of the extent of malnutrition or obesity in adults and elders. For healthy adults, most of the times, if not always, an increase in body weight is indicative of fatness or adiposity in direct proportion to body weight. In diseases of renal (kidney) hepatic (liver) and cardiovascular (heart and circulatory system) origin, an increase in weight is indicative of fluid retention and accumulation. Similarly, a decrease (in body weight) may be due to anorexia (decreased appetite in fevers or other situations); malabsorption (malabsorption syndrome) or a spurt in metabolism (hyperthyroidism). Alterations in body weight in pregnancy are usefully interpreted as indications of maternal nutritional standing.

It is customary to express the weight of children in terms of percentages in various percentiles of standards or as plane percentages, representing three degrees of malnutrition. Evaluation and interpretation of weight measurements must be made keeping in view the length and size of the frame, proportion of fat, muscle and bone. Also, a close clinical examination should precede weight measurements so as to exclude the possibility of pathological increase in weight due to edema and spleen enlargement (Figs. 11.2, 11.3 and 11.4).

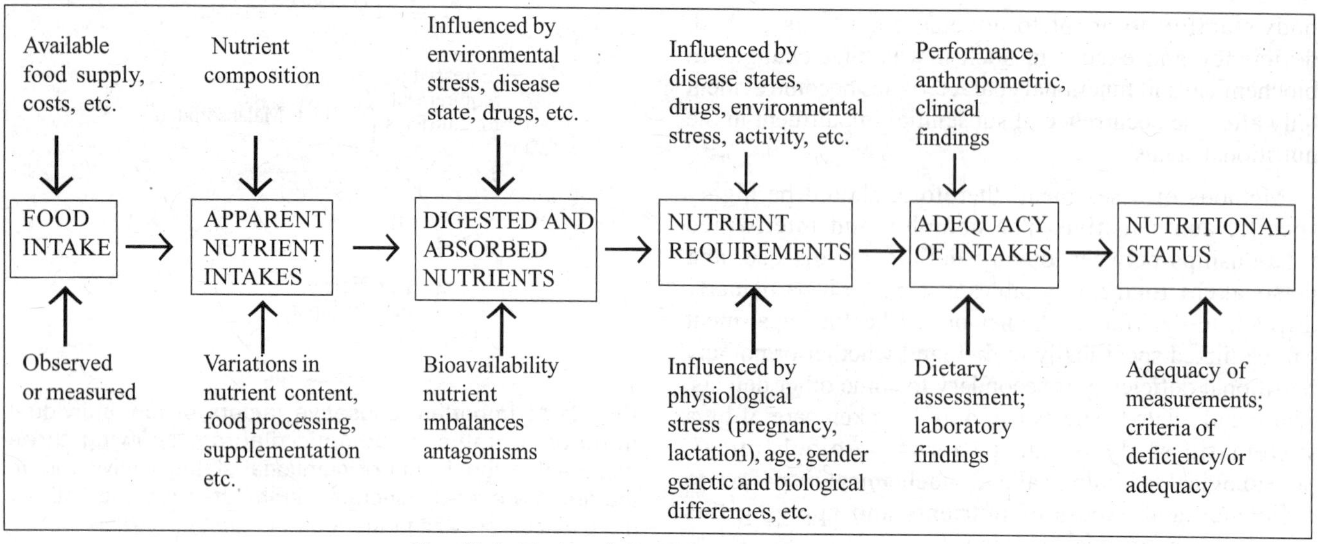

Fig. 11.2: Factors influencing nutritional status

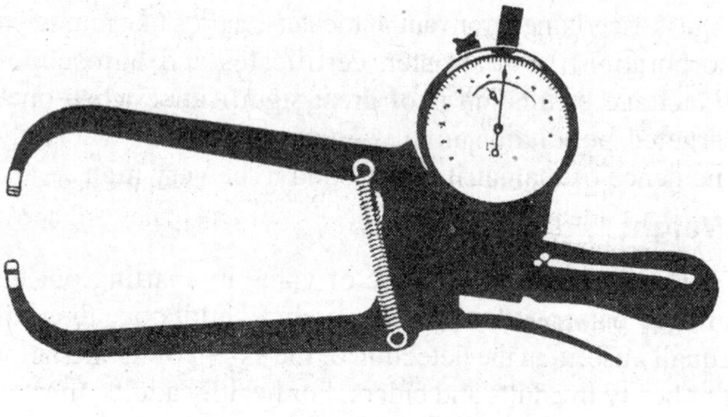

Fig. 11.3: Harpenden skin-fold calipers

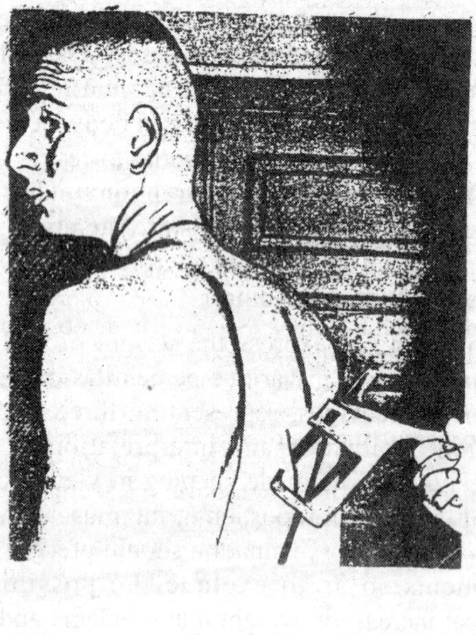

Fig. 11.4: Measurement operation with a skinfold calipers

Height

Significance of body length measurement in young children and of height measurement in older ones and adults, is well documented and recognized. Height of a person—contributed by various components, viz. legs, pelvis, spine and skull—varies as per its genetic make up; the full realization of genetic potential depends upon dietary adequacy. That is why backward social milieu and economic deprivation dictated chronic malnutrition affect height.

Body Composition

Different indices of body composition, measured by various techniques, give a fairly good idea of the nutritional status of a person. Direct (by the application of Archimide's principle) or indirect (by skinfold thickness measurements) body density (or specific gravity) measurements are related to percent body fat and give the degree of adiposity of the subject. For instance, a body specific gravity of 1.048 corresponds to 25 percent fat but when the specific gravity of an obese person is as low as 1.002, the body fat content increases to 49.8. Though viscera (brain, liver, heart, kidney and other internal organs) make up an appreciable part of the body weight yet by and large, it remains unaffected by malnutrition. Therefore, muscle and fat are the only soft tissues that register a quantitative regression with deficiency of protein and calories. Based on this fact, skin-fold thickness measurements are made with calipers, applied at constant pressure, on selected body sites viz. triceps, biceps, subscapular, abdominal, hip pectoral and calf areas. Measurements involving three skinfold measurements are considered more reliable than a solitary one. However in assessment works of preliminary nature, triceps thickness measurements are most widely undertaken by applying calipers on the outer skinfold (Fig. 11.4) of the back upper arm, midpoint between the shoulder tip and the elbow. Thus information concerning the amount and distribution of human subcutaneous fat, and hence of caloric reserves, is obtained by body composition studies. A rough estimate of protein status can be made by measuring body weight, since body weight for height has been used as a crude indicator of total body protein. Reference standards for body weights at various heights have been successfully used for roughly estimating the body protein content and energy balance. Also by making use of mid upper arm circumference (midway between the tip of acromion and the olecranon) and skinfold thickness over the mid triceps (midway between acromion and the olecranon) or over the subscapular (about 1 cm below the inferior angle of the scapula) are measured using a flexible steel or fiber glass tape and Herpenden calipers respectively. Since the mid upper arm circumference is made up of muscle and fat over the constant humerus, the skinfold thickness factor (reflecting fat) when subtracted from mid upper arm circumference gives the remainder as mid upper arm muscle circumference (MAMC), an index of total body protein as under. Mid upper arm muscle circumference (cm)—0.3142 triceps skinfold thickness (cm) = MAMC (cm).

Head Circumference

Since long, pediatricians (child specialists) have been using head circumference as a standard procedure to detect pathological conditions accompanied by a large head, e.g., in hydrocephalus, or too small a head, as in microcephaly.

From nutritional stand point too, head circumference measurement is valuable, for it directly relates to brain size and, to a small extent, to the thickness of the scalp tissue and the skull. An increase in head circumference is almost essential during the first year of age, indicating the age related increase in brain size with little nutritional or health influence. Interestingly, the dependence of head circumference on nutritional status becomes slightly evident in the second year of life when nutrient related decreases in brain size, thickness of scalp, soft tissues and the skull occur in protein energy malnutrition (PEM). However, the effect is much less than that on the chest circumference which registers a greater decrease in its circumference in response to PEM (Fig. 11.5).

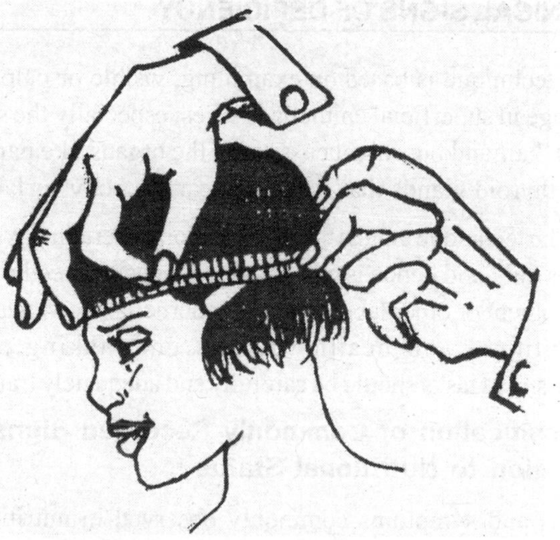

Fig. 11.5: Measurement of head circumference

Chest Circumference

It has been observed that circumference of the head and the chest are almost the same at six months of age after which the skull grows slowly as compared to the chest (Table 11.1). The chest circumference ratios of less than one can be attributed to growth failure and fat wasting of the chest wall, and is taken as a community indication of PEM during early years of childhood. Similarly, skinfold thickness measurements at triceps and arm circumference are also used to estimate muscle mass and caloric insufficiency.

The convenience and simplicity of these methods lie in the fact that almost all such measurements can be undertaken with the help of a weighing machine, a flexible steel or fiberglass tape and calipers, even outside the laboratory on the locations of survey/field work.

Table 11.1: Head and chest circumference measurements in first five years of life

Age (months)	*Head (cm)*	*Chest (cm)*
Birth	35.0	35
3	40.4	40
6	43.4	44
12	46.0	47
18	47.4	48
24	49.0	50
36	50.0	52
48	50.5	53
60	50.8	55

CLINICAL SIGNS OF DEFICIENCY

The technique is based on examining, visible or palpable change in superficial epithelial tissues; especially the skin, eyes, hair and buccal mucosa; or in the organs like parotid and thyroid glands that are quite near the body surface.

The technique entails the examination of certain physical signs only and hence is quick and inexpensive, needing no equipment or other laboratory paraphernalia. However, the nutritional and health workers undertaking such assessment tasks should be carefully and adequately trained.

Classification of Commonly Recorded Signs in Relation to Nutritional Status

Signs and symptoms commonly observed in nutritional survey, have been classified into the following three groups by World Health Organization's (WHO's) expert committee on medical assessment of nutritional status.

Group I: Signs that are considered to be of value in nutritional assessment. The signs are highly probable to indicate the deficiency of one or more nutrients in the tissues in the recent past.

Group II: Signs that need further probing and investigation.

Group III: Signs not related to nutrition.

This classification facilitates a nutritional worker in the most useful selection of signs to record in a particular field study, whether preliminary in nature, comprising rapid clinical screening of the community for sure signs (group I), or in a study advanced in nature, where evaluation of less certain signs (group II) also becomes necessary. Ability to recognize and eliminate signs unrelated to nutrition (group III), spares the workers a considerable time and effort removing confusion in interpretation and evaluation (Table 11.2).

Table 11.2: Classification list of signs used in nutrition surveys

Area of examination	*Group 1: Sign known to be of value in nutrition*	*Group 2: Sign that need further investigation*	*Group 3: Some signs not related to nutrition*
1. Hair	Lack of luster Thinness and sparseness Dyspigmentation of proximal part of hair Flag sign Easy pluckability		Alopecia Artificial discoloration
2. Face	Diffuse depigmentation Nasolabial dyssebacea Moon face	Molar and supraorbital pigmentation	Acne vulgaris Acne rosacea Chloasma
3. Eyes	Xerosis conjunctivae Xerophthalmia (including keratomalacia) Bitot's spots Angular palpebritis	Conjunctival infection Circumcorneal infection Circumcorneal and scleral pigmentation Corneal vascularization Corneal opacities and scars	Follicular conjunctivitis Blepharitis Pingueculae Pterygium Pannus
4. Lips	Angular stomatitis Angular scars Cheilosis	Chronic depigmentation of lower lip	Chapping from exposure to harsh climates
5. Tongue	Edema Scarlet and raw tongue Magenta tongue Atrophic papillae	Hyperaemic and hypertrophic papillae Fissures Geographic tongue Pigmented tongue	Aphthous ulcer Leukipkai

Contd.

Contd.

6. Teeth	Mottled enamel	Caries Attrition Enamel hypoplasia Enamel erosion	Malocclusion
7. Gums	Spongy, bleeding gums	Recession of gum	Pyorrhea
8. Glands	Thyroid enlargement Parotid enlargement	Gynecomastia	Allergic or inflammatory enlargement of thyroid or parotids
9. Skin	Xerosis Follicular hyperkeratosis, types 1 and 2 Petechiae Ecchymoses Pellagrous dermatosis Flaky paint dermatosis Scrotal and valuval dermatosis	Mosaic dermatosis Intertriginous lesions Thickening and pigment-tation of pressure points	Folliculosis Ichthyosis Acneiform eruptions Miliaria Epidermophytosis
10. Nails	Koilonychia	Brittle, ridged nails	
11. Subcuta-neous tissue	Edema Amount of fat		
12. Muscular and skeletal system	Intramuscular or sub-periosteal hematomas Craniotabes Frontal and parietal bossing Ephiphyseal enlargement (tender or painless) Beading of ribs Knock knees or bow legs Diffuse or local skeletal deformities	Winged scapula Deformities of thorax	Funnel chest Kyphoscoliosis
13. Internal systems:			
a. Gastro-intestinal	Hepatomegaly ascites		Splenomegaly
b. Nervous	Mental confusion Sensory loss Motor weakness Loss of position sense Loss of vibratory sense Loss of ankle and knee jerks Calf tenderness	Psychomotor change Condition of ocular fundus	
c. Cardio-vascular	Cardiac and peripheral vascular dysfunction Pulse rate	Blood pressure	

* Expert Committee on Medical Assessment of Nutritional Status. Tech. Rep. Series, No. 258, World Health Organization, Geneva, 1963, pp. 57-58.

Brief Description of Related Clinical Signs

The clinical signs, believed to be of dietary origin, are recorded systematically by following a common practice of examining subjects from head to foot as discussed hereunder:

Eyes: Dryness of cornea and conjunctiva, are the most commonly noticed symptoms, usually associated with vitamin A deficiency. A more severe deficiency manifests itself as Bitot's spots followed by a completely opaque cornea (xerophthalmia).

Eyes also become red due to an infiltration of cornea by blood vessels in riboflavin deficiency.

Membranes: Prevalence of anaemia can be inferred by observing the colour of the mucous membranes, e.g., the colour of the mucous membrane, on the underside of the eyelids where inadequate blood supply makes it look pale in colour in an anaemic individual as compared to a healthy, non-anaemic one where the membrane is not pale but highly coloured.

Skin: The condition of skin also reflects, many a time, the nutritional status of the individual. However to draw correct inference it becomes imperative to distinguish such conditions from age related changes taking place in the skin.

For instance, dermatitis symptoms of varying forms and extent are indicative of certain vitamin deficiencies. Whereas lesions on area of skin exposed to sunlight suggest niacin deficiency, roughness and hardness of papillae at the base of the hair follicle may appear as a consequence of vitamin A and essential fatty acid deficiency. The dermatitis occurs primarily in thighs, chest and back. Pyridoxine and/or riboflavin deficiencies cause nasolabial dermatitis. A dry inelastic skin is observed after dehydration. Essential fatty acid deficiency manifests as eczema in infants.

Mouth and Teeth: Angular stomatitis (cracks at the corners of the mouth) and cheilosis (vertical cracks followed by redness, swelling and ulceration in areas other than the corners of the lips) indicate riboflavin deficiency. A magenta colour of the tongue is also due to this deficiency.

Loss of papilla on the tongue and a scarlet and raw appearance of the tongue are associated with niacin deficiency.

Colour: Soft, spongy and bleeding gums are hallmarks of L-ascorbic acid (vitamin C) deficiency.

Poor periodontal tissue and loss of teeth and persistent backaches occur due to porous nature of teeth and bones (as in osteoporosis), a low serum calcium and high phosphorus/calcium ratios (more than one) in the diet.

The presence of mottled tooth enamel is frequently seen in high fluoride ingestion, especially in areas where drinking water supplies contain high fluoride (more than four parts per million) levels.

Other Tissues: A decreased intake of iodine with or without high intake of goitrogens (mostly present in vegetables of Brassica family) manifests itself as cretinism in infants (where mother's nutriture has been affected during pregnancy) and thyroid enlargement in other age groups.

Other symptoms related to thiamine deficiency and protein malnutrition include edema, especially of lower extremities. Protein malnutrition also causes depigmentation, lack of luster and a decrease in the diameter of hair.

Lack of vitamin D induces bowed legs and rickety rosary (beading of ribs especially at the junction with the breast bones). Iron deficiency can be gauged from cupping of the nails. Neurological symptoms associated with vitamin B_{12} and thiamine deficiencies are recognized by evaluating the reflexes of lower extremities.

Clinical signs, as it was made clear in the beginning of this discussion, result from long term nutritional deficiencies.

DIETARY ASSESSMENTS

Qualitative and quantitative assessment of food intake, is a technique used for the assessment of nutritional status, as it furnishes useful indications about dietary inadequacies. By undertaking dietary surveys of individuals or groups their dietary deficient or excessive intakes can be identified. However definite conclusions are not drawn unless low or high intakes, as registered by dietary surveys are accompanied by corresponding biochemical and/or physical indices, corroborating the deficient or excessive daily dietary intakes. But when dietary data pertaining to a particular nutrient intake is matched by corresponding biochemical changes and clinical signs, the dietary intake values serve to confirm the dietary diagnosis and lays down the basis of a dietary treatment regimen. Aforementioned limitations apart, limitations related to individual variabilities in digestion absorption and utilization (bioavailabilities) of nutrients also matter. Moreover a dietary assessment study reflects the current or recent nutrient intake, whereas much of the clinical evidences and anthropometric measurements, indicate long term nutriture. Biochemical changes, occupy a somewhat midway position, whereby such changes occur after some time lag when the deficient intakes continue for quite sometime. However, the lag period needed for the perceptible sign to appear takes a far greater time compared to the occurrence of biochemical changes. That probably explains the discrepancies arising between dietary and clinical findings, e.g., continuation of deficiency symptoms for sometimes after a switch over to an improved diet. Conversely, absence of biochemical or clinical signs of a deficiency on the face of a lower dietary intake and nutrients reserves may be a reflection on the time required for nutrient reserves to get depleted, after the decline of dietary quality and quantity.

Evaluation of food intake data is made by transforming it into energy, carbohydrate, protein, fat, minerals and vitamin intake values by using food composition table. This also incorporates an element of error in the nutrient intake data as the food composition values cannot be very precise and accurate for different foodstuffs at different places.

Dietary assessments are made by direct methods by which 'individual food intake per day', are calculated by a number of methods, such as 24-hour recall or three-day recall method and 'weighted food record' method. To extract the relevant information from illiterate or not so well educated subjects, the interviewer should be familiar with the ethos, culture and food patterns. Similarly, to estimate the qualitative food intake the nutritional investigator must not only understand the system of measures used in the area under study but also should standardize them.

After having obtained the information on composition and pattern of dietary intake, its translation into nutrient intake values is done in the following manner.

First estimate nutrients consumed in a day by using standardized food composition table. Then, dietary deficiency or excess for one or more nutrients can be assessed by comparing the values obtained with corresponding recommended dietary allowance (RDA) values.

Given hereunder is a brief resume of dietary assessment methodology.

Methodology for Dietary Surveys

Dietary surveys can be planned to determine food consumption of families or of individuals. Family food consumption or household consumption, as it is more appropriately called, is an estimate of the total amount of food used by an entire household for a fixed period of time, usually one week. The most commonly used methods are the food account, food list and food record.

Food Account

The food account is a record of all food purchased or produced for family consumption over a period of several weeks. The length of time depends on the complexity of the diet since no record is made of food already in the household or of that remaining at the end of the study period. When the diet is relatively monotonous or only a few food supplies are routinely stored in the home, a period of two weeks is often satisfactory since under these conditions food purchases tend to represent food consumed within a brief period of time.

Food List

The food list is essentially a recall method. The homemaker is asked to estimate by weight, retail unit or household measure, the quantity of food used by the entire household during the previous week. The method requires a well trained interviewer who can help the homemaker recall by daily menu or purchases all food used by the household. The food list is advantageous in that only one visit to the household is necessary, because it requires a little time and effort on the part of the homemaker. Cooperation usually is good. Accuracy of the food list is judged to be satisfactory for this purpose and errors tend to be due to omission of food items or incorrect estimation of amounts of food used.

Food Record

This method involves a weighed inventory of foods at the beginning and close of the study period, usually one week, together with a day-by-day record by weight of food brought into home during the week. Records of plate and kitchen wastes are sometimes, but not always, included. This method is time consuming and therefore more expensive than the food list. At least two visits to the home are required of the interviewer and considerably more time is demanded of the homemaker. Accuracy of the method is relatively high although it is generally believed that food list is an equally satisfactory and much less expensive means for obtaining household food consumption data.

Weighed Household Consumption

In some cases it is both feasible and advisable to obtain household food consumption by daily weighing of food prepared and served in the home. This method usually required that an investigator be present in the home at the time when food is prepared. The method has the advantage of providing more precise information than can be obtained by recall or record. It is perhaps the best approach to use in rural or small village situations where much food is obtained from home gardens or local barter and where retail measures or weights are uncertain. However, the method requires a greater investment in time and personnel than other techniques and is seldom used unless it is certain that data of comparable validity cannot be obtained by other means.

Surveys of house food consumption are designed to yield essentially two kinds of data, namely economic consumption, that is, the monetary value of food entering the home or food available for consumption; and/or physiological consumption, the food actually eaten by the family. In any case certain kinds of accessory information must be obtained, such as the number of individuals usually fed from the family food supply, the number of meals eaten away from home, and the number of guests entertained during the study period.

Individual Food Intake

Evaluation of individual nutritional status leading to identification of vulnerable groups within a population group requires study of food consumed by a given individual. Four methods are commonly used to determine individual food consumption; estimation by recall, food record, dietary history and weighed intake.

Estimation by Recall

Recall of food intake is almost always for a 24-hour period only, and for this reason it is generally designated the 24-hour recall. The subject is asked to recall all food consumed during the previous day and to estimate quantities in ordinary measures or servings in order to increase accuracy of quantities of food consumed, the subject may be provided with measuring cups or other devices to aid in estimation. Information obtained by this method is not necessarily representative of usual intake of an individual. The method, therefore is most useful when relatively large numbers of subjects are involved and provides a qualitative and a quantitative description of groups dietary patterns. The 24-hour recall can serve as a basis for educational programmes or gross evaluation of dietary intake of large groups. It is not valid as an accurate measure of food intake of one individual. When large numbers of subjects are involved, the method, is considered, to be indicative of the dietary pattern characteristic of the group. Because of ease of obtaining data, the 24-hour recall has gained in usage. Recently the use of periodic 24-hour recall of the same individual was described as a means of continuous monitoring of food consumption patterns.

Food Record

This method requires that the subject keeps a record of food eaten for varying lengths of time, usually three to seven days. Quantities of food are estimated in common household measures. Accuracy of the method depends largely on the diligence and integrity of the subjects and on the subject's ability to estimate quantities of food. The method appears to be a fairly accurate estimate of individual food consumption over a specific period of time.

Weighed Intake

A very accurate record of food consumption can be obtained by having a subject or a trained person weigh all food consumed during a given period of time. This method of obtaining food consumption data is obviously expensive and time consuming and consequently is rarely used in nutrition surveys. In spite of the accuracy of data obtained on quantities of food consumed, the method is limited in other ways. Because of the tediousness of the procedure, subjects are prone to try to find shortcuts and thus to change from their usual eating patterns.

The weighed food intake, however, is standard procedure in a laboratory-controlled metabolic study, and although a few surveys have involved weighted data, this method most often is limited to research studies. Under these circumstances, it is the researcher rather than the subject who bears the burden of the tedious procedure.

Diet History

The diet history is designed to discover the usual food intake pattern over a relatively long period of time and is most often obtained by interview. A series of food records kept at intervals over a period of months or years yields data comparable to the diet history but obviously is more expensive procedure both in terms of time and personnel. The diet history often is used for studies of food habits or in clinics or hospital dietetics, and seldom used as research tools.

Since all known methods for obtaining dietary data have certain advantages as well as limitations, the choice of method should depend on the population sample to be surveyed and the specific use for which the data is intended.

In addition to the choice of method, the investigator must decide how the collected data will be handled. It may be necessary to know only the general pattern of food. Food intake or the range of nutrient intake for a population and the specific food groups from which nutrients are obtained. In certain epidemiological studies, the pattern of eating throughout the day can be as important as total nutrient intake. Furthermore, the consumption of food in commercial establishments and the use of highly processed convenience foods in the home have increased. It is becoming more and more important to assess the contribution of food consumed from these sources and their effects on total nutrient intake.

ROLE OF VITAL AND HEALTH STATISTICS IN NUTRITIONAL ASSESSMENT

Mortality and morbidity ratios are affected by many factors including environmental conditions of sanitation and the extent of immunization and medical care. Infants are especially vulnerable to environmental stresses and neglect. There is evidence suggesting that the high mortality rate observed among children one to four years of age in many areas of world is the result of the interaction between malnutrition and infectious diseases. Many workers have reported that deaths that had been attributed to diarrhea or parasitic infection among children under five years of age are, infact, caused by or associated with malnutrition. It is generally accepted that the mortality rate in the preschool age range of one to four years may serve as a rough index of malnutrition in a community.

The occurrence of high mortality rates in a community, therefore suggests that for each child who dies in early life, many others live who are being handicapped by incipient malnutrition. Unfortunately, accurate health and vital statistics are not available for various populations in our country, and even when statistics are available, the investigator can estimate only that a nutritional problem exists. The identification of the problem requires more specific evaluation.

ECOLOGICAL AND FAMILY FACTORS THAT DETERMINE NUTRITIONAL STATUS

a. Ecological Factors

1. Travel and communication.
2. Drinking water.
3. Health care services.
4. Electrification.
5. Sanitation.
6. Educational facilities.

b. Family Factors

1. Family composition.
2. Literacy level of family members.
3. Socio-economic profile of the family.

BIOCHEMICAL EVALUATION

Biochemical evaluation of nutritional status entails determining quantitative levels of nutrients or their metabolites in blood or urine samples. Such an evaluation provides valuable indications regarding their normal deficient or excessive dietary intake, absorption, utilization and excretion are obtained.

Characterization of the state of biochemical processes occurring in tissues and organs is carried out either by chemically analyzing the tissue specimens (bioptates), or indirectly, by performing chemical analysis of biological fluids like blood and urine. The latter analysis (of biological fluids) is easier to carry out as the samples are obtained by almost non-invasive procedures. The blood, consisting of cells and plasma, is the circulation fluid tissue of the organism. Concentration of various biochemical substances in blood, as also the cellular metabolism of blood, reflects to a reasonable extent the general metabolic trends in the organism and help in assessing the metabolic changes in other tissues. Further, the formed elements of blood, responsible for various important functions, are also estimated by determining the corresponding biochemical indices. Likewise, plasma or serum determinations, not only convey valuable informations on the functioning of blood (transport, regulatory, homeostatic and other functions) but also infer inklings about the metabolic transformations occurring in other tissues. Biochemical examination of urine, for instance, enables us to judge the excretory and ureopoietic functions of the kidney along with the metabolic status of different tissues and organs of the body.

It is a well known fact that signs and symptoms of a nutrient deficiency do not become manifestly evident after the digestion of a deficient diet. There usually is an intervening period during which the nutrient reserves tend to absorb the blow inflicted by nutrient(s) depleted diet. Symptoms of deficiency appear thus only after a sizeable depletion of nutrient(s) reserves. A developing deficiency is diagnosed therefore, before the clinical manifestation of signs and symptoms because the concerned biochemical parameters show up the change before the appearance of clinical symptoms. However, during recovery process, the biochemical changes normalize well before the disappearance of clinical signs.

Biochemical tests, which are based on knowledge of the metabolism and utilization of nutrients, are a useful adjunct to anthropometric and clinical assessment. They confirm suspicions of existing long-term deficiencies, are the most objective measures of nutritional status, and provide an early warning of clinical deficiency symptoms. Body measurements and clinical assessments reflect long-term and previous nutritional status, but biochemical analyses reflect the most recent situation, status of stores, or functional effects.

Most biochemical measurements are static indicators of concentrations of nutrients which are affected by a multitude of biological and technical factors. Over the past ten years there has been increased interest in functional indices of nutritional status. Areas of functional competence likely to be affected by malnutrition are cognitive ability, disease response, reproductive competence, physical activity and work performance, and social behaviour performance. The true significance of nutritional deficiency is in the impairment of these types of functions.

Inadequate intake, inefficient digestion, disturbances in metabolism, or altered excretion of nutrients shows up quickly in the chemical composition of body fluids. Blood and urine, therefore, provide an accessible window on current nutritional status. Most nutrients and/or their metabolites can be detected in either or both of these fluids. A sample of blood, for instance, contains all the substances that are currently circulating to every cell in the body. A urine sample contains wastes and byproducts that indicate how those substances have been used in the cells. For example, a low urinary level of a particular substance may reflect inadequate intake, abnormal metabolism, or malabsorption from the digestive tract (in which case, the fecal content of that substance will be abnormally high, a situation that can be detected by different biochemical tests). A high urinary level, on the other hand, may suggest an excessive supply of certain nutrients or physiological abnormalities.

Generally, decreased levels of nutrients or their metabolites in blood and urine reflect depleted tissue reserves of the nutrient in question. However, this is not always the case. Under certain conditions, vitamin A stores in the liver may not be released into the blood, and blood levels of the vitamin will be abnormally low even though tissues are not depleted.

Analysis of nutrient levels in various body tissues such as liver or muscle would also provide this information, but that would involve the discomfort of having a tissue sample removed, as well as a certain amount of risk. For this reason, routine biochemical assessments utilize less invasive techniques, biopsies being requested only as a last resort or to confirm other findings implicating particular organs.

Blood Analyses

Measurements of the constituents in the blood provide clues about the level of nutrients in the body. Concentrations of some nutrients—vitamins, protein, lipids, and some minerals and other substances—can be measured directly.

Blood samples taken after an overnight fast are preferred, since concentrations of many nutrients are affected by meals and some also exhibit a diurnal variation. Concentrations in the blood can be altered by factors other than nutrition. For example, in patients with infection, serum iron is low because iron moves out of the blood and into the tissues, not because of iron deficiency per se.

In addition to directly measuring the concentrations of nutrients in blood, the concentrations of compounds which require specific nutrients for their proper function can be measured. For example, iron is an essential component of hemoglobin and if not present in sufficient amounts in the body, will result in less hemoglobin being produced. Therefore, measuring hemoglobin will provide information regarding iron status. Furthermore, if the precursor of hemoglobin, erythrocyte protoporphyrin, is not used to make hemoglobin, its concentration in blood increases. If not enough hemoglobin is being produced due to lack of iron, red blood cells are smaller and less red than normal (microcytic and hypochromic). This can be detected when the red blood cells are examined under a microscope. One of the most frequently used tests of nutritional status, hematocrit, is a ratio of the packed cell volume to the total volume of the sample. In patients with iron deficiency anemia the red blood cells get smaller and fewer in number, the packed cell volume goes down and the hematocrit is lower than that of a healthy person. All of these changes can be caused by problems other than iron deficiency; therefore, other measurements must be used to confirm the diagnosis of iron deficiency anemia.

Another method of measuring the nutritional status of some nutrients, usually vitamins, is to measure the activity of enzyme systems which require that specific nutrient as an essential cofactor for the reaction. Thiamin status is frequently measured using this technique. While direct measurement of thiamin or its phosphate ester in blood is now possible, the most useful and reliable method of assessing thiamin status is to measure the activity of the enzyme transketolase in red blood cells. A sample of blood is added to an incubation mixture which contains all components necessary for the reaction except thiamin. The amount of thiamin present will affect how much of the substrates are used or how much product is produced. Similarly, glutathione reductase activity is used to evaluate riboflavin status.

A knowledge of the regulatory mechanisms controlling each nutrient is important for accurate interpretation of biochemical results. For example, abnormal serum calcium levels do not usually result from a dietary deficiency of this mineral; rather, they are more likely to reflect a disturbance in one or more of the interconnected mechanisms that maintain calcium homeostasis, such as vitamin D, or they may be secondary to protein status.

Urine Analyses

Analysis of urine can detect normal or abnormal amounts of some nutrients or of their metabolites. Direct analysis can be done for a number of substances; glucose and albumin are among the most common. In addition, tissue reserves of water-soluble nutrients can be estimated by means of a "load" or "saturation" test: For example, administration of a large dose of ascorbic acid is followed by measuring the urinary excretion of vitamin C. With adequate tissue reserves of the vitamin, a large percentage of the administered dose will be excreted. Conversely, if the body's tissue reserves are low, a high percentage of the loading dose will be retained in the body, and therefore less will appear in the urine.

Indirect, functional measures are also employed in urinalysis. For example, a "loading" dose of tryptophan, which is converted to nicotinic acid, may be administered before urine is collected for evaluation of vitamin B_6 status. Vitamin B_6 is required in the conversion of xanthurenic acid to nicotinic acid (niacin), a step in the normal metabolism of tryptophan. Therefore, in patients with B_6 deficiency, a load dose of tryptophan will create an accumulation of xanthurenic acid, which will be excreted in the urine because there is insufficient vitamin B_6 available to convert it further to nicotinic acid.

Collection of urine samples is, surprisingly, more difficult than collection of blood samples. Although the momentary discomfort of drawing blood is avoided, the inconvenience factor is substantially increased. Ideally, biochemical tests are performed on a 24-hour sample of urine, which reflects the quantitative daily output of many substances rather than the relative output at any one time of day. Few subjects are willing to take the time and care required to collect 24-hour, or even 12- or 6-hour, urine samples. In most cases, a single specimen must suffice, from which quantitative estimates of daily excretion are calculated in reference to excretion of creatinine.

Thus conclusion on nutritional assessment of individuals or population groups are drawn by obtaining information from one or more 'assessment technique application' on the target group depending upon the purpose of assessment (Tables 11.3 and 11.4).

Table 11.3: Laboratory tests useful for the assessment of nutritional status

Nutrient	*Laboratory test* *Commonly used*	*Adult normal or acceptable values*	*Special or less used*
Vitamin A	1. Serum retinol level 2. Plasma retinol-binding protein level	>30 ug/dL 30-40 ug/dL	Serum carotene level
Vitamin C	1. Serum ascorbate level 2. Leukocyte ascorbate level	>0.3 mg/dL >15 mg/dL cells (>20 ug/10^8 cells)	Whole blood ascorbate level Saturation test Urinary ascorbate level Tyrosine load test
Vitamin D	1. Serum 25-hydroxycholecalciferol level 2. Serum Ca level 3. Serum P level 4. Serum alkaline phosphatase level	>20 mg/dL 9-11 mg/dL 3-5 mg/dL <40 King-Armstrong units <15 Bodansky units	Serum 1-25 dihydroxycholecalciferol level X-ray and radiographic examinations
Vitamin E	1. Serum vitamin E level 2. Erythrocyte hemolysis test	≥0.7 mg/dL <10% hemolysis	Erythrocyte vitamin E level
Vitamin K	1. Prothrombin test	11-18 sec.	Clotting factors
Thiamin	1. Erythrocyte transketolase stimulation 2. Urinary thiamin excretion	<15% ≥65 ug/g creatinine	Blood thiamin level Thiamin load test
Niacin	1. Urinary 2-pyridone/N'-methylnicotinamide ratio	>1.0	Erythrocyte levels of nicotinamide mononucleotide
Folic acid	1. Serum folic acid level 2. Erythrocyte folic acid level	≥6.0 mg/mL 160 mg/mL cells	Deoxyuridine suppression Formiminoglutamic acid excretion
Vitamin B_{12}	1. Serum vitamin B_{12} level	200-900 pg/mL	Schilling test
Riboflavin	1. Erythrocyte glutathione reductase stimulation 2. Urinary riboflavin excretion	<1.20 ≥ 80 ug/g creatinine	
Vitamin B_6	1. Erythrocyte AST activity 2. Erythrocyte AST-PLP stimulation coefficient 3. Plasma pyridoxal phosphate level	>1.1 IU/mL cells 2.0 >5.0 mg/mL	Erythrocyte ALT activity Xanthurenic acid excretion following a tryptophan bad Urinary vitamin B_6 excretion Urinary 4-pyridoxic acid excretion Methionine load test
Pantothenic acid	1. Urinary excretion level	≥ 2.0 mg/g creatinine	Blood pantothenic acid level Coenzyme A blood level Coenzyme A-dependent blood enzymes
Biotin	1. Urinary biotin excretion level 2. Blood biotin levels	30-60 ug/24 h 120-240 mg/dL	Biotin-dependent blood enzymes
Essential fatty acid deficiency	1. Serum triene/tetraene ratio	<0.4	

Contd.

Contd.

Zinc	1. Serum zinc level 2. Plasma copper : zinc ratio	80-120 ug/dL <2.0	Urinary zinc excretion Hair zinc level Erythrocyte zinc level Neutrophil zinc level
Copper	1. Serum copper level	75-125 ug/dL	Urinary copper excretion Hair copper level
Selenium	1. Serum selenium level	> 12 ug/dL	Erythrocyte selenium level Blood glutathione peroxidase activity
Iodine	1. Serum protein bound iodine 2. Urinary iodine excretion	4.8 ug/dL > 50 ug/g creatinine	Free and total plasma thyroxine levels

Table 11.4: Some functional tests for biochemical assessment of nutritional status

Sr. No.	*Nutrient deficiency*	*Name of the test*	*Laboratory determination*	*Basis of the test*
1.	Vitamin B_6	Tryptophan load test	Estimation of urinary Xanthurenic acid	In vitamin B_6 deficiency tryptophan owing to the failure of being converted to niacin, is alternatively converted to xanthurenic acid causing its blood load and urinary excretion.
2.	Vitamin A	Retinol load test	Estimation of circulating levels of retinol binding protein (RBP)	Vitamin A deficiency inhibits the release of RBP from liver, but a high dose (Retinol load) releases the stranded surplus from liver.
3.	Folic acid	Histidine load test/FIGLU test	Estimation of urinary form-imino-glutamic-acid (FIGLU)	A decreased conversion of FIGLU to glutamic acid (due to folic acid deficiency) results in its high level in blood and excretion in urine.
4.	Vitamin B_{12}	Isoleucine load test	Estimation of urinary methylmalonic acid	In vitamin B_{12} deficiency, methylmalonic acid, an intermediate of isoleucine metabolism becomes the stranded metabolite and hence excreted in the urine. Conversion of methylmalonic acid to succinic acid is vitamin B_{12} dependent.
5.	Vitamin C	Vitamin C saturation test	Estimation of urinary vitamin C excretion	A poor vitamin C status leads to tissue desaturation and uptake to vitamin C by tissues and with small excretion in urine. A normal status however, cause small absorption and more excretion.

STUDY QUESTIONS

1. Explain the terms nutritional assessment, nutritional status, nutritional monitoring and nutritional surveillance and their importance in applied nutrition programmes.
2. Write a comprehensive essay on the effectiveness of anthropometric status measurement in nutritional assessment.
3. Explain briefly the methodology of dietary assessment and its relevance in nutritional assessment.
4. Explain, how static and functional biochemical indices infer valuable informations pertaining to nutritional status?
5. Comment critically on the statement—Assessment of clinical signs and symptoms, if undertaken skillfully and methodically, convey valuable indications about a person's nutritional status.

CHAPTER 12

Water and Electrolyte Balance

> *Chapter Outlines*
> - Introduction
> - Body fluid regulation
> - Electrolytes
> - Electrolyte balance
> - Acid-base balance
> - Role of aldosterone in fluid and salt balance
> - Disturbances in fluid-electrolyte and acid-base balance
> - Study questions

INTRODUCTION

Single-cell organisms receive their nutrients directly from the environment and discard waste products directly into it. In multicellular organisms, the situation is not so simple. There too, each cell needs nutrients and produces wastes, but most of the cells are not directly in contact with the environments.

Body fluids serve as a medium for carrying nutrients to and waste products from the cells and also for carrying the chemical communicators that coordinate and compliment activities among cells.

Whereas the fluids present within the cells are called intracellular fluids, all the body fluids that are not present inside the cell are collectively known as extracellular fluids. These fluids make up about one quarter of a person's body weight. The most abundant is interstitial fluid, which directly surrounds most cells and fills the spaces between them. It makes up about 17 percent of body weight. Another body fluid is blood plasma, which flows in the arteries and veins. This makes up about 5 percent of body weight. Other body fluids that occur in lesser amounts are urine, lymph, cerebrospinal fluid, aqueous humor, and synovial fluid. All body fluids are aqueous solutions. Water is the only solvent in the body.

The blood plasma circulates in the body through a closed and intricate system of blood vessels, and is in contact with the other body fluids through the semipermeable membranes of the blood vessels. Therefore, blood can exchange chemical compounds with other body fluids and, through them, with the cells and organs of the body.

There is, however, only a limited exchange between blood and cerebrospinal fluid, on the one hand, and blood and the interstitial fluid of the brain, on the other. This limited exchange between blood and interstitial fluid of the brain is referred to as the blood-brain barrier. This is permeable to water, oxygen, carbon dioxide, glucose, alcohols, and most anesthetics, but only slightly permeable to electrolytes such as Na^+, K^+ and Cl^- ions. Many larger molecular weight compounds are also excluded.

The blood-brain barrier protects the cerebral tissue from detrimental substances in the blood and allows it to maintain low K^+ concentration, which is needed to generate the high electrical potential essential for neurotransmission.

Body fluids have special importance for the health care professionals. Samples of body fluids can be taken with relative ease using either non-invasive or slightly invasive techniques. The chemical analysis of blood plasma blood serum, urine, and occasionally of cerebrospinal fluids is of major importance in diagnosing diseases.

An adult weighting 60-65 kg has a total free water of about 45 liters. On anatomic and functional grounds, total body water can be divided into two main categories, namely, (1) the fluid found within the cells, the intracellular fluid (ICF), and (2) fluid outside the cellular membrane, the extra-cellular fluid (ECF). Out of the 45 liters of water, about 30 liters constitute ICF and 15 liters make the ECF. The latter may be divided for practical purposes into four categories: (a) blood-plasma (the fluid within the blood vessels) approximately 3 liters; (b) interstitial fluid in tissues interstices between the blood vessels and the cells (lymph is included in this category), (c) the fluid of the dense connective tissue cartilage and bone which, in reality, is a continuation of interstitial fluid but because of the compactness of collagen fibers and of the bone matrix it is penetrated extremely slowly by water which equilibrates rapidly in the rest of the interstitial fluid, and (d) the transcellular fluid—extra-cellular fluids not included in the other categories. These are separated from the ECF—water by an epithelial membrane and include the cerebrospinal fluid, cavity fluids of the eye, the pleural, pericardial and peritoneal fluids, fluids within the ducts of digestive glands, etc. About 12 percent is constituted by the latter three; (b) (11 liters), (c) and (d) (1 liter).

Except for the transcellular fluids, the distribution of water is very specific and is decided by two factors viz. (1) water is freely diffusible throughout the entire body, and (2) solutes are relatively restricted in their movements (either physically as with plasma proteins or actively as in the case of electrolytes). Because of these factors water moves in such a direction that osmotic equilibrium is achieved. Any disturbance in body water therefore results in movement of water by osmosis until equilibrium is attained. Osmosis is one of the chief physicochemical factors in fluid and electrolyte balance in the body. It is defined as the process whereby solvent molecules (usually water) move through the semi-permeable membrane to the more concentrated solution till the concentration of the solute(s) become equal on both sides. Cell membranes function as semi-permeable membranes to regulate water balance in living systems.

Other factors that regulate the movement of water are 'obligatory' movement of water with salts and 'facultative' movement of water under the influence of antidiuretic hormone (ADH). Movement of electrolytes under the influence of adrenal cortical hormones called mineralocorticoids, like aldosterone also affects the movement of water. In addition, oncotic pressure, i.e., osmotic pressure of colloidal plasma proteins, though of a low magnitude of about 28 mm Hg (as only 0.49% of whole plasma) has a profound influence on the maintenance of blood volume.

Apart from the total amount of water (total body water), there is also the need for maintaining constancy of fluid volume, concentration of electrolytes and colloids and the osmolalities of different body fluids within limits.

The rate of turnover of water is quite high as the water of the fluids is continuously being renewed. A normal human adult should have an average obligatory intake of 1600 ml of water required to meet the obligatory loss of 1600 ml and an extra facultative intake of 900 ml to compensate for the facultative loss through the kidneys.

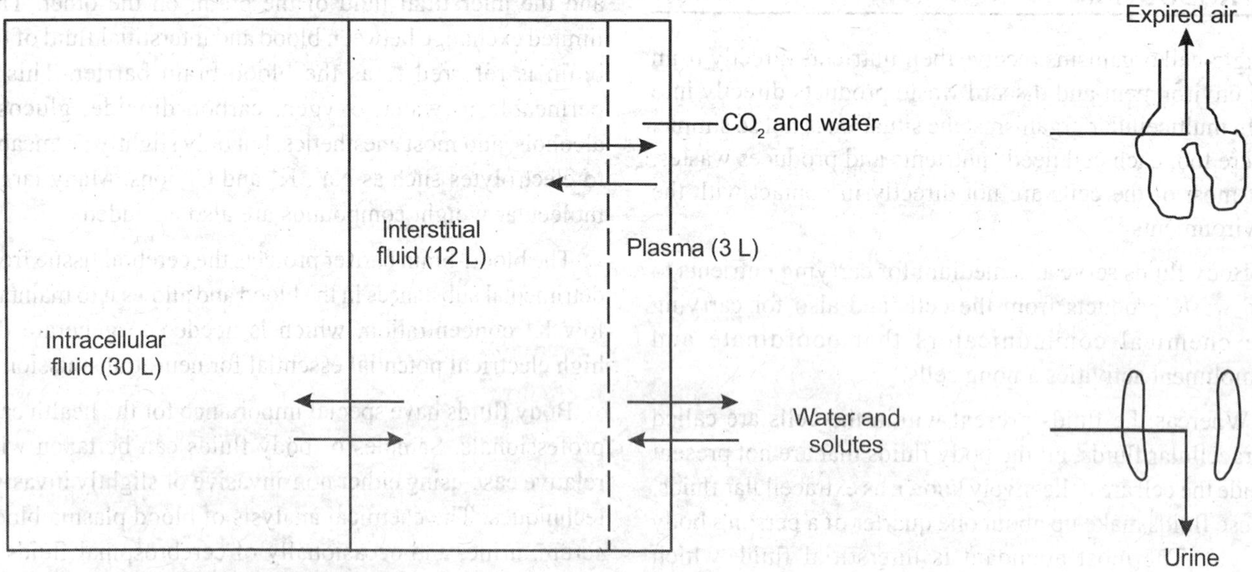

Fig. 12.1: Fluid compartments of the body and interchanges from one compartment to another

BODY FLUID REGULATION

Thirst is the sensory impression that motivates the ingestion of water. It is caused mainly by an increase in the effective osmolality of the body fluids. Ingestion of water reduces and restores back the osmolality to normal levels.

Water is continuously lost from the body in the expired air and from the skin. The sum of these losses is termed as "insensible loss" of water and is about 600 ml to 1000 ml per day in an average adult. This water does not have any substantial amounts of solutes in it.

The exchange of water and solutes between the body fluids and the lumen of the gastrointestinal tract is large. It is contributed by the saliva and secretions of the stomach, liver, pancreas and intestinal mucosa. Though the volumes of these secretions may as high as 8 liters per day under ordinary circumstances, the net loss from the body is negligible.

The cardiovascular-renal system maintains fluid homeostasis by directly regulating the amount and composition of urine. About 80% water of glomerular fluid in the kidneys is reabsorbed into plasma by proximal tubules and is referred to as "obligatory absorption" which is not under hormonal control. The remaining 20% is called "facultative absorption" and is under the hormonal control of ADH. The ADH secretion is believed to be due to stimulation of specific osmoreceptors which respond to changes in crystalline osmotic pressure. These osmoreceptors set up nerve impulses which reflexly stimulate the hypothalamus and through it the pituitary. At normal blood osmotic pressure, the receptors discharge steadily and so maintain a steady secretion of ADH. Increased secretion results from decreased fluid volume, shock and stress. Decreased osmolality, increased fluid volume and alcohol-intake decrease the secretion of ADH thereby allowing the kidneys to excrete a dilute urine.

ELECTROLYTES

Electrolytes are distributed in solution in all biological fluids; blood, lymph, digestive juices, urine, etc. Of the cations Na^+, K^+, Ca^{2+}, Mg^{2+}, those that are predominant are sodium and potassium. The chief cation of plasma and other ECF is sodium while that of ICF is potassium. The important anions are Cl^-, HCO_3^-, $H_2PO_4^-$, HPO_4^{2-}, SO_4^{2-}, protein and organic acid ions. The chief anions of plasma and ECF are chloride bicarbonate while that of ICF is phosphate. While all the ions are osmotically active, the maximum contribution comes from Na^+ and Cl^- ions. Sodium chloride contributes about 80% to the osmotic pressure of plasma. It constitutes about 245 millimoles for a total of 300 millimoles of osmotically active substances in plasma. Hence the importance of common salt (NaCl) in fluid and electrolyte balance is paramount (Table 12.1 and Fig. 12.2).

Table 12.1: Fluid balance

Intake			Output		
	Obligatory	*Facultative*		*Obligatory*	*Facultative*
Drinking	600	900	Kidneys	600	900
Food	700	0	Skin	400	0
Oxidation (Metabolic water)	300	0	Intestines	200	0
			Lungs	400	0
Total	1600	900		1600	900
Total: 2500 ml			Total: 2500 ml		

With light activity and no visible perspiration.

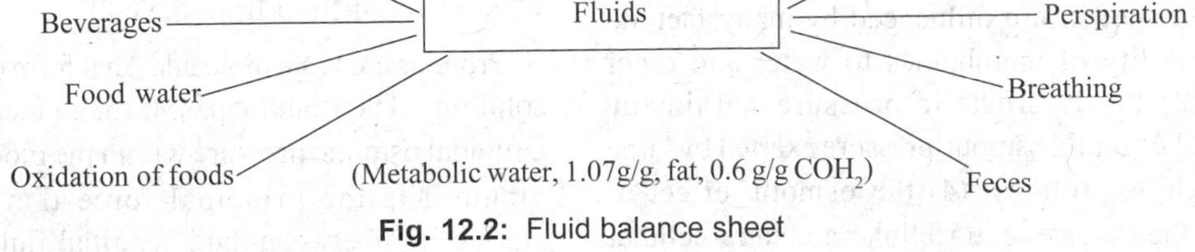

Fig. 12.2: Fluid balance sheet

The quantity of Na^+ in plasma and lymph determines the volume of these fluids and hence Na^+ is referred to as the kingpin of ECF. One of the reasons for this might be hydration of Na^+ ions which is 1.66 times greater than that of K^+ ions. Intake of salt or its intravenous injection increases the volume of fluids and may even cause tissue edema. Loss of Na^+ as in sweating, vomiting or diarrhoea causes decrease in plasma and ECF volume. In fact, was it not for Na^+ (as common salt) tissues will not hold water without salt. While Na^+ causes retention of water, K^+ which is chemically so close to Na^+ tends to decrease fluid water having a diuretic effect.

Composition of Body Fluids

Electrolyte composition of normal human plasma in respect of some important ions is given below:

Na^+ — 130-140 mEq/l

K^+—3—5 mEq/l

Cl^- as —NaCl—95—110 mEq/l

HCO^-_3—22—30 mEq/l

Of the three main body fluids-intracellular fluid, interstitial fluid, and blood plasma—Figure 12.3 shows the average concentration of the substances dissolved in these three fluids, blood plasma and interstitial fluid have similar compositions (the main difference is that the blood has a higher protein concentration), but intracellular fluid is quite different. On the cation side, the intracellular fluid has a high concentration of K^+ and a low concentration of Na^+; in the other two fluids (blood plasma and interstitial fluid), these concentrations are reversed (with high Na^+ and low K^+). Intracellular fluids also has a higher Mg^{2+} concentration. On the anion side, there is virtually no Cl^- inside cells, while this is the most abundant anion outside the cells. On the other hand, the concentration of phosphate (mostly HPO_4^-) and, to a lesser extent, of sulfate, are much greater inside the cells. As might be expected, the protein concentration is much higher inside the cells.

ELECTROLYTE BALANCE

The movements of water and solutes from one compartment to another are influenced by many factors: (1) the permeability of membranes to water and other substances; (2) the hydrostatic pressure within the capillaries; (3) the colloid osmotic pressure exerted by large molecules such as proteins; (4) the osmotic effect of electrolytes in the fluids of extracellular and intra-cellular

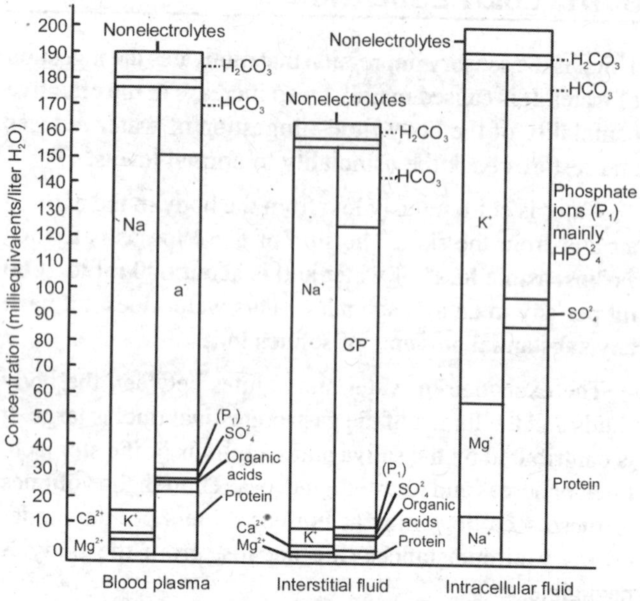

Fig. 12.3: Electrolyte composition of body fluids

fluids; (5) the lymph flow; (6) the mechanisms for active transport; (7) the competition of substances for carriers to transport materials across cell membranes; and (8) the hormonal and nervous controls influencing each of these factors.

Water can move in and out of cells by osmosis, which is the passage of fluid from the less concentrated to the more concentrated side of the membrane. Osmotic pressure is the difference in the force exerted on each side of the membrane. Thus, the solution that is more concentrated exerts a pull on the water in the more dilute solution.

Sodium has little effect on the osmotic pressure between the capillaries and the interstitial fluid because its concentration in the two fluids is about equal. However, sodium is the principal cation in intercellular fluid and potassium in intracellular fluid so that these electrolytes effect important osmotic controls between these fluid compartments. A reduction of extracellular sodium, for example, results in the entrance of fluid into the cell, whereas an increase in extracellular sodium results in the withdrawal of fluid from the cell.

Proteins are large molecules that form colloidal (gluelike) solutions. They cannot pass through membranes and exert colloidal osmotic pressure within the blood vessels. Plasma albumin is the principal force that maintains fluid equilibrium between the interstitial fluid and the plasma.

The plasma albumin exerts a constant pull of fluid from the interstitial fluid to the plasma. Thus, the colloid osmotic pressure opposes and balances the flow of materials out of the capillaries that is exerted by filtration pressure. When the concentration of plasma albumin is reduced, the osmotic pressure is reduced and the fluid remains in the tissues spaces.

Mechanisms of Water Balance Regulation

The sensation of thirst is one means whereby the body meets its water need. When the ionic concentration of the extracellular fluid is increased, the cells in the thirst center of the hypothalamus become dehydrated and the desire to drink water is initiated.

Water reabsorption from the renal tubule is modified according to the extracellular fluid concentration. This depends upon the osmoreceptor system, which is effective in two ways. One of these is the change in osmotic pressure that occurs in the interstitial fluid of the renal medulla. The loops of Henle of the renal tubules extend into the medulla. Because rapid, active absorption of sodium and chloride occurs, the interstitial fluid of the medulla has a high concentration of sodium and chloride and hence exerts increased osmotic pressure. As the tubular fluid passes into the collecting ducts located in the medulla, water is rapidly absorbed from the ducts.

Water reabsorption by the tubules is also controlled by the secretion of antidiuretic hormone by the posterior pituitary gland. Osmoreceptors especially in the supraoptic nuclei of the hypothalamus are sensitive to increases in the osmolarity of the extracellular fluid. Under conditions of increased concentration, impulses are initiated that stimulate production of ADH. The hormone enters the circulation and passes to the kidney where it increases the permeability of the distal and collecting tubules so that the amount of water that is reabsorbed is greatly increased. If the concentration of electrolytes is low, no stimulation of the osmoreceptors occurs and hence the hormone is not produced. The cell permeability is then decreased so that more water will be excreted, thereby restoring normal electrolyte concentration (*See* Fig. 12.4).

Regulation of Ionic Balance

The regulation of sodium concentration in the extracellular fluid is better understood than that of other ions, but it is believed that the mechanisms that control the concentrations of other electrolytes are similar. These mechanisms are under nervous and hormonal control.

A low concentration of sodium in the extracellular fluid stimulates the secretion of aldosterone and, to a lesser extent, other mineralocorticoids by the adrenal cortex. The sequence for the stimulation of the adrenal is believed to be as follows: with a drop in blood pressure of the juxtaglomerular cells, the kidney is stimulated to produce renin, an enzyme, which in turn acts on a globulin substance in blood, angiotensinogen, to convert is to angiotensin I, an inactive substance. An enzyme in the plasma converts angiotensin I to angiotensin II; the latter substance in the blood circulation stimulates the production of aldosterone by the adrenal cortex. Upon reaching the renal circulation,

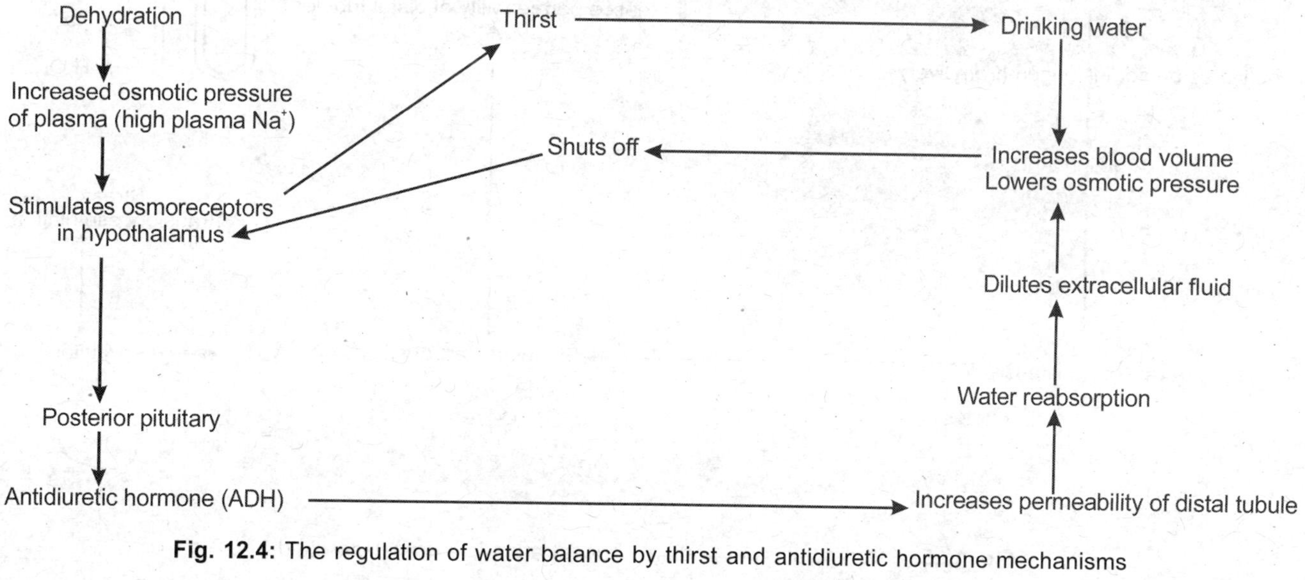

Fig. 12.4: The regulation of water balance by thirst and antidiuretic hormone mechanisms

aldosterone increases the permeability of the distal and collecting tubules so that more sodium is reabsorbed into the peritubular capillaries. When the extracellular sodium concentration in high, the adrenal cortex stops secreting aldosterone, and thus greater amounts of sodium will be excreted. When sodium is reabsorbed it carries positive electrical charges which draw negative ions, principally chloride, through the tubular membrane. Thus, the reabsorption of chloride closely parallels that of sodium (*See* Fig. 12.5).

Potassium ions are passively secreted into the distal and collecting tubules. This secretion is greater when the potassium content of the extracellular fluid is high. The retention of sodium under the influence of aldosterone is accompanied by an increased loss of potassium.

ACID-BASE BALANCE

Acid-base balance refers to the regulation of the hydrogen ion concentration of body fluids. Normal metabolic processes result in the continuous production of acids that must be eliminated. The mechanisms for maintaining body neutrality are so efficient that the healthy individual does not need to give any thought whatsoever to the nature of his or her diet insofar as acid-producing or alkali-producing elements are concerned.

Many pathologic conditions, however, are characterized by serious disturbances in acid-base balance; for example, acidosis in uncontrolled diabetes mellitus, or fasting for weight reduction, following severe dehydration, and in renal failure. Through the study of physiology and biochemistry the student has gained an understanding of electrolyte and fluid balance, the chemistry of respiration, and the regulation of acid-base balance. Several references at the end of the chapter may be consulted by the student who desires a review or more extensive study than is provided in the following brief summary.

A pH ranging from 0 to 6.9 indicates that the substance is acidic. Foods such as lemon juice. The acid in the stomach is even more acidic. Between 7.1 or 14 the pH range is basic or alkaline. Substances such as baking soda (sodium bicarbonate), and most tap water are basic, a pH

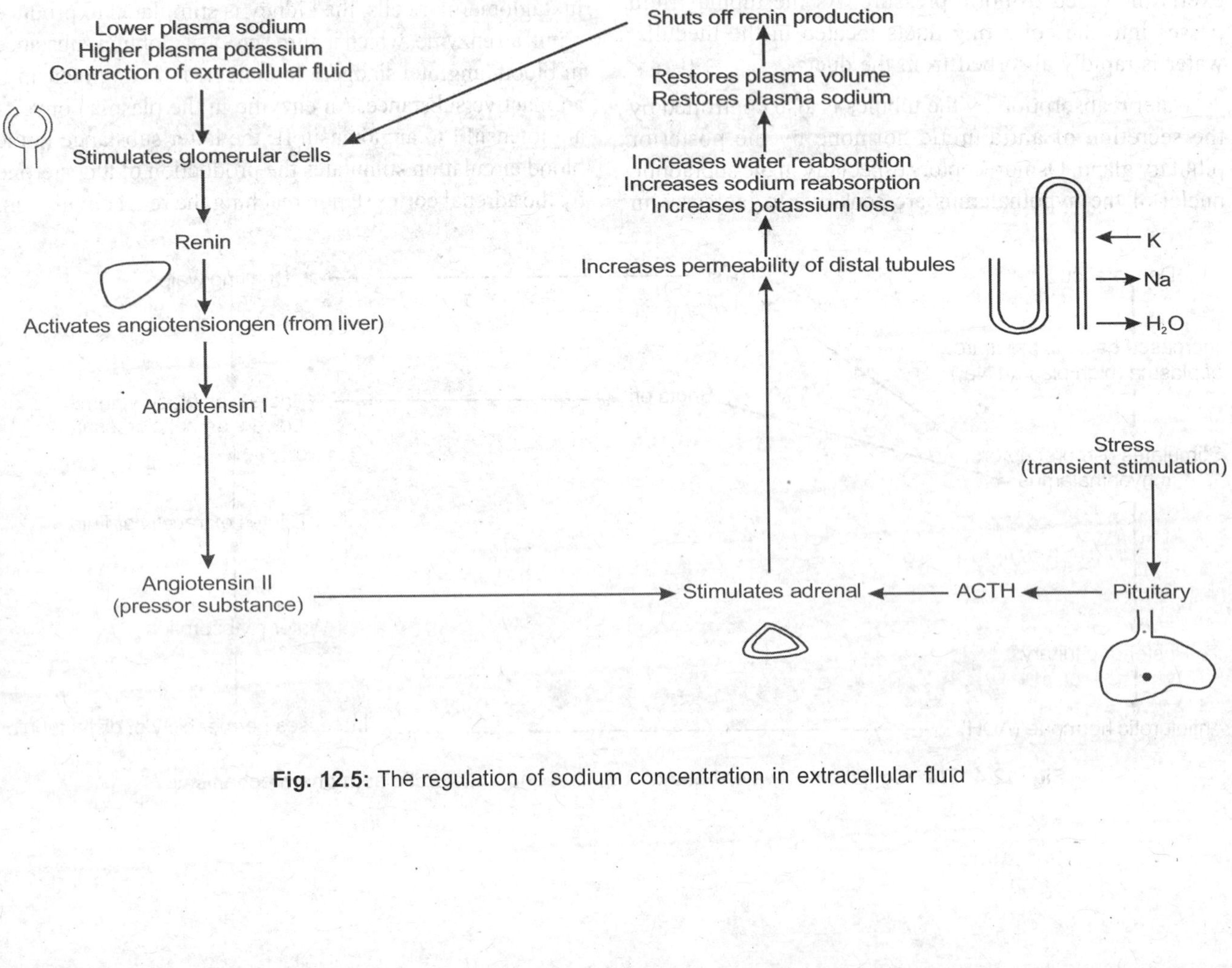

Fig. 12.5: The regulation of sodium concentration in extracellular fluid

of 7.0 is neutral. pH of blood plasma is maintained within 7.35 to 7.45 and extremes of pH compatible with life are 6.8 and 7.8.

Acids Formed in Metabolism

The principal end products of metabolic activities are acid, chiefly carbonic acid. The oxidation of carbohydrates, fatty acids, and amino acids in the tricarboxylic acid cycle yields carbon dioxide and water; carbonic acid is the hydrated form of carbon dioxide. Intermediate products in metabolism are also acid, such as lactic and pyruvic acid formed in carbohydrate metabolism, keto acids formed in fatty acid oxidation, and amino acids resulting from the hydrolysis of proteins. Urea synthesis is an acid-producing process, and nucleoproteins give rise to uric acid. Sulfuric acid is formed in the body from the sulfur-containing amino acids and phosphoric acid from the phospholipids and phosphorproteins.

Acid and Alkaline Ash Foods

If the cations (Na^+, K^+, Mg^{2+} and Ca^{2+}) remaining in the body on the metabolism of a food exceed the anions (PO_4^{2-} and Cl^-), the food is said to produce an alkaline ash and the excess cations will allow the body to retain more bicarbonate ions, thus producing an alkaline reaction. Vegetables, fruits, milk, and some nuts yield excess cations.

Meat, fish, poultry, eggs, cheese, cereals, and some nuts when metabolized yield an excess of anions that are not removed from the body immediately. These foods are said to produce an acid ash. The excess anions carrying a negative charge must be balanced approximately with some cations. This yields an acid reaction because less bicarbonate, which also carries a negative charge, can exist in the body. The excess bicarbonate ions form carbonic acid, increasing the acidity.

Fats, sugar and starches contain no mineral elements and are metabolized quickly to carbon dioxide and water which are rapidly removed from the body. These foods, therefore, do not form excess cations or anions which would disturb the neutrality regulation.

Although lemons, oranges, and certain other fruits contain some free organic acids that give them a taste of acid (sour), they yield an alkaline ash because the body quickly oxidizes the anions of the acid to carbon dioxide and water and leave excess cations that are removed more slowly from the body. Plums, cranberries, and prunes contain aromatic organic acids that are not metabolized in the body, and therefore they increase the acidity of the body fluids.

The Regulation of Body Neutrality

The reaction of the body fluids is kept within a narrow range by the following mechanisms:

1. Dilution is an important defense against the effects of the metabolic acids. The total volume of body fluid, representing about two thirds of body weight, is so great that the considerable amounts of carbon dioxide produced result in only a slight increase in the bicarbonate concentration because of the distribution throughout the fluid system.
2. Acid-base buffer systems are an important mechanisms for the regulation of acid-base balance. A buffer is a substance that will react chemically with either acids or alkalies so that there is not a marked change in the pH of the solution. The bicarbonate-carbonic acid (HCO_3^-/H_2CO_3) system is one important buffer of the blood in maintaining neutrality. The ease and speed with which the body can get rid of carbon dioxide obtained from this buffer mixture constitute one of the first lines of defense. The plasma bicarbonate is an indicator of the alkaline reserve of the body. Serious disturbances may occur if the alkaline reserve is depleted to a low level. Other buffer systems include the following:

$$\frac{\text{Protein}}{\text{H. protein}} \quad \frac{HPO_4^{2-}}{H_2PO_4^-} \quad \frac{Hb^-}{HHb} \quad \frac{HbO_2^-}{HHbO_2}$$

3. In addition to its buffer action, hemoglobin aids in the transport of carbon dioxide from the cells to the lungs, where it can be excreted from the body in the expired air. This loss represents part of the functioning of the bicarbonate-carbonic acid buffer system.
4. The respiratory rate regulates the losses of carbon dioxide and the intake of oxygen. If the hydrogen ion concentration is increased, the respiratory center in the brain causes an increase in the rate of pulmonary ventilation. The increased respiratory rate increases the loss of carbon dioxide, and the hydrogen ion concentration of the body fluids returns to normal. If the hydrogen ion concentration is lowered, the respiratory center is inhibited and the rate of ventilation is reduced; thus, the carbonic acid concentration of the body fluids rises.
5. The kidney makes the final adjustment that keeps the body pH within normal limits. The glomerular filtrate has a pH of 7.4, but the kidney can excrete a urine that

is as acid as pH 4.5 or as alkaline as pH 8; normally, the average urine pH is 6.0. Bicarbonate ions are filtered into the tubular fluid and their loss from plasma represents loss of alkali. Hydrogen ions are secreted into the tubules, and their loss from plasma represents a loss of acid. When the hydrogen ions of the plasma are increased, the secretion of the hydrogen ions into the tubular fluid also increases and exceeds the loss of bicarbonate, thus permitting the return of plasma to its normal pH. The urine excreted is then more acid. Conversely, in alkalosis by the hydrogen ion secretion into the tubules is decreased, thus allowing greater loss of bicarbonate. The urine then becomes more alkaline.

The kidney cannot excrete strong acids such as HCl and H_2SO_4. The hydrogen ions secreted into the lumen of the tubule are excreted by combining with disodium phosphate to form monosodium acid phosphate. By excreting practically all of the phosphate as acid phosphate ($H_2PO_4^-$, instead of HPO_4^{2-}) only one phosphate is lost instead of two, thus reducing by half the number of milliequivalents of fixed anions that are excreted; this permits the return of more fixed anions to the circulation.

The kidney is also able to synthesize ammonia from glutamine and other amino acids. The ammonia combines with hydrogen ions to form the ammonium ion (NH_4^+), which can then replace cations such as sodium or potassium.

Acidosis and Alkalosis

The acid-base balance of the body can be upset of an increase in hydrogen ions, a loss of hydrogen ions, an increase in base, or a loss of base. In each instance the treatment can be instituted only after evaluation of symptoms that are present, the determination of the pH and the carbon dioxide content of the blood plasma, and the cause of the imbalance (*See* Fig. 12.6).

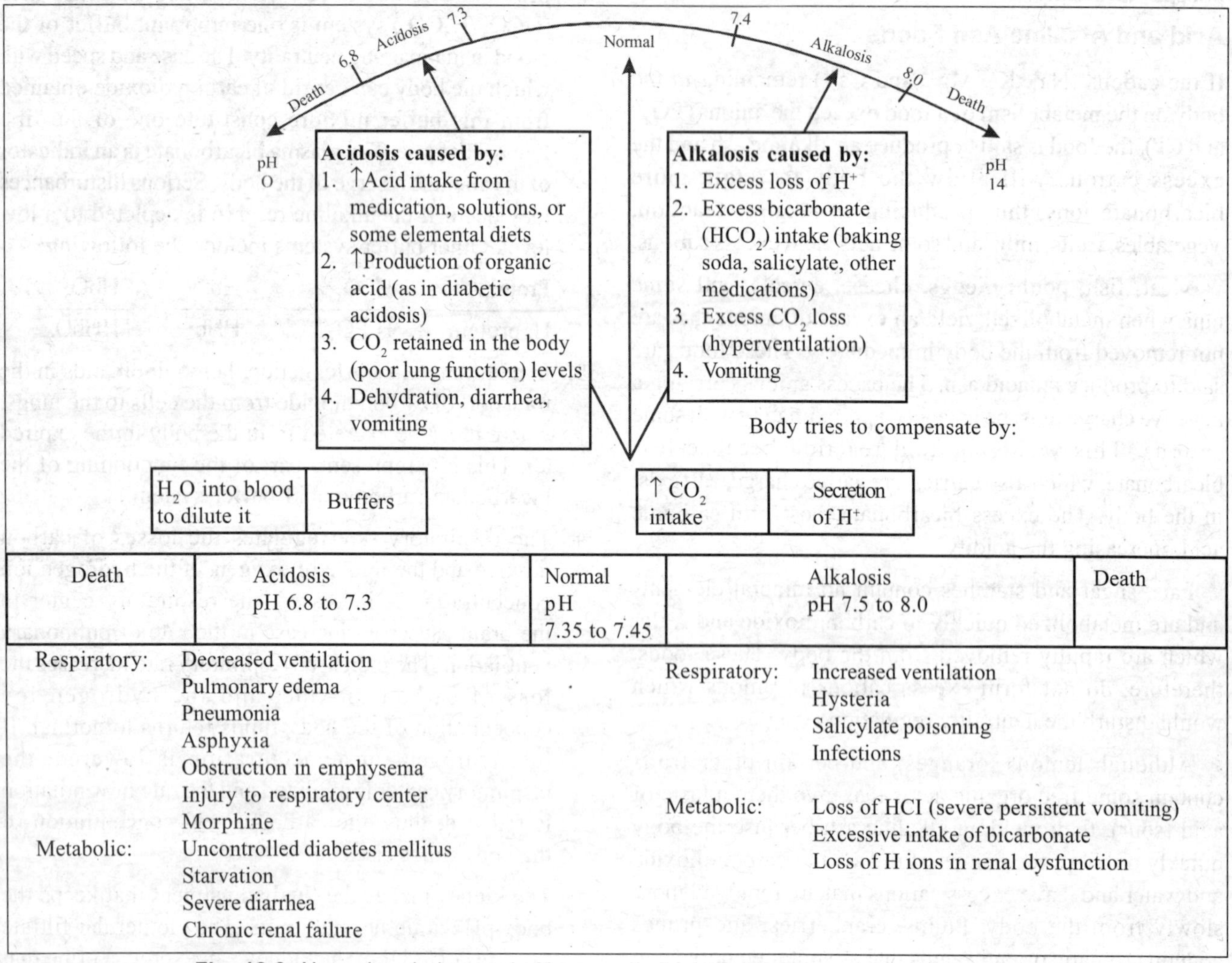

Death	Acidosis pH 6.8 to 7.3	Normal pH 7.35 to 7.45	Alkalosis pH 7.5 to 8.0	Death

Respiratory: Decreased ventilation, Pulmonary edema, Pneumonia, Asphyxia, Obstruction in emphysema, Injury to respiratory center, Morphine

Metabolic: Uncontrolled diabetes mellitus, Starvation, Severe diarrhea, Chronic renal failure

Respiratory: Increased ventilation, Hysteria, Salicylate poisoning, Infections

Metabolic: Loss of HCI (severe persistent vomiting), Excessive intake of bicarbonate, Loss of H ions in renal dysfunction

Fig. 12.6: Normal and abnormal pH ranges in body fluids (Two schematic diagrams)

Acidosis is a condition in which the hydrogen ion concentration is increased or there is an excessive loss of base (mineral cations); the ratio of bicarbonate to carbonic acid is less than 20:1, and the pH is below 7.35. Alkalosis is a condition in which the hydrogen ion concentration is decreased or the base is increased; the ratio of bicarbonate to carbonic acid is greater than 20:1, and the pH is above 7.45.

With changes in concentrations of hydrogen ions and base, the lungs and kidneys attempt to compensate. Ventilation by the lungs is increased when there is an increase in hydrogen ions, and the kidney attempts to adjust by excreting a more acid urine and conserving base with the synthesis of more ammonia. When there is an increase in base, the respiration is depressed, and the hydrogen ions are retained and more base is excreted by the kidneys. If these adjustments succeed in keeping the bicarbonate-carbonic acid ratio at 20:1, the pH remains at 7.35 to 7.45; the acidosis or alkalosis is said to be "compensated". When the pH is outside these limits, the acidosis or alkalosis is "uncompensated".

Respiratory acidosis or alkalosis results from an abnormality of the control of the normal CO_2 tension. Hypoventilation such as that seen in pneumonia; pulmonary edema, suppression of breathing as with morphine, and asphyxia lead to acidosis. The kidneys partially compensate by increasing the excretion of hydrogen ions and the synthesis of ammonia, thereby increasing the return of bicarbonate to the blood.

Respiratory alkalosis occurs when there is over ventilation of the lungs so that excessive amounts of carbonic acid are lost. This may result from hysteria, from salicylate poisoning, in fevers and infections, and at high altitudes. By reducing the excretion by hydrogen ions and the synthesis of ammonia and by increasing the excretion of sodium, the kidney compensate in part.

Metabolic acidosis or alkalosis refers to changes resulting from faulty intake or output of acids or bases other than carbonic acid. Metabolic acidosis occurs in a variety of circumstances: The rapid production of ketones in uncontrolled diabetes mellitus; the inability of the kidney to excrete acid phosphates in chronic renal failure; the ketosis of starvation; or the loss of bicarbonate and sodium with severe diarrhea. Ventilation of the lungs is greatly increased. The synthesis of ammonia by the kidney may increase ten-fold in an effort to conserve base.

Metabolic alkalosis occurs when there is a severe loss of hydrochloric acid as a result of vomiting, or by the ingestion of soluble alkalinizing salts such as sodium bicarbonate.

ROLE OF ALDOSTERONE IN FLUID AND SALT BALANCE

As per previous discussion the cardiovascular—renal system maintains fluids and electrolyte balance by directly regulating the content and composition of urine and the balance in the kidneys between filtration and reabsorption is under hormonal control, the reabsorption of water being promoted by vasopressin, a small peptide hormone manufactured in the hypophysis. In the absence of this hormone, only the proximal tubular reabsorb water—not the distal tubular or the collecting tubular. As a consequence, without vasopressin too much water passes into the urine. Patients with *diabetes insipidus* suffers from this condition. In the presence of vasopressin, water is also reabsorbed in these parts of the nephrons; thus vasopression causes the blood to retain more water and produces a more concentrated urine. The production of urine is called diuresis. Any agent that reduces the volume of urine is called an antidiuretic. For this reason vasopression is also called ADH for antidiuretic hormone.

Usually, the vasopressin level in the body is sufficient to maintain the proper amount of water in tissues under various levels of water intake. However, when severe dehydration occurs (caused by diarrhea, excessive sweating, of insufficient water intake), another hormone also helps to maintain proper fluid level. This hormone, aldosterone, controls the Na^+ ion concentration in the blood. In the presence of aldosterone, the reabsorption of Na+ ions is increased. When more Na^+ ions enter the blood, more Cl^- ions follow (to maintain electroneutrality) and, to solvate these ions, more water. Thus, increased aldosterone production enables the body to retain more water. When the Na^+ ion and water levels in the blood return to normal, aldosterone production stops. The process is schematically summarized in Figure 12.7.

Blood Pressure

Blood pressure is produced by the pumping action of the heart. The blood pressure at the arterial capillary end is about 32 mm Hg. This pressure is higher than the osmotic pressure of the blood (18 mm Hg). The osmotic pressure of the blood is caused by the fact that more solute are dissolved in the blood than in the interstitial fluid. At the

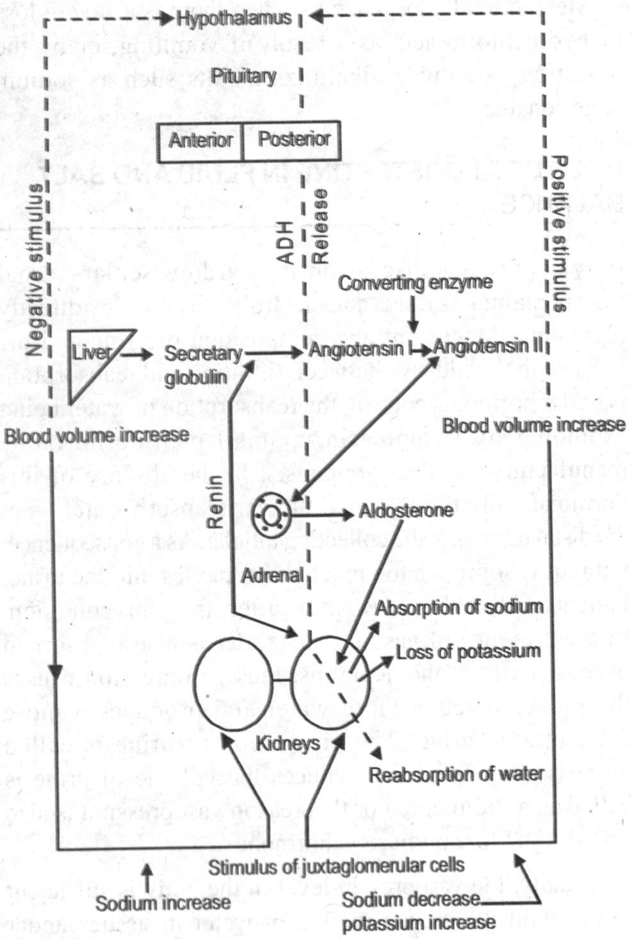

Fig. 12.7: A schematic diagram showing the mechanism of salt and water regulation

capillary end, therefore, nutrient solutes flow from the capillary into the interstitial fluid and from there into the cell. On the other hand, in the venous capillary the blood pressure is about 12 mm Hg. This is less than the osmotic pressure, and so solutes (waste products) from the interstitial fluid flow into the capillaries.

The blood pressure is maintained by the total volume of blood, by the pumping action of the heart and by the muscles that surround the blood vessels and provide the proper resistance to blood flow. Blood pressure is controlled by several very complex systems, some of them acting within seconds and some that take days to respond after a change in blood pressure occurs. For example, if a patient hemorrhages, three different nervous control systems begin to function within seconds. The first to respond are baroreceptors in the neck, which detect the consequent drop in pressure and send appropriate signals to the heart to pump harder and to the muscles surrounding the blood vessels to contract and thus restore pressure. Chemical receptors on the cells that detect less O_2 delivery or CO_2 removal also send nerve signals. Finally, the central nervous system also reacts to oxygen deficiency with a feedback mechanism by slowing down aerobic metabolism.

Hormonal controls act somewhat more slowly and may take minutes or even days. The kidneys secrete an enzyme called renin, which acts on an inactive blood protein called angiotestinogen, converting it to angiotensin, a potent vasoconstrictor. The action of this peptide increases blood pressure. Aldosterone also increases blood pressure by increasing Na^+ ion and water reabsorption in the kidneys.

Finally, there is a long-term renal-blood control for volume and pressure. When blood pressure falls, the kidneys retain more water and salt, thus increasing blood volume and pressure.

A large number of people in India have high blood pressure (hypertension). Epidemiologic studies have shown that even milk hypertension (diastolic pressure between 90 and 104 mm Hg) brings about the risk of cardiovascular disease. This can lead to heart attack, stroke, or kidney failure. Hypertension can be effectively managed with diet and drugs. As blood pressure is under a complex control system, so hypertension must be managed on more than one level. Recommended dietary practices are low Na^+ ion intake and abstention from caffeine (coffee) and alcohol.

DISTURBANCE IN FLUID-ELECTROLYTE AND ACID-BASE BALANCE

As discussed above water balance is carefully controlled by thirst by adrenal gland, the hypothalamus and the kidney. This balance of mechanisms, hormones, and renal blood pressure as illustrated in Table 12.2 Water balance and sodium balance are closely related, because body water must always contain a certain concentration of sodium. The more sodium the body holds, the more water is must also hold. This is part of normal balance.

When sodium, the other electrolytes, acids or bases lose their proper balance in the body fluids, a life-threatening emergency can quickly develop. These imbalances usually occur in diseases and treatment depends on the disease. Fluid and electrolyte imbalances can result in or be caused by dehydration (too little water) or edema (extra water held in part of the body where it does not belong). They can also lead to an imbalance in acids and bases in the body. The substances named in Table 12.2 get affected in fluid and electrolyate imbalance.

Table 12.2: Affected substances in fluid and electrolyte balance	
Bicarbonate	*Organic acids*
Calcium	pH
Chloride	Potassium
Glucose	Proteins
Lipids	Sodium
Magnesium	Sulfate

There is some evidence that an electrolyte/fluid imbalance may play a role in the development of cataract.

Dehydration

Dehydration occurs when the tissues of the body lose needed water. It is one extreme of fluid imbalance; edema (below) is the other.

Water may be lost with or without a loss of the electrolytes. *Hypertonic dehydration* is a condition that occurs when, proportionately, more water is lost than electrolytes. This happens in burn patients, in diabetes, in excessive sweating (as from a fever), or after a long period without water. The concentration of electrolytes in the blood becomes too high. Muscle weakness, paralysis, and abnormal heart and lung functions are some of the symptoms. Treatment depends on the cause, but will include replacing the lost fluids.

Hypotonic dehydration occurs when, proportionately, more electrolytes are lost than water. This is a result of severe vomiting and diarrhea, some hormone deficiencies, kidney disease, and extreme sodium deprivation. Symptoms depend on the electrolytes most affected but will include muscle changes and sometimes mental disorientation or convulsions.

Finally, isotonic dehydration occurs when fluids and electrolytes are lost in the same proportion as they exist in body fluids. This type of dehydration many result from blood loss, mild diarrhea, or vomiting.

Edema

Edema means the swelling caused by excess fluids in body tissues. Edema was once called dropsy.

Many conditions may lead to edema. If something goes wrong with the 'thermostat' system that regulated fluid and sodium balance (the system described in Table 12.3), the body may conserve more water than it should.

Another cause of edema may be an imbalance in the osmotic pressure. Briefly, osmotic pressure in the blood, for example, is the pressure needed to retain water inside the blood. As the number of particles increases, more water pushes in through the walls of the blood vessels. Water comes from the cells and the interstitial fluid. It helps to keep the concentration of water-to-particles normal throughout the body.

Normal osmotic pressure in the blood is 280 to 290 milliosmoles per kilogram (mOsm/kg) of plasma. Some foods and dietary formulas cause the pressure to rise to over 600 mOsm and this high level can affect fluid balance.

Osmotic pressure is important in every cell of the body. It is dependent on water, but also on the ability of particles to enter or leave the cell. This ability, in turn, depends on the permeability of the cell membrane, that is, the ability of particles to move from one side of the cell membrane

Table 12.3: Regulation of fluid balance

Stimulus	*Mechanism*	*Response*	*Comments*
Total body water content drops 1%-2%	Thirst	Water is consumed	
Extracellular fluids volume drops	Sensed by cells in hypothalamus	Release of antidiuretic hormone (ADH)	ADH causes the kidneys to conserve sodium and water. These substances are then reabsorbed back into the body.
Blood pressure in the kidneys drops	Sensed by cells in the kidney	a. Enzyme *renin* is released b. Renin makes *angiotensin* c. Angiotensin triggers the adrenal glands to release the hormonal aldosterone	Angiotensin causes the tubules in the kidney to narrow. This increases renal blood pressure. Aldosterone causes the kidney to save sodium. The increased osmotic pressure causes water also to be conserved.

* These are mechanisms that turn 'on' when water and sodium levels are low. They turn 'off' automatically (except in disease) once balance is restored to a certain point.

to the other. If membrane permeability is damaged, there will be an imbalance in osmolarity. Fluid will accumulate in the wrong areas and edema will result. The damage depends on the cause.

Heart failure can result in edema; pulmonary edema (fluid around the lungs) is often part of congestive heart failure and makes it difficult for both heart and lungs to function. Edematous swelling may also occur following infections (fluid surrounds and cushions the affected area), bacterial poisons, venom (from snake bites or bee stings), or electrolyte imbalances that cause the body to hold excess sodium.

Kidney disease causes increase in fluids, which cannot be excreted because the kidneys do not function, to build up in the peritoneal cavity (the spaces between organs in the abdomen, enclosed by the peritoneal membrane). This type of edema is called ascites. Ascites, or excess fluid in the peritoneum, also can result from too little protein in the blood. Osmotic pressure goes down when there is not enough protein, and fluid has seeps from the blood to the interstitial spaces in the peritoneum. This is also common in liver diseases, especially alcoholic cirrhosis.

Treatment of edema varies. Persons with liver damage usually begin a diet that strictly controls electrolytes. Fluids and protein; edema is only one sign of many complex problems. Persons with kidney failure may begin dialysis and a diet tightly controlling the same nutrients in slightly different ways. Edema that results from a simple excess sodium content in the body may be treated with a low-sodium diet. Edema resulting from venom or infection usually requires close medical attention, with nutrition playing a lesser role unless malnutrition is also a problem.

One of the major situations that need a specific fluid or electrolyte-controlled diet is discussed below as an illustrative example.

Diarrhea of Malnutrition

Malnourished children in poor countries rarely die of their malnutrition. They usually die from diseases or infections that their bodies are simply too weak to fight. In places where water may be contaminated, diarrhea (gastroenteritis) is a real risk and can quickly cause death, especially in children, since fluid and electrolyte balance, acid and base balance, are quickly and seriously upset. The World Health Organization (WHO) estimates that at least 5 million children die every year simply from diarrhea. In response, WHO has developed an oral rehydration therapy that any trained person can administer to persons with severe diarrhea. It is a mixture of fluid, electrolytes, and sugar that when mixed and administered to a person, can help restore a normal fluid and electrolyte balance save lives. The WHO rehydration solution is a mixture of:

3.5 grams (2/3 tsp) sodium chloride (table salt).

2.5 grams (2/4 tsp) sodium bicarbonate (backing soda).

1.5 grams (1/3 tsp) potassium chloride.

[The primary ingredient in many salt substitutes; also available in pure from a pharmacist].

20 grams glucose (or 40 grams—3-1/3 tbsp—of sucrose or table sugar).

1 liter of boiled or sterile water.

Some professionals recommend that 2 grams of sodium be used in mild diarrhea instead of 3.5 grams. The fluid may help in an emergency, but anyone with severe or chronic diarrhea should receive medical attention as quickly as possible.

STUDY QUESTIONS

1. Name the daily sources of water and the routes of excretion. How do hormones regulate water and electrolyte homeostasis? Explain the elaborate process briefly.
2. Give a brief description of the water compartments of the body in terms of size and electrolyte composition.
3. Describe briefly regulatory mechanisms of fluid and electrolyte balance and abnormalities related to them.
4. How can specific dietary interventions help correct the fluid and electrolyte abnormalities in dehydration, edema and malnutrition related diarrhea.
5. Explain elaborately the terms: acidosis and alkalosis.

CHAPTER 13

Food Spoilage, Food Poisoning, Food Preservation and Food Hygiene

Chapter Outlines

- Food perishability
- Microbial food spoilage
- Food borne illness: The sources and management
- Food preservation
- Food additives
- Food toxins of natural origin
- Food hygiene
- Study Questions

FOOD PERISHABILITY

Food, as we all know, is produced by living organisms, animal or plants. Owing to this fact, food is mainly composed organic substances. When such food is in the making in the living plant or animals, these organic substances are involved in a variety of complex and carefully controlled chemical reactions which occur in the presence of specific enzymes. When a food crop is harvested or flesh providing animal is slaughtered, many of these reactions stop. However, the enzymes present remain still active and continue catalyzing reactions which, at times, adversely affect the quality of food, therefore, an abundant proportion of food is perishable or prove to spoilage and in the natural course of events becomes inedible fairly quickly. As a matter of fact, food spoilage occurs mainly as a result of chemical reactions involved in the process of keeping and ageing, or through the action of microorganisms, or through a combination of both. A knowledge of the intricacies of food spoilage enables us to take steps to prevent or minimize spoilage. Apart from chemical and microbial spoilage; contamination with dirt, chemicals, or damage by animal/insect pests also play a part in spoilage. In developing countries like India, a fairly high percentage (30-40%) of different foodstuffs is wasted due to spoilage of one or the other kind. Not to stop at this, ingestion of such food courses infection and toxicity in the affected population due to the presence of disease causing microorganisms or the toxins present in them or produced by them produce their adverse effect.

Growth stops when a fruit is plucked from the branch but it remains alive and ripening continues. Once ripe, it deteriorates rapidly due to the combined action of enzymes and microorganisms.

Likewise, in a slaughtered animals, the initial changes are beneficial as it causes tenderization and flavouring. These changes are termed as 'hanging' or 'conditioning'. However, if meat is kept for a long time at room temperature the spoilage occurs due to chemical changes involving protein breakdown and fat oxidation and rancidity. Similar changes occur in fish albeit with greater intensity and shorter time, the reason being fish a cold-blooded creature and its enzyme operate instantly and at room temperature. Once chemical changes occur, microorganisms also start thriving and growing to complete the story of spoilage, infection and toxicity or poisoning.

The greatest health risk from food consumption arises when it gets contaminated by bacteria and, to a lesser extent, by molds, fungi, yeasts and viruses. Microbial growth can render a product unacceptable in three ways. First, the food may become spoiled as a result of enzymatic decomposition of the product, or by an increase in microbial numbers, or the release of compounds that result in unappetizing flavours, colours and aromas. Second, microorganisms can release toxins into the food during their growth. Ingestion of such toxin containing foods results in a brief yet serious illness. The onset of such illness occurs only a few hours after the toxic principles gain entry into the body and establish contact with susceptible tissues. Such a food borne illness is known as food poisoning or food intoxication. Third, food may become unfit for human consumption due to the presence of viable pathogens. The food can establish an infection after having been ingested along with food that becomes the vehicle carrying pathogens into the host where they (pathogenic bacteria) reproduce and cause disease. Such food borne outbreaks of diseases are known as food infections.

Foods with properties that really support distinctive microbial growth are called perishable and the foods that can be kept longer without microbial growth are called either non-perishable or semi-perishable. One of the most important factors affecting perishability is the amount of moisture in the food. The amount of moisture in the food that is available for growth is called the water activity level. Apart from this; pH, available oxygen supply and nutrient balance, all influence the likelihood of spoilage, food poisoning and infection. The prevention of food borne illnesses is made possible by a number of food preserving methods. Natural preservation can be the result of protective husks, skins, shells or membranes. The high acidity of many foods prevents microbial growth and antimicrobial agents such as lysozyme and fatty acids are also effective. Other methods include drying, refrigeration, freezing, irradiation, canning and the use of chemical preservatives. The generation of organic acids in food by fermentation not only increases the shelf life of its products but also results in flavours, aromas and fixtures not found in the starting food material.

The greatest health risk from food is contamination from bacteria and, to a lesser extent, from molds, fungi, yeasts, and viruses. Though these microbes can all cause food borne illness, yet mostly microbial contamination is the cause of most food infection and food poisoning incidents.

MICROBIAL FOOD SPOILAGE

The microorganisms principally responsible for food spoilage are moulds, bacteria and yeasts.

Moulds: Moulds are a form of fungi. Unlike yeasts and bacteria they are multicellular organisms. They grow as fine threads or filaments which extend in length and eventually form a complex branched network or mat called mycelium. At this stage mould growth on foods is easily visible as a 'fluff'. Moulds also produce spores, or seeds, and these can be carried considerable distances by air currents and in this way infect other foods. Mould spores are almost always present in the atmosphere and large numbers may be literally 'floating around' in food premises.

Most moulds require oxygen for development and this is why they are usually found only on the surface of foods. Meat, cheese and sweet foods are especially likely to be attacked by moulds. In alkaline or very acid foods (pH below 2) mould growth is usually inhibited although some moulds will grow even under these conditions. Moulds grow best at a pH of 4-6 and a temperature of about 30°C; as the temperature decreases so does the rate of growth, although slow growth can continue at the temperature of a domestic refrigerator. Mould growth does not occur above normal body temperature but it is very difficult to kill moulds and their spores by heat treatment. To ensure complete destruction of all moulds and their spores sterilization under pressure is necessary (i.e. at above 100°C). Alternatively, the food may be heated to 70-80°C on two or more successive days so that any spores germinating between the heat treatments will be destroyed.

Certain moulds produce poisonous substances known as mycotoxins which can be harmful if eaten. The mould Aspergillus flavus which can grow on groundnuts (i.e. peanuts) and cereals produces aflatoxin which causes serious illness if eaten. Moulds grow on other foods, including cheese and bread, and these are usually regarded as being unattractive but not harmful. It is possible, however, that they may contain dangerous mycotoxins and so it is safer not to eat them.

Bacteria: Bacteria are simple single-cell organisms. They are minute living particles either spherical (cocci), rod-shaped (bacilli) or spiral (spirella). It is difficult to get any idea of the size of bacteria but 10^{13} of them (i.e. about 2000 times the population of the world) would weigh only about a gram. Bacteria and their spores are widely distributed. They are present in the soil, in the air and in and on human and animal bodies. Uncooked food of all descriptions will almost certainly be contaminated with bacteria. In fact, they occur so universally that it is exceedingly difficult to get away from them!

Bacteria grow by absorbing simple substances from their environment and when they reach a certain size the parent organism splits to form two new ones. In favorable circumstances this fission may occur every 20 minutes or so and in 12 hours one bacterium can provide a colony of some 10^{12} bacteria.

When bacteria multiply in or on food their presence becomes obvious when they are present to the extent of 10^6 - 10^7 per gram of foodstuff. Bacteria grow most readily in neutral conditions and growth in usually inhibited by acids. Some bacteria, however, can tolerate fairly low pH. For example, *Lactobacilli*, which cause souring of milk with the production of lactic acid, and *Acetobacter*, which convert ethyl alcohol to acetic acid, flourish in acid conditions. Some bacteria will only grow in the presence of oxygen whereas others, known as anaerobes, will only grow in its absence.

Bacteria grow best within a given temperature range and in their vegetative stage (i.e. when they are actually growing) all of them can be killed by exposure to a temperature near to 100°C and at this temperature they are destroyed instantly. Bacteria, like moulds, can form spores. The heat resistance of bacterial spores varies from species to species and with the pH of the surrounding medium.

The most common food spoilage organisms are mesophilic bacteria which originate in warm-blooded animals but are also found in soil, water and sewage. Mesophilic bacteria grow best at about normal body temperature between 30 and 40°C and do not grow below 5°C. Psychrophilic bacteria, which have their origin in air, soil and water, grow best at a somewhat lower temperature–about 20°C–although some of them are quite happy at considerably lower temperatures. Such psychrophilic bacteria can grow quite easily at the temperature of a domestic refrigerator. A small group of bacteria can grow at temperatures upto 60°C and these are known as thermophilic bacteria. The spores of thermophilic bacteria can be very heat resistant.

Bacteria are not necessarily harmful to man and the species. Escherichia coli exists in vast numbers in the human gut. Some bacteria present in the gut are positively beneficial because they synthesize some absorbable B group vitamins and vitamin K from the contents of the large intestine. Bacteria which do not harm to man are, nevertheless, capable of spoiling food.

Yeasts are microscopic unicellular fungi but, unlike moulds, they reproduce themselves by budding, i.e., by the formation of a small off-shoot or bud which becomes detached from the parent yeast cell when it reaches a certain size and assumes an independent existence. Yeasts can also form spores but these are far less heat-resistant than mould spores and bacterial spores. Yeasts occur in the soil and on the surface of fruits. For example, the presence of yeasts on the skin of grapes is the reason why grape juice ferments to become wine. Yeasts can grow in quite varied conditions but the majority prefer acid foods (pH 4-4.5) with a reasonable moisture content. Most yeasts grow best in the presence of oxygen between 25 and 30°C. Some yeasts can grow at 0°C and below. Yeasts and yeasts spores are easily killed by heating to 100°C.

Yeasts are used for making bread (and other fermented goods), beer and vinegar. They cause spoilage of many foods including fruit, fruit juices, jam, wines and meat. Although they may spoil food yeasts are not pathogenic, i.e., they do not cause diseases such as food poisoning. Microorganisms attack food because they require energy and raw materials to support their metabolic processes and explosively rapid growth. In other words, like us, they need food–only more so. Microorganisms break down the complex molecules of the foods on which they are growing and convert them into smaller absorbable molecules. If microbes are allowed to grow unhindered their presence on food often (but not always) becomes apparent to the eye and especially in the case of meat, to the nose.

Microbial growth usually ceases when the food has become really foul because the microorganisms themselves can no longer tolerate the conditions they have created. Organic acids are among the substances produced during microbial breakdown of food and these accumulate and eventually suppress further microbial growth. Given time, another species of microorganisms may appear which is able to tolerate the more acidic conditions and attack on the food will then continue.

Vegetables and fruits have dry, relatively non-porous skins and their cell juices are mildly acidic. They are thus more likely to suffer from the growth of moulds and yeasts than from attack by bacteria. Yeast and mould spores are always present in the air but intact fruits and vegetables are not at great risk. However, if they are over-ripe or damaged, so that cell fluids leak onto the surface, mould or yeast growth is highly likely. If other conditions are favourable the food will deteriorate quickly. It is well known that 'one rotten apple in a barrel' can have a devastating effect. The reason is, of course, that the rotting specimen generates many millions of voracious microbes which quickly attack adjacent wholesome apples.

Fruits and vegetables will remain in good condition for the maximum possible time if they are clean, kept cool and handled with care.

Meat spoilage is mainly caused by bacteria and mould, although meat is not immune from attack by yeasts. Healthy carcass meat should be free from bacteria. In practice, the surface is usually contaminated from the hide and intestines when the animal is slaughtered and when the carcass is cut up. Poultry is particularly prone to bacterial contamination and the skin and interior surfaces usually harbour great numbers of bacteria.

When microbes grow on the surface of meat they break down the protein molecules and grow to form a film of bacterial slime. Carbon dioxide, hydrogen and ammonia are formed and the surface layer of meat becomes grayish-brown in colour owing to conversion of myglobin to metmyoglobin. As putrefaction continues hydrogen sulphide, mercaptans and amines, all of which are foul-smelling, are formed and collectively demonstrate the inedible state of the meat.

FOOD BORNE ILLNESS: THE SOURCES AND MANAGEMENT

The risk of having food poisoning is common, partly because the food industry goes all out to increase the shelf life of products. Longer shelf life of products at room temperatures allows more time for bacteria in foods to multiply. Some bacteria grow even at refrigeration temperatures. Partially cooked and some fully cooked products pose a special risk because refrigerated storage may only slow but not prevent bacterial growth.

Food poisoning risk is even increasing as we rely more heavily on centralized kitchens outside the home to prepare our foods. As the foods are usually prepared in central kitchens or processing plants and transported to individual stores, if a food product is contaminated in the central kitchen or processing plant, consumers over a wide area can suffer food poisoning.

Table 13.1 enlists the various kinds of illnesses caused by microbial food poisoning.

Thus specific toxin producing bacteria and other microbes cause food poisoning. These organisms cause health problem either directly, by invading the intestinal wall, or indirectly, be producing a toxin in the food that later harms us.

Salmonella organisms in contaminated food deliver a direct hit to the intestine, causing food-borne infections. The staphylococcus bacterium produces a toxin, which in turn causes a food-borne intoxication. Many different types of bacteria cause food poisoning, such as Bacillus, Campylobacter, Clostridium, Escherichia coli, Listeria monocytogenes, Vibrio, Yersinia enterocolitica Salmonella and Staphylococcus. Because each teaspoon of soil contains about two billion bacteria, we are constantly at risk for food poisoning. Luckily, only a small number of all bacteria, actually pose a threat. Determining which microbe has caused a food-poisoning incident entails identifying the clinical features of the poisoning, the incubation period for symptoms, and the food source (Table 13.1).

Steps to Prevent Food Borne Illness

We can greatly reduce the risk of poisoning by following some very important rules:

- Wash hands thoroughly with hot, soapy water before handling food. Always wash hands after handling raw meat, fish, poultry, or eggs.
- When grocery shopping, select frozen foods and perishables, such as meat, poultry, or fish, last. Always put these products in separate plastic bags so that drippings don't contaminate other foods in the shopping carton. Then, don't let groceries remain in a warm car or scooter dicky, this allows bacteria to grow. Refrigerate or freeze food promptly.
- Don't buy or use food from containers that leak, bulge, or are severely dented. Don't buy or use food from jars that are cracked or have loose or bulging lids. Don't taste or use food that has a foul odur or that spurt liquid when opened. The deadly Clostridium botulinum toxin is probably present.
- Wash thoroughly all counters, cutting bonds, dishes, and other equipment in hot soapy water, and rinse. Do this both before and after coming in contact with raw meat, fish, poultry and eggs, to rid Salmonella present.
- Wash fresh fruit and vegetable carefully to remove dirt.
- If possible, cut foods to be eaten raw on a clean, plastic cutting board reserved for that purpose. If the same board must be used for both meat and other foods, cut the items to be eaten raw before cutting any potentially contaminated items, such as meat.

Table 13.1: Microorganisms and parasites that cause foodborne illness: their source, symptoms and means of prevention

Microorganism	*Source*	*Symptoms*	*Means of prevention*
Bacteria			
Staphylococcus aureus	Live in nasal passages and in cuts on skin. Toxin is produced when food contaminated by bacteria is left for extended time at room temperature. Meats, poultry, egg products, tuna, potato, and macaroni salads, and cream-filled pastries are likely targets.	Onset: 2-6 hours after eating. Diarrhea, vomiting, nausea, and abdominal cramps. Mimics flu. Lasts 24-48 hours. Rarely fatal.	• Sanitary food-handling practices. • Prompt and proper refrigeration of foods. • Keep cuts on skin covered.
Salmonella	Found in raw meats, poultry, eggs, fish, milk, and products made with these items. Multiplies rapidly at room temperature. The bacteria themselves are toxic.	Onset: 5-72 hours after eating. Nausea, fever, headache, abdominal cramps, diarrhea and vomiting. Can be fatal in infants, the elderly, and the sick.	• Handling food in a sanitary manner. • Thorough cooking of foods. • Prompt and proper refrigeration of foods. • Watch cross contamination.
Clostridium perfringens	Widespread in environment. Generally found in meat and poultry dishes. Multiply rapidly when foods are left for extended time at room temperature. The bacteria themselves are toxic.	Onset: 8-24 hours after eating (usually 12 hours). Abdominal pain and diarrhea. Symptoms last a day or less, usually mild. Can be more serious in older or already ill people.	• Sanitary handling of foods, especially meat and meat dishes, gravies, and leftovers. • Thorough cooking and reheating of foods. • Prompt and proper refrigeration.
Clostridium botulinum	Widespread in the environment. However bacteria produce toxin only in low-acid, anaerobic (oxygen-free) environments, such as in cans of green beans, mushrooms and spinach. Honey may carry spores.	Onset: 12-36 hours after eating. Symptoms include double vision, inability to swallow, speech difficulty, and progressive paralysis of the respiratory system. OBTAIN MEDICAL HELP IMMEDIATELY BOTULISM CAN BE FATAL.	• Using proper methods for canning low acid foods. • Avoiding commercial cans of low acid foods that have leaky seals or are bent, bulging, or broken. • Toxin can be destroyed after can or jar is opened by boiling contents hard for 20 minutes, but discard if suspect toxin is present because of off-odors.
Campylobacter jejuni	Found on poultry and beef and can contami-	Onset: 3-5 days after eating, or longer.	• Thorough cooking of foods.

Contd.

Contd.

	nate meat and milk. Chief foods sources are raw poultry and meat and unpasteurized milk.	Diarrhea, abdominal cramping, fever and sometimes bloody stools. Lasts 2-7 days.	• Handling food in sanitary manner. • Avoiding unpasteurized milk.
Listeria monocytogenes	Found in soft cheeses and unpasteurized milk. Resists acid, heat, salt and nitrate well.	Onset: 4-21 days. Fever, headache, vomiting and sometimes even more severe symptoms. May be fatal.	• Thorough cooking of foods. • Handling food in a sanitary manner. • Avoiding unpasteurized milk.
Yersinia enterocolitica	Common in nature; carried in food and water. They multiply rapidly at both room and refrigerator temperatures. Generally found in raw vegetables, meats, water, and unpasteurized milk.	Onset: 2-3 days after eating. Fever, headache, nausea, diarrhea, and general malaise. Mimics flu and appendicitis. An important cause of intestinal distress in children.	• Thorough cooking of foods. • Sanitizing cutting instruments and cutting boards before preparing foods that are eaten raw. • Avoidance of unpasteurized milk and unchlorinated water.
Viruses *Hepatitis A virus*	Chief food sources: foods that are handled a lot during preparation and then eaten raw (such as vegetables).	Onset: 30 days Jaundice, fatigue, may cause liver damage and death.	• Sanitary handling of foods. • Use of pure drinking water. • Adequate sewage disposal. • Adequate cooking of foods.
Parasites *Trichinella spiralis*	Found in wild animals whose meat eaten after hunting.	Onset: Weeks months. Muscle weakness, fluid retention in face, fever, flu-like symptoms.	• Thoroughly cooking.
Aniskis	Found in raw fish.	Onset: 12 hours. Stomach infection, severe stomach pain.	• Thoroughly cooking of fish.
Tapeworms	Found in raw pork and fish.	Abdominal discomfort, diarrhea.	• Thoroughly cooking of all animal products.
Mycotoxins *A group of toxic compounds produced by molds, such as aflatoxin*	Produced in foods that are relatively high in moisture. Chief food sources: beans groundnuts and grains that have been stored in moist place.	May cause liver and/or kidney disease.	• Checking foods for visible mold and discarding those that are contaminated. • Proper storage of susceptible foods.

- Cook animal foods thoroughly, internal temperature for poultry should reach 82°C; for fish 77°C; and for eggs the yolk should at least be semisolid and the white hard. A good general precaution is to eat no raw animal products. This includes any use of raw or undercooked eggs. Many people are poisoned each year by eating raw seafood. Undercooked pork can allow infection by the parasite that causes trichinosis.
- Once a food is cooked, cool it rapidly (to 4°C) within 2 to 4 hours if it is not to be eaten immediately. Greater surface area allows quicker cooling, so separate foods into several pans. Don't recontaminate cooked food through contact with raw meat or juices that might be on your hands, cutting boards, or dirty utensils.
- Reheat leftovers to 74°C and reheat gravy to rolling boil to kill potential clostridium perfringens bacteria present. Stopping at an acceptable eating temperature is not good enough.
- Keep hot foods hot and cool foods cold. Avoid time and temperature abuses. Store food below 4°C or above 60°C. Food poisoning microbes thrive at more moderate temperatures between 16°C to 32°C.
- Avoid coughing and sneezing over foods, even when you are healthy. Cover cuts on hands. This helps stop staphylococcus aureus from entering your food.
- Make sure the refrigerator stays below 4°C. Generally keep it as cold as possible without freezing the milk.
- Consume only pasteurized milk and pasteurized cheese. This is especially important for pregnant women because very toxic bacteria and viruses that thrive in unpasteurized milk can harm the foetus.
- Completely remove moldy portions of food or don't eat the food. When in doubt throw the food out. Mold growth is prevented by properly storing foods at cold temperatures and using the foods within a reasonable length of time.

Microbes that cause food poisoning commonly enter food through cross-contamination (usually from improper food handling) and grow because they are maintained at temperatures favourable to them. Many foods contain problem microbes. Most food poisoning incidents could be eliminated through sanitary food-handling procedures and appropriate storage (Fig. 13.1).

FOOD PRESERVATION

Microorganisms are present in the air, in dust, soil, sewage and on the hands and other parts of the body. They are so widely distributed that their presence in or on food is inevitable unless special steps are taken to kill them. If food is to be kept in good condition for any length of time it is essential that the growth of microorganisms be prevented. This can be done either by killing them and then storing the food in conditions where further infection is impossible or by creating an environment which slows down or stops their growth.

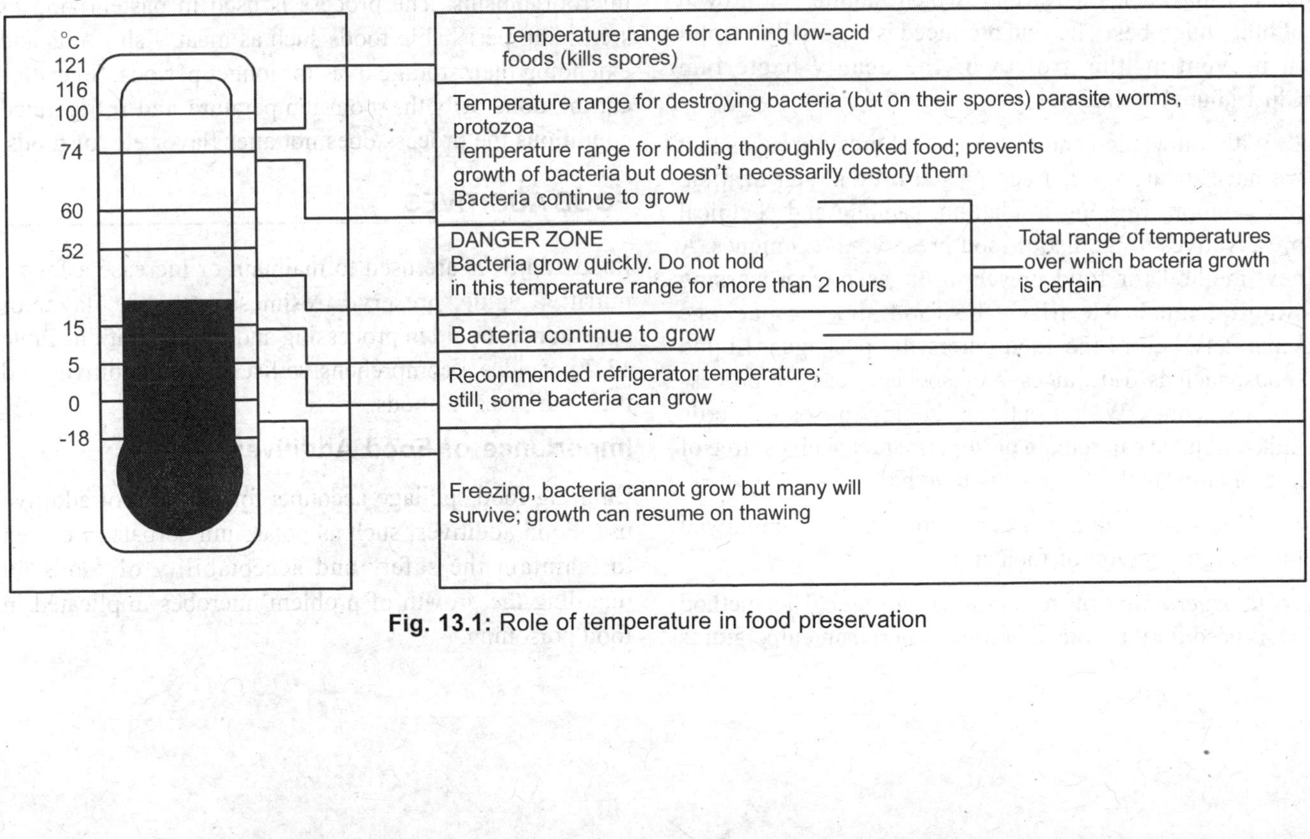

Fig. 13.1: Role of temperature in food preservation

The ability to preserve food in good condition for long periods is an undoubted boon. The amount of food wasted is reduced and the incidence of food poisoning kept low. A wider range of foods is available including foods 'out of season' and foods from overseas that could not be transported and stocked in former times. The widespread use of preservatives, refrigerators, 'deep freeze' equipment and canned and dehydrated food has made it easy for the consumer or caterer to have available a wide range of wholesome food at all times of the year.

In addition to suppressing the growth of microorganisms an effective method of food preservation must retain, as far as possible, the original characteristics of the food and impair its nutritive value as little as possible.

For centuries, salt, sugar, smoke, fermentation, and drying have been used to preserve food. Most preserving methods work on the principle of decreasing the water– the amount of water not bound to other components in the food. Salt and sugar decrease free water by binding to it. The process of drying drives off free water. Bacteria need abundant stores of water to grow. However, yeasts and molds can grow with less water.

Decreasing the water content of some rather high moisture foods, however, would cause them to lose essential characteristics. To preserve such foods, such as cucumber pickles, sauerkraut, milk (yogurt) and wine fermentation has been traditional alternative. Selected bacteria are used to ferment or pickle food. The fermenting bacteria make acids and alcohol, which minimize the growth of other microbes. The acid produced is especially helpful in preventing the growth of the deadly bacterium Clostridium botulinum.

With knowledge and technological breakthroughs that we have today, we can add pasteurization, sterilization, refrigeration, freezing irradiation, canning and chemical preservatives to the list of food preserving techniques. A new method for food preservation–aseptic processing simultaneously sterilizes the food and the package separately before the food enters the packages. Liquid foods, such as fruit juices, are especially easy to process in this manner. With aseptic packaging, boxes of sterile milk and juice can remain on supermarket shelves, free of microbial growth, for months together.

In India, the common preservation processes employed for the preservation of food are:

1. *Refrigeration (low temperature storage)*: This method is used for the storage of food material at temperatures just above freezing point between +1 to 10°C. It has the effect of slowing down the growth of organisms, but of course doesn't destroy them. It is used for short terms storage.
2. *Freezing*: This process is used to store food material at temperature lower then -18°C. It reduces the activity of microorganisms to almost zero, and also reduces the reaction rate of chemicals to a very low level. Most frozen material has a life of 3 months and above.
3. *Drying*: It is one of the earliest preservation processes and has been used since man discovered fire. It involves the reduction in moisture content of food material to a level below 10 percent by weight. It has the effect of inhibition on the growth of many microorganisms though they are not, necessarily killed.

The use of naturally occurring chemicals (salt, sugar, etc.) together with smoking and drying form the important basis of food preservation. The main objective of chemical additives are to inhibit microbial growth (rarely to kill) and to inhibit oxidation of animal fats, vegetable oils and dairy products.

Thermal preservation: In order to kill microorganisms, the application of heat is generally required, and for food material containing pathogens, this is many a time the only way to ensure safety for the consumer.

Radiation preservation: Irradiation is the ability of radiations such as gamma rays and fast electrons to destroy microorganisms. The process is used in pasteurizing or sterilizing perishable foods such as meat, fish, fruits and extending their storage lives for longer periods. Since this can be done at both, room temperature and refrigerated conditions the process does not alter flavor etc. of foods.

FOOD ADDITIVES

Food additives are used to maintain or increase a food's nutritive value, preserve freshness, enhance flavor or appearance, or aid in processing and/or preparation. Table 13.2 provides a comprehensive list of food additives and their purposes in foods.

Importance of Food Additives

Limiting food spoilage accounts for the bulk of additive use. Food additives, such as potassium sorbate, are used to maintain the safety and acceptability of foods by retarding the growth of problem microbes implicated in food poisoning.

Table 13.2: Types of additives

Anticaking	Formulation aids; carriers, binders, fillers, plasticizers	Processing aids: clarifying, clouding, catalyst, flocculants, filter aids, crystallization inhibitors
Antimicrobial	Fumigants	Propellants
Antioxidants	Humectants	Sequestrants
Colour and adjuncts	Leavening	Solvents and vehicles
Conditioners	Lubricants and release agents	Stabilizers and thickeners
Curing and pickling	Non-nutritive sweeteners	Surface active agents
Dough strengtheners	Nutritive sweeteners	Surface-finishing agents
Drying agents	Oxidizing and reducing agents	Synergists
Emulsifiers	pH control	Texturizers
Enzymes		
Firming agents		
Flavour enhancers		
Flavouring agents		
Flour treating		

Additives are also used to inhibit some enzymes that lead to undesirable changes in color and flavor in foods, but do not cause anything so serious as food poisoning. This second type of food spoilage occurs when enzymes in a food react with oxygen; for example, when apple and peach slices darken or turn rust color as they are exposed to air. Antioxidants are a type of preservatives that retard the action of oxygen-requiring enzymes on food surfaces. These preservatives are not necessarily novel chemicals. They include vitamin E, vitamin C, and a variety of sulfites.

They are also added to improve flavor and color, leaven, provide nutritional fortification, thicken and emulsify food.

Additives are components limited in foods to at the most 1/100 of the highest amount that causes no observable effect when consumed by animals.

Classification of Food Additives

Food additives are classified into two types: those that are (intentionally) directly added to foods and those that have (incidentally) indirectly entered foods.

Directly Added Food Additives

Additive knowingly (directly) incorporated into food products by manufacturers.

Indirectly Added Food Additives

Additives that gain access to food products indirectly from environmental contamination of food ingredients or during the manufacturing process.

Sugar, salt, corn syrup and citric acid etc. constitute the bulk (98%) of all additives by weight.

Common Food Additives

A list of food additive categories appears in Table 13.2. Let us look at some of the major categories to understand exactly why food additives are used and to learn more about the specific substances that are used as food additives.

Acidic or Alkaline Agents: Acids, such as calcium lactate, have many uses in foods. As flavor enhancing agents, they impart a tart paste to soft drinks, and cheese spreads. As preservatives, they inhibit microbial growth. As antioxidants, they prevent discoloration and rancidity. They also adjust acid and base balance. Adding acids during food processing increases the margin of safety from botulism in naturally low-acid vegetable, such as beets.

Alkaline products, such as sodium hydroxide, can alter the texture and flavour of foods, including chocolate. In processing, alkaline products are sometimes used to produce a milder flavour by neutralizing the acids produced during fermentation.

Anticaking Agents: By absorbing moisture compounds such as calcium silicate, ammonium citrate, magnesium stearate, and silicon dioxide keep table salt, baking power, powdered sugar, and other powdered food products free flowing. These chemicals prevent the caking and lumping that would make powdered or crystalline products hard to use.

Antioxidants: These preservatives help delay food discoloration from oxygen exposure, such as that occurs when potatoes are diced. They also help keep fats from turning rancid. Two widely used antioxidants are BHA (butylated hydroxyanisole) and BHT (butylated hydroxytoluene). Vitamin E and related compounds also serve as antioxidants.

Sulfites too are widely used as antioxidants in foods. They are, actually a group of sulfur-based chemicals—sulfur dioxide, gas, sodium and potassium bisulfate, and sodium and potassium metabisulfite. After ingesting sulfites, people who are very sensitive to them may have difficulty in breathing, wheeze, vomit, have hives, diarrhea, abdominal pain, cramps, and dizziness. Now-a-days manufacturers are required to declare the presence of sulfites on labels of packaged foods containing at least 10 parts per million of sulfites. Potatoes are not covered by that regulation.

Colours: Colour additives do not improve nutritional qualities, but they can make foods more eye appealing. Food colourings cannot be used to deceive consumers, for example, by covering blemishes, or to conceal inferiority, or to mislead people in any way. Although colourings are arguably unnecessary additives. They are used to make food products attractive and appealing to the eye.

Controversy has surrounded the use of some food colours. Currently, the safety of using tartrazine is disputed. It has caused allergic symptoms, such as hives, itching, and nasal discharge in sensitive individuals, especially in people allergic to aspirin.

Emulsifiers: These products, by distributing and suspending fat in water, improve the uniformity, smoothness, and body of foods such as bakery goods, ice cream and candies. In mayonnaise, for example, egg yolks act as emulsifiers in holding together the oil and the acids, such as vinegar or lemon juice. Lecithin, derived from soybeans, acts as an emulsifier in chocolate and margarine. Monoglycerides and diglycerides, found also as by-products of fat digestion, are used as emulsifiers in cake mixes.

Flavours and Flavouring Agents: Naturally occurring and artificial agents can impart more flavour to foods. These agents include extracts from spices and herbs, as well as man-made agents. You probably have recognized flavours of some spices and of liquid derivatives of onion, garlic, cloves, and peppermint in foods. To meet the demand of industry, manufacturers have developed synthetic flavours that not only taste like natural flavours, but also have the advantage of stability. Often artificial flavours, such as butter or banana flavours, have the same chemical composition that makes up part of the natural flavour.

Flavour Enhancers: These substances—monosodium glutamate (MSG), for example—help bring out the natural flavours of foods. Some people are sensitive to MSG and experience flushing. Chest pain, facial pressure, dizziness, sweating, rapid heart rate, nausea, vomiting and high blood pressure after exposure. Because MSG is often used in Chinese food, reactions have been called Chinese restaurant syndrome. The onset of symptoms occurs about 10 to 20 minutes after ingestion and may last from 2 to 3 hours. People who find themselves sensitive to MSG should avoid it.

Infants are more sensitive to MSG because they have not yet developed a complete blood-brain barrier. This means they cannot fully exclude such substances as MSG.

Humectants: These chemicals, such as glycerol, propylene glycol and sorbitol, are added to foods to help retain proper moisture, fresh flavour and texture. They are often used in candies and shredded coconut.

Leavening Agents: Air and steam can be used to create a light texture in breads and cakes; however, carbon dioxide bubble are much more reliable for this purpose. Common leavening agents that produce carbon dioxide gas include yeast, baking powder, and baking soda. Baking soda needs to react with acids to generate carbon dioxide. Baking powder can be used in either acid or alkaline conditions.

Maturing and Bleaching Agents: Compounds such as bromates, peroxides, and ammonium chloride hasten the natural aging and whitening processes of milled flour. This shortens the delay in using flour in baked products. Otherwise, freshly milled flour lacks the qualities necessary to make a stable, elastic dough, and otherwise requires several months to be useful in baking.

Nutrient Supplements: Vitamin and mineral supplements are added to foods to improve their nutritional quality. Sometimes they replace nutrients lost in processing, as occurs when enriching flour, vitamin A is added to margarine and to some forms of milk. Vitamin D is added to some dairy products. Potassium iodide is added to salt, and calcium to some flours. Breakfast cereals often contain a variety of added nutrients.

Preservatives: There are many types of preservatives. Some inhibit microbial growth, others function as antioxidants or sequestrants. Sodium benzoate, sorbic acid, and calcium propionate are common preservatives. Sorbic acid is a potent inhibitor or molds and fungal growth. Calcium propionate, a natural part of some cheeses, inhibits mold growth.

Nitrates—and the related form, nitrites—are used as preservatives, especially to prevent growth of Clostridium botulinum. Sodium and potassium nitrates and nitrites are used to preserve meats, such as bacon, ham, salami, and hot dogs. Nitrates and nitrites have been used for centuries—in conjunction with salt—to preserve meat. An added effect of nitrates is their reaction with myoglobin pigments in meat to form a bright pink colour. This gives the characteristic appearance to ham, hot dogs, and other cured meats.

Nitrate consumption from both cured foods and natural vegetables has been associated with the synthesis of nitrosamines in the stomach. Nitrosamines are potent cancer-causing agents, particularly for the stomach and esophagus. Actual risk appears to be low, however, except for people who secrete little stomach acid (some elderly people, for example). It is that consumers take for granted a margin of microbial safety gained from nitrite use in cured meats. People often serve these meats cold or at least underheated. Consequently government agencies have chosen not to ban nitrate or nitrite use in foods, but rather to change manufacturing practices to lower amounts of performed nitrosamines.

The addition of vitamin C to cured meats, such as bacon, is one way to reduce the amount of nitrosamines formed in foods. This is a common practice today. Other antioxidants, such as vitamin E, also inhibit synthesis of nitrosamines.

Alternative Sweeteners: Currently, saccharin and acesulfame are the only non-nutritive sweeteners used in foods. Since aspartame yields energy, it is considered a nutritive sweetener. Saccharin is carcinogenic to rats when administered over two generations. The cancers are found primarily in the bladder. However, population studies of humans have not found an increased risk of developing bladder cancer from exposure to saccharin.

Stabilizers and Thickeners: Theses additives impart a smooth texture and uniform colour and flavour to candies, ice creams, and other frozen deserts, chocolate milk, and artificially sweetened beverages. Commonly used substances are pectins, vegetable gums (such as guar gum and carrageenan), gelatins and agars. They work by absorbing water. Without stabilizers and thickeners, ice crystals form in ice cream and other frozen desserts, and particles of chocolate separate from chocolate milk. Stabilizers are also used to prevent evaporation and deterioration of flavorings used in cakes, puddings and gelatin mixes.

Sequestrants: These compounds include EDTA and citric acid. They bind many free chemical ions, and by doing so, reduce the ability of ions to cause rancidity in products containing fat.

In general, if one consumes a variety of foods in moderation, the chances of food additives jeopardizing one's health are minimal. Paying attention to one's body, if one suspects an intolerance or sensitivity, consultation with your physician for further evaluation is necessary. Remember that, in the short run, one is more likely to suffer from either poor food handling practices that allow bacteria to grow in food or from consuming raw animal foods, than from eating additives. Excess kcalories, saturated fat, and other potential "problem" nutrients pose the greatest long term risk.

FOOD TOXINS OF NATURAL ORIGIN

Foods contain a variety of naturally occurring toxic substances. Following are some of the more important examples (Table 13.3):

Mushrooms—some species are poisonous.

Safrole—found in, mace and nutmeg; causes cancer.

Solanine—found in potato shoots and green spots on potato skins; inhibits nervous system action.

Aflatoxin—found on moldy grains and peanuts; causes cancer. One should rigorously inspect peanut butter to ensure that it's safe for consumption.

Avidin—found in raw egg whites; binds biotin, preventing its absorption. Cooking inactivates avidin.

Goitrogens—found in raw rutabagas, turnips, brussels sprouts, broccoli and soybeans; inhibit thyroid hormone metabolism. Cooking destroys them.

Thiaminase—found in raw fish and mussels; it destroys the vitamin thiamin. Cooking inactivates thiaminase.

Protease inhibitor—found in raw soybeans; inhibits digestive enzymes.

Saponins—found in alfalfa sprouts; destroy red blood cell membranes.

Tannins—found in tea; bind calcium and iron.

Oxalic acid—found in spinach; binds calcium.

Herbal teas—containing senna or comfrey; can cause diarrhea and liver damage.

Nitrates—found in spinach, lettuce and beets; can be converted into the carcinogen nitrosamine.

Table 13.3: Various naturally occurring toxins present in foods along with a brief mention of their deleterious effects

Almonds, lima beans, kirsch, fruit stones and seeds	Cyanogens which produce cyanides	Inhibition of respiratory system with possible fatal consequences
Nutrimeg, mace, back pepper, parsley celery seed	Myristicin	Headaches, cramps, nausea, hallucination
Green or sprouting potatoes	Solanine and chaconine	Stomach upsets, nervous effects
Rhubarb (especially leaves)	Oxalic acid	Interference with calcium absorption
Alcoholic drinks	Ethanol (ethyl alcohol)	Personality changes, vomiting, unconsciousness subsequent 'hangover'
Cabbage and other brassicas	Goitrogens	Interference with iodine absorption by thyroid gland
Most raw beans (especially soya)	Protease inhibitors	Interference with protein digestion and absorption
Bread and other cereal products	Phytic acid	Complexes with iron and calcium and may interfere with their absorption
Raw beans	Heamagluttenins	Cause red blood cells to cling together
Mushroom of Amanita variety	Amanitin	Inactivates metabolic enzymes causing severe illness with possible fatal results
Some shellfish	Alkaloid related to stychnine	Severe and sometimes fatal illness
Fish especially puffer fish and scombroid fish (e.g., tuna, mackerel and bonito) if not fresh	Various toxins derived from food eaten by fish	Severe digestive upset
Mustard	Sanguinarine	Fluid retention (dropsy)
Turnips, celery, parsley	Psoralens	Genetic mutations
Tea, coffee, cola drinks	Caffeine	Diuretic and stimulant
Some cheeses, yeast extract, red wines	Tyramine	Increased blood pressure, migrain. Interferes with some antidepressant drugs

Browning products—found in toasted grains; can cause genetic changes by causing alterations in DNA.

FOOD HYGIENE

The subject of food hygiene deals with how treatment of food affects the health of the consumer. High standard of hygiene minimize food spoilage and help to ensure that when food is eaten it is as wholesome and free from pathogenic bacteria as far as possible.

Many factors may affect the quality and wholesomeness of food. The important ones are:

a. The way in which it is grown or, in the case of animals, they are reared and fed.

b. The design and cleanliness of farm building, slaughterhouses and factories in which it is processed.

c. The premises, equipment and conditions in which it is stored.

d. The care taken by food handlers to avoid contamination from other foods.

e. The personal hygiene of food handlers.

It is not possible to deal with all these matters here. The last two points listed, however, are of concern to all food handlers and, indeed, to all those who have an interest in food hygiene and safety.

The basic principles of good food hygiene practice can be summarized as follows:

1. Avoid contamination of food by bacteria.
2. Prevent the multiplication of any bacteria which somehow gain access to food.
3. Destroy any remaining bacteria, wherever possible, by thorough cooking.

These three foundations of food hygienic practice are detailed below.

Avoid Contamination

i. Keep raw and cooked food separate. The same working surfaces and equipment should not be used for both raw and ready-to-eat foods. Surfaces and equipment used for raw foods (including vegetables) should be thoroughly cleaned afterwards.

ii. Keep animals out of food areas and make sure that birds and insects do not have access.

iii. Dispose of waste food promptly.

iv. Do not use washbasins for food-preparation or food-preparation sinks for washing hands.

v. Maintain high standards of personal hygiene. Thorough handwashing is essential especially after handling raw meat or using a toilet. Clean towels or disposable towels or hot-air driers should be used for hand-drying to prevent reinfection of clean hands by dirty towels.

vi. Clean protective clothing (including head covering) should be worn in food areas and should be removed while leaving those areas.

vii. Hands should be kept away from bacteria-rich areas of the body including the mouth and nose. It is for this reason that smoking by food handlers is prohibited by law. Soiled handkerchiefs and uncovered wounds are other potent sources of infection.

Prevent Multiplication of Microorganisms

i. Keep foods cold or hot. Avoid the temperature zone 5-65°C in which bacteria flourish. Food should be in this temperature danger-zone for as little time as possible.

Cook Food Thoroughly

ii. Cooling times and temperatures must be sufficient to ensure that all bacteria and their toxins are destroyed. If bacteria present in food (or their spores) are not killed when the food is cooked they may multiply when it is cooling through the 'danger-zone', or if it is kept in this temperature zone before being served.

iii. Meat and poultry should be completely defrosted before cooking. If this is not done some bacteria or bacterial spores may survive the cooking process.

Essentiality of Food Hygiene in Present Context

There are many reasons for the increase in food poisoning in India over recent years, but some of the more important ones are as follows:

1. *A great increase in community feeding*: Large scale catering, whether in hospitals, schools, canteens, or restaurants, means that a single infected food can produce many cases of food poisoning.

2. *Varied menus and rapid food service*: In order to have a wide menu and be able to produce dishes quickly food may be precooked and kept warm until it is required or it may be reheated rapidly and perhaps inadequately in a microwave oven or under an infrared grill when it is ordered.

3. *Increased use of convenience foods*: Although factory processing are carefully controlled and carried out under hygienic conditions, one source of infection can

lead to the contamination of thousands of prepacked items. In addition, the use of convenience foods, especially meat products, which are eaten cold or only warmed and not-heated enough increases the risk of food poisoning.

4. *Increase in factory farming*: The intensive rearing of poultry and animals increases the possibility of large scale infection of such food supplies, especially by Salmonella.
5. *Rapid increase in consumption of take-away meals*: Such food may be kept warm for long period or briefly reheated in the home thus allowing rapid bacterial growth. For example, 'take-way' rice may be contaminated with Bacillus cereus.
6. *Changing pattern of shopping and food storage in the home*: A weekly, rather than a daily, shopping routine means that food has to be stored for greater periods of time. Incorrect storage conditions may encourage the growth of bacteria. Increasing use of freezers means that meat, especially poultry, needs to be thawed before it is cooked. Incomplete thawing followed by normal cooking may not kill all bacteria, especially in the center of the food.
7. *Increased use of packed meals*: The incidence of food poisoning is much higher in summer than in winter largely because of inadequate refrigeration. The increasing tendency to have a packed meal, often including cooked meat in sandwiches, in the middle of the day increases the risk of food poisoning in summer.
8. *Use of staff untrained in hygiene in catering establishments*: Large-scale handling of food by staff not trained or conscious of hygiene requirements is a major source of infection. In such circumstances cross-contamination, that is the transfer of bacteria from a contaminated source to an uncontaminated source, can easily occur and spread the risk of infection.

Many times salmonella are responsible for most food borne illness account for 70-80 percent of all cases. Clostridium perfringens is next in importance, accounting for 15-25 per cent. Outbreaks of food borne illness caused by this organism often involve food which has been prepared in bulk and hence tend to affect a large number of people.

STUDY QUESTIONS

1. Explain the concepts of ‘Food Perishability’, ‘Food Poisoning’, ‘Food Safety’ and ‘Food Hygiene’.
2. What role do microorganisms play in food perishability and food poisoning? Explain briefly.
3. What valuable tips a food scientist would give to a consumer to prevent poisoning?
4. Give an introductory account of the process of ‘food preservation’—a process that is employed increasingly these days to prevent perishability of foods.
5. What are ‘food additives’? What purpose do they serve in foods? Give a brief account of common food additives.
6. Elaborate on food toxins of natural origin.
7. Write a note on the statement: ‘Food hygiene is an essential prerequisite to food safety’.

CHAPTER 14

Important Considerations for Meal Planning

Chapter Outlines

- Meal planning
- Important considerations for meal planning
- Meal planning in a nutshell
- Study questions

MEAL PLANNING

Doing meal planning, not only involves selecting foods that provide optimum nutrition but also blending of colour texture and flavour of different food items. Planning meals, therefore, is both a science and an art. A good, nourishing meal should also please the eye of the consumer as some body has very aptly said: 'We eat with our eye'. The skill and expertise of meal planning come through inspiration, thought and practice. Besides, one also needs to know the basic facts about the nourishing abilities of various foodstuffs.

In planning family meals, several things, including money, time, energy, knowledge, skills and abilities, human and material resources; all influence the quality (nourishing ability), palatability (taste) and presentation (the way in which a meal is served) of the food prepared.

The central aim of meal planning is to fulfill the nutritional needs of each member of the family within the constraints of time, energy and money available; to make the meals appetizing and serve them in appealing, eye catching manner, mainly, because a majority of people do not eat things they do not like in sight smell and taste even if they are rich in nutrient composition. Therefore, such preparation methods needs to be used which retain nutrient value of foods without compromising their palatability. Further meals have to be planned in keeping with the budget of the family. A seasoned meal planner goes for a nutritionally rich diets which do not necessarily contain expensive milk and meat products as the major dietary ingredients. Hence the watchword of meal planning is to plan within family means.

IMPORTANT CONSIDERATIONS FOR MEAL PLANNING

Since a plethora of factors affect meal planning, it is always desirable to make the following considerations while planning meals.

Nutritive Adequacy

A good meal is one that provides not only the macronutrients (carbohydrates, proteins and fats) in requisite amounts but also furnishes micronutrients (vitamins and minerals) in adequate proportion to each member of the family. Therefore, the age, gender; physiological state and occupation of the family members have to be taken into consideration and reckoning while planning meals for the family.

One convenient way to work out the energy requirements of a family is to assess the needs of women and children in relation to those of average man by taking the energy consumption of an average male sedentary worker (energy requirement 2400 kcals) as one unit, referred to as 'Adult consumption unit' and abbreviated as cu-unit. Table 14.1 enlists the coefficients of caloric requirement in terms of cu-unit. Table 14.2 gives an account of the classification of the activities based upon occupation.

Table 14.1: Coefficient for (In term of Adult Consumption Units) computing calorie requirement of different groups

Group	*Cu-Units*
Adult male (sedentary worker)	1.0
Adult male (moderate worker)	1.2
Adult male (heavy worker)	1.6
Adult female (sedentary worker)	0.8
Adult female (moderate worker)	0.9
Adult female (heavy worker)	1.2
Adolescents - 12 to 21 years	1.0
Children - 9 to 12 years	0.8
Children - 7 to 9 years	0.7
Children - 5 to 7 years	0.6
Children - 3 to 5 years	0.5
Children - 1 to 3 years	0.4

Table 14.2: Classification of activities based on occupations

Sedentary:	
Male:	Teacher, Tailor, Barber, Executive, Shoemaker, Priest, Retired Personnel, Landlord, Peon, Postman, etc.
Female:	Teacher, Tailor, Executive, Housewife, Nurse, etc.
Moderate:	
Male:	Fisherman, Basket-maker, Potter, Goldsmith, Agricultural labor, Carpenter, Mason, Rickshaw-puller, Electrician, Fitter, Turner, Welder, Industrial labor, Cooli, Weaver, Driver, etc.
Female:	Servant (maid), Cooli, Basket-maker, Weaver, Agricultural labor, Beedi-maker, etc.
Heavy:	
Male:	Stone-cutter, Blacksmith, Mine-worker, Wood-cutter, Gang man, etc.
Female:	Stone-cutter

In dealing with the energy intake of a group of mixed age and sex composition, the number of "consumption units" in the group is first calculated. For example, a family consisting of father doing sedentary work and mother and two children aged 10 and 6 years has an 'adult man' equivalent or consumption units of 3.2 (i.e., 1.0 + 0.8 + 0.8 + 0.6) and the daily energy requirement of the family would be 2400 × 3.2 or 7680 kcals. If it is necessary to draw up a diet schedule for the family, foods supplying calories should be provided. If analysis of the existing diet of the family indicates that the total caloric intake per day is below this level, attempt should be made to make good the deficiency.

While drawing up either a new diet schedule or correcting inadequacies in the existing diets, it is safer to err on the side of excess by 100 to 200 kcals to allow for waste of all kinds. The relation between energy requirement and such factors as body weight (in case of adults) activity, age should be borne in mind. However, body weight adjustments are not to be made in case of growing children, the level recommended for the age should be provided (even if the body weight is lower than normal) in such cases.

Whereas most of the caloric requirement has to be met by carbohydrates and facts, a small proportion of the requisite energy should also come from proteins. Normally, the caloric contribution from the different macronutrients should be as under: Carbohydrates 60-70%; fat 20-30% and proteins 10%.

Although meal protein may differ from population to population, it should be made pertinent that the diet planned does not lead to protein or iron deficiency. Likewise, exclusion of milk products, either by compulsion or by choice, should be avoided as far as possible, lest it would result in calcium deficiency. Generally speaking, inclusion of one or more foods from each food group, tends to prevent most dietary imbalances.

Specific nutritional requirements for various phases of life span may be satisfied by including more units or serving from the food groups that contribute those specific nutrients. For instance a teenager may need six units from first food group to meet his protein needs for growth and maintenance compared to and adult who would require only three. Elderly person, having a problem in chewing and mastication of foods may be provided with carrot salad in grated form, the other members of the family may be served raw carrot sticks. Salads may be served raw and without oil seasoning to an obese family member, other members of the family may partake of salads seasoned with oil.

Emphasis on Time and Energy Budgeting: Easy to Cook Meals

Time and energy budgeting requires planning of menus for several days well in advance and shopping once in a week. Using innovative and scientifically tenable preparation methods that save on energy and time without compromising nutritive and palatability characteristics. One may also consider planning some convenience foods especially when the home maker is also a working person. Even the leftovers from the previous meal can be handled meaningfully.

For instance, boiled rice as leftovers can be used in khichri or some rice pudding. A thoughtful meal planner always thinks of enhancing the nutritive value of certain foods by sprouting or fermenting certain foods.

Even for a housewife it is never advisable to plan and cook meals that comprise a number of dishes with each taking long preparation time, for spending too much time in the kitchen would make her frustrated and irritating on one hand and leave many other household chores undone or halfdone. A good and practical meal plan is the one that consumes minimum amount of time, energy and expenditure and yet does not lack in nutritive quality, flavour and taste.

Individual Likes and Dislikes

A common tendency that prevails amongst people is to select or reject certain foods on the basis of individual likes and dislikes. However, in order to plan meals in accordance with recommended daily allowances, foods from each group have to included and it doesn't become possible to exclude or include a given good item right away on this basis. Some ingenious ways, therefore, have to be found to take care of this aspect. One way to circumvent individual preferences is to change the form of the food rather than completely omitting it. Milk for instance, if not liked as such may be given in the form of curd, cheese or any other sweet dish. Likewise, soyabeans, if not acceptable as beans, may be consumed in the form of soyaflour to make chapattis mixed with wheat flour. It should remain the endeavour of the meal planner to devise new ways of using available foods so as to make the menu acceptable and healthful.

Variety in Meals

Variety in meals is obtained by combining foods in various ways. It promotes acceptability and ensures better nutrition. Variety is brought about by affecting changes in colour, shape, texture, flavour and method of preparation of a food as also by varying the choice of foods within each group on day-to-day basis.

Colour: The meal planner should show sensitivity towards colour combinations of various food items by avoiding meals that are all white or of one colour tone. Attractive colour combinations are appealing to the eye and inviting to the palate.

Texture: To bring variation in texture it should become customary to include crisp and chewable food items along with soft foods.

Flavour: Different flavours impart variety to the meals and enhance their appeal. As all spicy or all bland foods in a meal make it monotonous, it becomes desirable to blend bland foods with those that are intensely flavoured.

Preparation: To avoid the loss of nutritive value and enhance palatability a variety of preparation methods including boiling, banking and roasting should be used. Likewise, by using various foods combinations, e.g., dosa, idle, roti, khichri, the nutritive value and completeness of the meal are increased.

Preparation Skill: Skill in food preparation plays no less role in making a meal acceptable and inviting. The skill is acquired by keenly observing and judiciously emulating persons having good culinary skills and wide experience in food preparation. By making ingenious food combinations like adding ground gram dal (besan) to methi leaves thereby diluting the better flavour of the latter and making it more acceptable or, for that matter, making finished vegetable more enjoyable by adding grated coconut. In general, strong flavours of one food are moderated by mixing them with another one with milder flavour or with other ingredients.

Meal Planning as Prerequisite for Satiety Values: Foods rich in proteins and fats have a higher satiety value vis-à-vis carbohydrate abundant foods.

Qualitative Aspects of Meals: In case the two consecutive meals are space apart. There is need to plan a meal abundant in carbohydrate and protein. However, a shorter interval before the two meals calls for a meal rich in carbohydrates.

Food Availability

Dietary habits of a community in earlier times of inequity, economic deprivation and inadequacies in food preservation, transport and distribution; were dictated by production and availability of foods in that area. However, with the scenario fast changing and fruits of development reaching the common man and means of preservation, transport and public distribution improving; even the scarcely available and most perishable foods are becoming increasingly available over large distance and almost all the seasons.

Hence food availability is becoming a matter of choice then compulsion and lesser constraints on food availability front are making the task of a meal planner less cumbersome. However, in a population milieu comprising largely of poor and lower middle class, a delicate balance has to be maintained between availability, cost and nutritive value. Therefore factors like seasonal availability of foods must be given due consideration.

Seasonal Foods: Some foods from each food group are available in each season in almost every area. Inclusion of seasonal foods in the meal scheme scales down the cost of meal making and makes such foods easily available. Also, over indulgence in unseasonable foods (especially fruits and vegetables), calling them happy outcomes of scientific development and prosperity is also fraught with apprehensions for going against the grain of nature.

Economic Considerations

Nourishment through foods is fundamental need of life and to make the foods available a significant part of the family resources are earmarked for this purpose. If the allowance allocated for food is low, it is all the more important to plan meals with sagacity and care so that adequate nutrition is ensured for each member of the family in the meals. That also should have variety and choice. Many a time, if not always, in low income groups the food choice becomes further restricted to cereal foods only. This makes it imperative to supplement the cereal foods with other food factors indispensable for a balanced diet. This no doubt, presents a challenge for a food planner. Nevertheless it is not a Herculean task. By having a sound knowledge of less expensive foods having high nutritive values, one can well affect a low cost meal planning. Such foods include cereal, pulse combinations as in khichri, paushthik roti, sprouted grains, butter milk, pickles and chutney.

Meal Planning in Keeping with Seasons: During cold weathers in winters, it is advisable to include heavy foods like soups in the meal planning and the summer meals must include certain lighter foods. However, the nutrient composition of a meal should remain the same as per the requirements of the subject or the target group.

Religion, Traditions and Customs

Food habits differ in various groups having different religious beliefs, customs and tradition. Hence a meal planner must bear these facts in mind while planning meals for communities or groups having different religions, traditions and customs.

Spacing in the Meals

Fix meal times so that family can be together, whenever possible. Plan snacks to include nutrients that are low in other foods for the day. Be particular in using high-carbohydrate, high-calorie foods for snacks to compensate for shortfall in energy intake through regular meals for the day. Generally whole day's meal consists of breakfast, lunch, dinner and in between snacks.

Breakfast

Breakfast is the opening meal of the day. As its importance is not properly understood and often foods selected are inadequate in its nutrient supply. Children often skip breakfast either due to shortage of time or attitude towards food. Because of longer duration between dinner of the previous night and the breakfast, the following morning, the blood sugar level goes down in the morning. If we don't supplement food breakfast around this time, it may be reflected in learning behavior, primarily in terms of ability to concentrate. Those who have regular breakfast are more apt in remembering things and don't suffer from memory lapses. A good breakfast contains protein rich foods like eggs, cheese, milk, whole pulses, nuts and legumes. Cereal preparations like parantha/puri, plain or stuffed sandwiches, porridge etc. are generally included in breakfast. The breakfast items vary from place to place depending upon the food availability and food consumption pattern. Wheat or maize preparation are common in the northern part, where parantha, puri, rice flakes are the usual preparations. Whereas idli, dosa and sambhar vada are relished in the south. A good breakfast should provide 1/3rd of a day's requirement for protein and energy.

Omission of breakfast as a part of strategy for reducing weight is not a good method as greater hunger in addition to physiological inefficiency is scarcely conducive to good disposition and well-being throughout the day. A breakfast may be light or heavy depending upon the activity and performance of a person.

The type of menu in incorporating breakfast too should depend upon individual likes and dislikes, family food pattern, customs, habits etc.

Lunch

Lunch is often considered as a poor meal, especially for those who generally take lunch away from home. About 1/3rd of a day's requirement should be met by lunch meal. A good lunch must provide protein and protective foods apart from starchy or energy yielding foods. Lunch, whether served at home or packed and carried to the work place, or purchased there itself, should be planned or chosen with care and wisdom; for a fixed meal plan is difficult to draw and execute. Consistent neglect of this important meal may affect the individual's performance at work place, behavior with colleagues and attitude towards life. The lunch should be planned in relation to other needs so that it supplies a fair share of the day's nutrient through the food selected.

Dinner

Dinner is considered as the main meal of the day in many families, where all the family members collect together for their meals. Hence the meal is different in number and type of dishes. It should fulfil 1/3rd of a day's requirement for protein, energy, vitamins and minerals. In its true sense the items planned for dinner should not be heavy in nature as dinner being the last meal of the day is digested, absorbed and assimilated during the time when a person is invariably in a state of rest and asleep.

Snacks

Different types of snacks are available and consumed by the young and old in our country. They are often eaten in between the meals and they can fill up the gaps and makeup for the nutrient deficiency that may occur in a day's meal. A number of fried or roasted foods are consumed as snacks. Often, snack foods contain insufficient amounts of proteins, minerals and vitamins and hence it is a folly to become entirely dependent on them for such nutrient replenishments. The best snacks are those that add needed energy to the diet already complete in other nutrients, or alternatively, supply the nutrients that are low in other foods.

Qualities of a Good Snack

1. It should supply light nourishment that can be cut down or omitted in the regular meal.
2. Its caloric content should be such that by partaking it the subject does not exceed his energy requirements.
3. It should not be eaten close to regular meals or in quantity that spoils the appetite for the regular meal.
4. It should be appetising and invigorating.

MEAL PLANNING IN A NUTSHELL

It is necessary to plan on a monthly basis. There are five main steps in meal planning:

1. Make a list of foods from each food group, that are available in the market.
2. Check the prices and decide which of the foods from each group fit in the food budget on the basis of the family size, physiological states, occupation and income of family members.
3. Estimate the day's needs for all the family members on the basis of the daily food guide and calculate the month's food needs from it.
4. Make a list of foods to be purchased monthly, fortnightly, weekly and even daily.
5. Plan menus to meet the daily nutritional requirements of the family.

It is possible that some changes have to be made towards the end of the week to use up foods which may not have a good quality. Sometimes an additional guest may result in change of menu.

For the home maker to prepare nourishing foods, the meal plan should be made with economy of time and energy in view. Making a food list ahead of time helps in budgeting shopping time. Some dishes may be made ahead of time, e.g., making halwa or laddu a day before. The plan must be related to facilities available for food preparation. With time, some kind of standardization occurs in the meal plans of each family, which helps in efficient management of meals.

STUDY QUESTIONS

1. What do you understand by the terms 'Meal Planning'? What are the advantages of a good meal planning?
2. What are the main considerations that an efficient meal planner must make to plan economic, nutritious and varied meals?
3. How do you make use of the concept of adult consumption units (ACUs) for computing caloric requirements of families or groups with varied activities and different stages of development?

CHAPTER 15

Meal Planning for Various Life Stages

Chapter Outlines

- Pregnancy and lactation
- Developments in the prenatal period
- Changes in the maternal tissue
- Nutrition during pregnancy
- Guidelines for meal planning during pregnancy
- Physiological changes in lactation
- Nutrition for the nursing mother
- Guidelines for meal planning during lactation
- Nutrition in the first 6 to 8 months
- Premature and very small babies
- Nutrition for 1-3 years old children (Pre-schoolers)
- Meal planning for 1-3 years old children
- Meal planning for school age children
- Growth and nutrient needs during adolescence
- Guidelines for menu planning for adolescents
- Tips on meal planning for vegetarians
- Benefits of good nutrition and health habits for body functioning
- Tips for healthy nutrition in general
- Study questions

Since nutritional needs change in the different stages of human life cycle to ensure optimum nutrition, meal planning for various physiological groups representing different stages of the life span is done as to ensure optimum nutrition.

PREGNANCY AND LACTATION

Pregnancy and lactation impose stress on expectant and nursing mothers respectively and thus both of them belong to the vulnerable groups nutritionally and healthwise. Between conception and birth, the single cell in the form of fertilized egg grows and develops into a 2.5 to 3 kg human, capable of survival in the world. At no other time in the human life span, development proceeds so rapidly and thus requires large amount of energy and nutrients for the expectant mother carrying the developing foetus.

DEVELOPMENTS IN THE PRENATAL PERIOD

There are three distinct prenatal developmental stages. The first, *blastogenesis*, occupied the first two weeks following fertilization. The fertilized egg (zygote) immediately divides into two cells, each of which then divides into two more, and so on. The zygote soon becomes a cell-lined hollow sphere, the *blastula*. While cell division is taking place, cell enlargement does not occur because there is as yet no source of nourishment for the zygote, which remains the same in overall size as the original ovum despite the rapid division of cells. As the cells continue to divide, two layers are distinguished. The inner cell mass will become the *embryo*, and the outer "feeding" layer, or *trophoblast*, will differentiate to form the *placenta*. At this point the blastula becomes attached to the wall of the uterus. The trophoblast penetrates the uterine lining and absorbs material from the lining to provide the first nourishment for the new organism.

Meanwhile the inner cell mass segregates into two spherical forms, separated by a thin cellular disc. This disc will become the embryo itself; one of the spheres becomes a yolk sac (which in humans does not contain yolk) and the other becomes a fluid-filled sac, the amnion, which will provide a protective environment as well as nourishment for the embryo.

In the *embryonic stage* the embryonic disc begins to differentiate into three types of cells, the *germinal layers*. The *ectoderm*, or outermost layer of cells, will form the brain, nervous system, hair, skin, and sensory organs. The *mesoderm*, or middle layer, will provide the body's supporting structures–bone; muscle; connective tissue; and parts of the cardiovascular, excretory, and reproductive systems. The innermost layer, or *endoderm*, will form the lining of the respiratory, urinary, and digestive tracts. Sixty days (eight weeks) after fertilization the embryonic stage is completed.

With the start of the third month, the embryo is considered a *foetus*. The *foetal stage* of development, which continues until birth, is a time of rapid growth. The specialized cells continue to divide and now also begin to grow in size.

The information that guides this dramatic progression from blastocyst to newborn baby is programmed in the genetic material carried by the egg and the sperm. Apparently there is a different genetic timetable for the development of each body system, and each is vulnerable to nutritional insult. Each system–muscular, skeletal, circulatory, and so on–develops at its own particular rate. Research on laboratory animals, for example, indicates that severe restriction of maternal protein intake during a critical period of nervous system development causes the offspring's brain to have fewer than the normal number of cells. The same short-term nutritional deficiency that might affect the growth of the nervous system may have little effect on another body system that is not a critical stage (Table 15.1).

Table 15.1: Time course of foetal development

System	*Time from onset*	*Transformation*
1. Dental	4-6 months	Hard tissue of primary teeth
2. Nervous	0-9 months	Survival reflexes present at birth
3. Muscles	5-6 weeks	Development of nerve muscles attachments
	8 weeks	Involuntary muscles function
	16 weeks	Muscle movement become palpable
4. Skin	4-5 months	Fat deposition 0.5-6%
5. Eyes	7 weeks	Nerves, eyelids, lens
	10 weeks	Eyelids fused out
	7-8 weeks	Eyes open but not mature
6. Ears	4-8 weeks	Structure develops
	16 weeks	Assumes specific appearance
7. Cardiovascular	6 weeks	Heart, the first foetal organ formed
	2 months	Circulation developed
8. Respiratory	6 weeks	Trachea, bronchi, lung structure develops
	12 weeks	Lungs take shape
9. Digestive	8 weeks	Lip formation
	12 weeks	Plate formation
	5 months	Digestive juices
10. Excretory	7 weeks	Bladder and urethra separate
	16 weeks	Kidneys take final shape
11. Reproductive	6 weeks	Gonads appear
	7-9 weeks	Gonads differentiate

Contd.

Contd.

12. Skeletal	2-8 weeks 12 weeks	Skeleton formation Bone starts to replace cartilage
13. Weight gain (i) by the foetus (ii)* by placenta and amniotic fluid	12 weeks 13-27 weeks 28-40 weeks	5 g 600 g* 1500 g 6000 g* 3000 g 7000 g*
14. Total weight gain by the mother	12 weeks 13-27 weeks 28-40 weeks	650 g 8500 g 11500 g

Nutrient needs throughout the embryonic stage are so small that only severe malnutrition on the part of the mother could have a significant effect. Foetal nutrient requirement, in contrast, increase during pregnancy and are greatest during the last trimester, when expansion of both the size and the number of cells is greatest. Brain, eyes, ears, heart and lungs are formed in embryonic stage.

When severe nutritional deficiencies continue throughout the pregnancy, every body system is in some way affected. In various studies, pregnant animals placed an extremely restricted diets have produced offspring of low birth weight, reduced brain-cell number and head size, and proportionate reductions in the size of various body organs.

Though it is unethical to perform deprivation experiments on pregnant women, yet specific data for nutritional needs in human pregnancy have accumulated as a result of studies involving natural and or accidental disruptions to population's food supply. The resulting data corroborate the results of animal studies: Severe nutritional defects early in the prenatal existence increase foetal mortality rates and affect physiological development; in the later months of pregnancy the primary effect is significantly to decrease overall growth and birth weight. Similarly, autopsies of stillborn infants have shown that those from low-income families were smaller in overall size and had smaller livers, adrenal glands, and other organs than those from higher-income and presumably better-nourished families.

Even microscopic examination of placental tissues has shown that infants who experienced prenatal growth failure, or are from low-income populations, had placentas of smaller size and fewer cells than those who were better nourished.

During blastogenesis and after, the embryo and placenta develop simultaneously. After implantation in the uterine wall, part of the embryonic mesoderm attaches as a lining to the trophoblast to become the *chorion*. The chorion sends numerous projections into the uterine lining, and from these develop the network of blood vessels that constitutes the foetal part of the placenta. These chorionic villi function in much the same way as the intestinal villi, providing the extensive surface area needed for nutrient transfer. While the embryonic portion of the placenta is being formed, the mother' body is responding. Glands and blood vessels within the uterine lining develop, and muscle fibers increase in size and strength (Fig. 15.1).

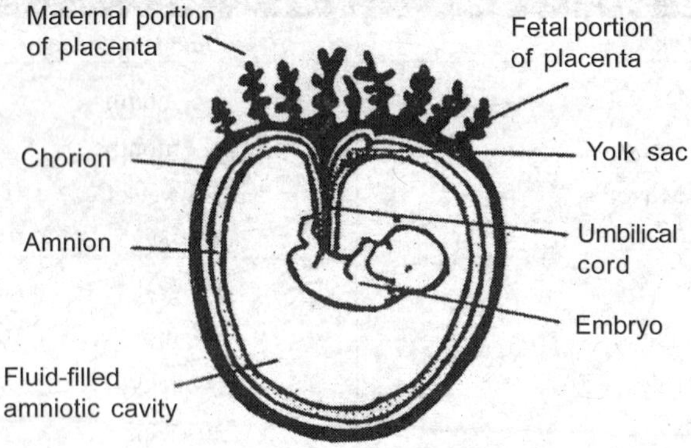

Fig. 15.1

Exchanges of nutrients and wastes take place in the placental as they do in the gastrointestinal tract: By passive transport, facilitated diffusion, and active transport across placenta membranes. Oxygen and nutrients pass from the mother to the foetus; carbon dioxide and metabolic wastes pass in the opposite direction, to be eliminated by the mother's body. What makes these transfers so complex is the involvement of two separate blood supplies–one from the mother and the other from the foetus.

There is no exchange of blood between the two, only an exchange of nutrients from one blood compartment to another. Maternal hemoglobin levels are vital to maintain the oxygen exchange system. Because 1.34 milliliters of oxygen are carried by each gram of haemoglobin, it is important for the mother to avoid iron deficiency, which would depress her haemoglobin levels and could possibly reduce the supply of oxygen available to her developing child.

Water and the fat-soluble vitamins diffuse to the foetal circulation. Amino acids, glucose, water-soluble vitamins, and such minerals as calcium, sodium, and iron are actively transported. The placental membranes have, at any one time, a limited carrying capacity for actively transported materials, and it is possible that excessive intakes of water-soluble vitamins (such as ascorbic acid) on the part of the mother may compete with transport of essential amino acids and impair growth and development. Placental membranes also ensure that nutrients needed by the foetus in higher concentrations than the mother requires, will not rush back into the mother's bloodstream.

Except for specific maternal antibody which is structurally able to penetrate and which provides important resistance to infection that lasts until six or more months after birth protein molecules do not cross the placenta, since they are too large to penetrate the cells of the placental villi. The foetus must synthesize its own proteins from the amino acids it receives from the maternal circulation.

In addition to serving as the conduit for these exchanges, the placenta supplements the mother's hormone production, becoming the primary source of progesterone and estrogen and the sole source of several hormones normally produced only during gestation: human chorionic gonadotrophin (HCG), human placental lactogen (HPL), human chorionic somatomammotrophin (HCS), and human chorionic thyrotrophin (HCT). Although much of this hormone production is stimulated by biochemical precursors produced by the foetus, the gestational hormones act primarily to regulate the mother's pregnancy and postpartum progress.

CHANGES IN THE MATERNAL TISSUE

The normal physiological adjustment process of pregnancy causes a number of changes in the mother's body, many of which are mediated by hormones. The more than 30 hormones secreted during gestation include some that are present only during that time and other, normally present, whose rates of secretion are altered. They are proteins or steroids that are synthesized from amino acid and cholesterol precursors in endocrine glands throughout the body. Those hormones with the most far-reaching effects are progesterone and estrogen, both of which are present in increased supply.

Progesterone, which acts on smooth-muscle tissue to produce relaxation, allows the uterus to expand as the foetus grows. Gastrointestinal muscles relax as well, slowing intestinal motility, with the obvious benefit to the foetus of additional absorption time and consequent increases in serum nutrient levels. Unfortunately, maternal constipation is often a side effect.

Progesterone also enhances fat storage, especially in the back, thighs and abdomen, with smaller amount deposited in mammary tissue. Generally increased fat storage throughout the body is not only physically protective of the foetus but also provides a potential energy reserve. Progesterone also heightens respiratory sensitivity, leading to hyperventilation, thus increasing the energy and oxygen supply available to the foetus and increasing the capacity to expire carbon dioxide.

Estrogen aids in expanding the uterus. By acting on components of connective tissue, it causes these tissues to become flexible enough to accommodate the shifts of bones and organs as they are displaced by the growing foetus and makes possible dilation at birth. But this same biochemical reaction also enhances fluid retention in connective tissue, which is common in pregnancy. At the same time, progesterone has a sodium-depleting effect. However, unless water retention is associated with hypertension and proteinuria (protein in the urine), there is no cause for concern. Normal fluid retention in pregnancy may even provide some benefits in parturition.

Other hormones have strictly metabolic effects. Thyroxine production is increased and, by a complex series of reactions, results in increasing maternal appetite as well as speeding the rate of breathing to provide additional oxygen for energy production from ingested food. As pregnancy progresses, the action of insulin becomes less efficient. Normally, this is not a problem, but in a diabetic or prediabetic mother, the output of insulin may be so low that glucose metabolism is impaired, with potentially serious effects for both foetus and mother. Cortisone, which is involved in the maintenance of blood glucose levels by stimulating gluconeogenesis from amino acids, is produced in greater amounts during the final days of pregnancy in response to increased estrogen production.

Other changes during pregnancy involve both blood volume and composition and kidney function. Expansion of maternal blood volume facilitates the transport of nutrients and metabolic wastes between mother and foetus. The highest plasma volume is reached at 34 to 36 weeks, when the mother's body contains 50 percent more plasma than when fertilization took place. As a result of this increase, the concentrations of many constituents in the blood (protein, water-soluble vitamins, minerals) are somewhat diminished. Kidney function is altered to accommodate the greater blood volume and increased amount of waste products. More blood flows through the kidneys, and the glomerular filtration rate is increased. There is, however, no related increase in the reabsorptive capacity of the kidney tubules, and as a result, substantial quantities of some water-soluble nutrients are flushed out of the mother's body along with normal metabolic wastes.

NUTRITION DURING PREGNANCY

(I) A women who is in a good stage of nourishment and therefore has enough reserves of nutrients will be able to meet the demands for nutrients of the baby growing within her. If she also continues to take nourishing food during her pregnancy, her own reserves also will not be used up. A good nutritional level will also minimize the risk of childbirth, and ensure a healthier baby. A pregnant woman gains about 11-12 kg in weight during pregnancy. Forty percent of this is due to the weight of the child placenta and amniotic fluid. Thus it is not far from reality to say that she has really to eat for two, for herself and for her child. If she does not do so, nutrients from her own body will be drawn upon and she is liable to develop anaemia, weakened bones (shown for example in bent legs) and vitamin A and B-group deficiency conditions. Thus it is obvious that she needs extra calories and extra protein. This is especially true if the pregnant women is working, or has to look after an already large family, since she will then have to do plenty of physical work and spend much energy on it. Several vitamins also are needed in greater amounts. More calcium is needed to form the bone and teeth of the child, and thus must come from taking more milk, fish, ragi, green leafy vegetables and dals. Iron is heavily drawn upon by the baby to make blood. It is also most important to build up the mother's iron reserves: a baby must be born with good iron stores, because mother's milk (which is the main food that it will get for several months) does not in any case carry much iron. Lacking iron reserves, many Indian babies soon become anaemic. Foods rich in iron which the pregnant women could take regularly are green leafy vegetables, bajra and ragi (most other cereals are poor in iron). Iron pills are also very effective in treating the anaemias of pregnancy.

(II) Folic acid and vitamin B_{12} are also especially important during pregnancy, and again it is perhaps simpler to rely on pills to provide them if one cannot afford to get them by buying a variety of natural foods. The other vitamins of the B-groups (thiamine, riboflavin and niacin) are needed in extra quantity; green leafy vegetables, groundnuts and dals can provide them. Vitamin C in the form of lemon juice, orange juice or amla, taken in the mornings, will help to overcome the nausea of pregnancy. Since eating large meals is difficult, the pregnant woman should train herself to eat frequently, and especially to take nutritious snacks containing the desirable foodstuffs between her regular meal times. Snacks made from combinations of these foodstuffs are especially useful, and some of these are listed in Table 15.2. She should also drink a lot of water so that the foods she eats are fully digested and utilised.

(III) While the placenta is capable of synthesizing some nutrients, such as glycogen and cholesterol, most nutrients are brought to the foetus by the mother's blood. If a nutrient is missing from her bloodstream, foetal development may be compromised. For example, if the amino acids needed for brain development are absent, brain growth is not normal.

Maternal malnourishment is a major cause of low birth weight. Babies who weigh less than 2.5 kg at birth are 10 times more likely to be mentally impaired than babies with normal weight and have a much higher risk of illness and death. It's up to the mother to provide the best possible environment for the body developing in her womb. The following are some of the nutrients considered especially vital to the growth of the foetus and the physiological changes occurring in the pregnant woman.

(IV) Nutrients that are Important in Pregnancy

Protein

Amino acids are the stuff of which life is made. Daily protein requirements increase during pregnancy. Pregnant women are advised to consume at least three servings of protein foods daily, in addition to their four servings of milk.

Iron

Both the foetus and the mother need iron to make red blood cells. Since it is almost impossible to obtain the iron required during pregnancy from food alone, iron is a recommended prenatal supplement.

Folic Acid

Folic acid is a vitamin required for cell division and development of the foetal nervous system. Research has shown that women who receive extra folic acid a month before conception and for the first few months of foetal development have a much lower risk of giving birth to a baby with neural tube defects such as spinal bifida. Because of its importance, folic acid is another recommended prenatal supplement.

(V) Calcium

Calcium is needed for the growth of bones and teeth. Blood calcium level is regulated by a number of hormones. So its level remains fairly constant. If dietary calcium is insufficient, calcium will be released from the mother's bones. That's why a woman is advised to consume four servings of milk and dairy products daily during pregnancy. Women who don't like milk should learn to disguise it in custards and milk-based soups. Prospective mothers, especially those who are still growing themselves, need not less than six milk servings per day.

Fiber

Although not considered a nutrient, an adequate intake of fiber is important during pregnancy to prevent constipation, which typically increases due to the action of progesterone, which relaxes smooth muscle, and compression of the colon by the growing uterus. Iron supplements, often prescribed during pregnancy, frequently contribute to constipation.

Fluids

As metabolic rate and blood volume increase, so does a woman's need for fluids. Six to eight glasses daily are recommended. Fluid intake should be even greater in hot environments and if the pregnant woman is exercising.

GUIDELINES FOR MEAL PLANNING DURING PREGNANCY

Guidelines to be used when planning menus for pregnant women:

1. Offer a varied and balanced selection of nutrient-dense foods. With such an increased need for so many nutrients, empty calories (fat, sugar and alcohol) are rarely an acceptable choice.
2. Though meat can be good protein source for non-vegetarians, vegetarians should include legumes and grains. Beans, peas, rice, and cheese should also be included in the menu.
3. Be sure to offer milk and other dairy products.
4. Use a variety of whole-grain and enriched breads, rolls, cereals, rice and other grain in menus.
5. Use assorted fruits and vegetables in all areas of the menu, including salads and desserts.
6. Be sure to have good sources of problem nutrients: Fiber, folacin, iron, vitamin B_6, and zinc (*See* Table 15.2).
7. Be sure to use iodized salt.
8. Be aware of diet-related changes and complaints during pregnancy.

The following complaints are common during pregnancy:

- Nausea and vomiting, commonly referred to as morning sickness (it can occur at any time of day), is due to hormonal changes and perhaps tension and anxiety. Generally mild and limited to early pregnancy, it is best controlled by eating small, frequent, carbohydrate-rich meals and by limiting drinking between meals. Women who feel nauseous do not enjoy the smell of cooking food.

Table 15.2: Problem nutrients during pregnancy and their sources

Nutrient	*Food sources*
Fiber	Bran, dried beans and peas, whole-grain breads and cereals, fruits and vegetables, nuts, seeds.
Folic acid	Organ meats, liver, legumes, dark green leafy vegetable, whole-wheat breads and cereals.
Iron	Red meat, liver, shellfish, poultry, dried fruit, beans, nuts, whole-grain and enriched breads and cereals.
Vitamin B_6	Green leafy vegetables, meats, poultry, fish, liver, legumes.
Zinc	Red meat, liver, poultry, fish, legumes.

- Pregnant women commonly report changes in taste and smell. They prefer foods saltier than previously and crave sweets and dairy products such as ice cream. They may have aversions to include caffeinated drinks, and meats in their diet. Their cravings and aversions do not necessarily reflect actual physiological needs.
- Constipation is not uncommon, due in part to the gastrointestinal tract slowing down and relaxing. It can be counteracted with increased fiber, fluid and exercise.
- Heartburn is a common complaint because of the growing uterus crowding the stomach. Also, the muscle that control the passage of food from the throat into the stomach relax, causing the acidic stomach contents to be regurgitated back into the throat. This condition is called heartburn, even though it has nothing to do with the heart. Possible solutions include eating small and frequent meals, eating slowly and in a relaxed atmosphere, avoiding caffeine, and not lying down after eating.

PHYSIOLOGICAL CHANGES IN LACTATION

The nine months of pregnancy are the prelude not only to childbirth but also to the nutritionally important period of lactation. The umbilical cord may be cut, but the nurturing bond between mother and child is not severed. A new system is ready to take over the lactating breast.

Many of the physiological changes occurring in the mother during pregnancy are preparation for lactation. During the first and second trimester, terminal tubules connected to the mammary milk ducts proliferate and group together to form what are known as lobules, or acinar structures, in which milk will be produced (*See* Fig. 15.2). Whether the breast is large or small, it will contain from 15 to 20 of these ducts, which connect the milk-producing centers to the nipples from which milk will be released. This is all the "equipment" that is required for successful nursing. Neither breast size nor shape has any influence on the ability of women to nurse. Almost all women who want to do breast feeding on infants; the focus should be on the development of the capability for lactation.

Microscopic studies of breast tissue have shown that the milk is produced in secretory (alveolar) cells which synthesize lactose, the predominant carbohydrate in milk. Progesterone, the primary pregnancy hormone, inhibits lactose production, thereby preventing significant milk accumulation during pregnancy. After birth however, progesterone levels fall; levels of prolactin, the lactation hormone, rise; and the mammary alveolar cells go into full operation for milk secretion. Prolactin is released by the hypothalamus in response to suckling by the infant. Suckling also stimulates production of oxytocin from the posterior pituitary gland. Circulation of oxytocin causes the muscle like cells in the breast to contract, which propels milk through the ducts for release through the nipple (Figs. 15.2 and 15.3).

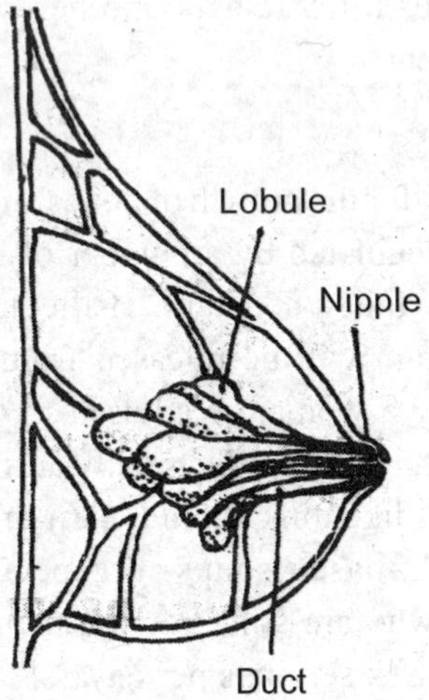

Fig. 15.2: Changes in the mammary gland in pregnancy

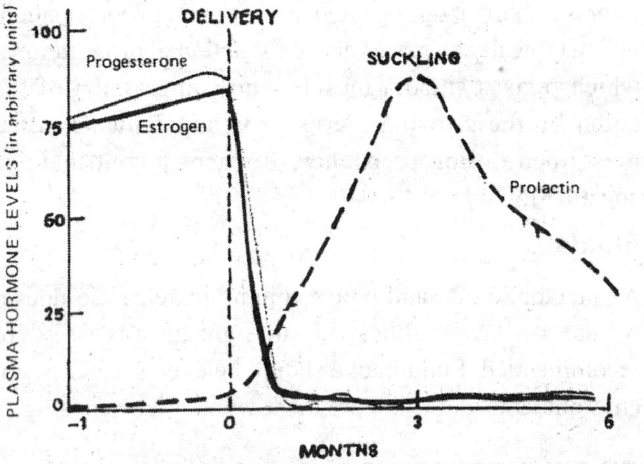

Fig. 15.3: Secretion of hormones before and after parturition (delivery)

In addition to lactose, three major milk proteins are synthesized by the alveolar cells: α-lactalbumin, β-lactalbumin and casein. Most of the amino acids contained in these proteins are taken up directly from the mother's plasma, although some of the non-essential amino acids are synthesized in the alveolar cells. Full lactation does not occur instantly at birth. For the first few days colostrom is secreted. Colostrom has slightly different concentrations of several nutrients than are present in mature milk.

NUTRITION FOR THE NURSING MOTHER

Pregnancy lasts for just nine months, but the duration thereafter of nursing a baby in India is often ever longer, and during this extended period a steady stream of nutrients in the form of breast milk is being put out by the mother and taken in by the hungry child. If the mother does not herself make up these nutrients from her food, to meet both her own needs and the extra quantities required to make breast milk, it is obvious that she will soon become drained of nutrients, and turn weak and exhausted. Many Indian mothers lose weight when nursing their babies, a sure sign that their food intake is not sufficient both in quantity and quality.

Proteins, calcium, phosphorus and iron are found to be present at a high level in mother's milk simply by drawing upon the stock in the mother's body. Significant amounts of mother's skeletal calcium are mobilized to provide 250-300 mg of calcium in the breast milk per day. What is even more remarkable is the germ free nature of the mother's milk.

However, all the nutrients cannot be drawn from the mother's body. If the mother's food does not contain some of them, the milk will also be poor in these and the child in turn will suffer. It has been found that levels of vitamin A, riboflavin, thiamine and vitamin C are all low in the breast milk of poor Indian mother because of her own poor intake.

In fact, when the mother starts to nurse, the new mother has about 2 to 4 kilograms of new fat stores deposited during pregnancy, which serve as a kind of back-up energy supply. These fat stores may be mobilized to provide approximately 200 to 300 kcal per day for about three months. It has been calculated that because human breast milk contains approximately 70 kcal/100 ml, and maternal efficiency in converting stored energy is at least 80 percent, the mother will need approximately 90 additional kcal for every 100 ml of milk she must produce. Thus, for 550 ml of milk, the average amount produced each day after lactation is established, the nursing mother needs nearly 600-650 kcal above her normal daily requirements. With 200 to 300 kcal available from existing fat stores, at least for the first three months, that will mean an additional 350-400 kcal per day that must be provided by the diet, or 200 kcal more than that during pregnancy. If lactation continues beyond three months, energy intake must be increased by an additional 200 to 300 kcal per day.

Even in countries like India where protein-energy malnutrition is common, however, protein levels in milk are not reduced, although total milk volume may be greatly diminished. The protein content of human milk remains remarkably constant despite the variations in maternal food intakes, leading to the conclusion that the essential amino acids are supplied from maternal stores if they are lacking in the mother's diet.

Breast milk also contains significant amounts of fat, mostly in the form of triglycerides but also including small amount of phospholipids, cholesterol, and free fatty acids. The levels of all lipids except fatty acids in breast milk appear to be independent of levels in the maternal bloodstream. Like carbohydrate and protein, the lipid content of breast milk is maintained even at the expense of maternal stores. It also contains fat soluble vitamins A and E and small amount if vitamin D, calcium, iron copper and other minerals.

Some general guidelines have been established regarding dietary allowances. The quality of the diet should be similar to that consumed during pregnancy, with additional energy intake to maintain lactation. At least half to one litre of milk, or its equivalent, should be consumed every day, either as a beverage or incorporated into other foods. High-quality protein and liberal amounts of fruits, vegetables, and grain products will ensure adequate provision of essential amino acids, vitamins, and minerals. Fluid intake is important; nursing women should consume 2 to 3 litre of fluid per day. Supplementation practices should parallel those that are necessary during pregnancy, especially for strict vegetarians. Iron supplementation should be continued for several months for all women to replenish maternal iron reserves which are usually depleted during pregnancy.

The nursing mother needs no special foods and need avoid no foods. Increased amount of food are needed, however, to provide the energy, protein, calcium and other nutrients that must be used for the infant's milk supply and the iron to replenish the mother's own depleted reserves. Energy intake should be monitored by the mother's weight status; as the baby grows older and is gradually weaned to other foods, less milk output will be there, and the amount of energy the mother needs will decline. Unless the mother decreases her own energy intake, she will have an undesirable weight gain.

So good and nourishing extra food eaten at frequent intervals in the form of snacks, is required to provide calories, proteins, vitamins and minerals. These snacks should include foodstuffs like milk, curd, dals, boiled or roasted groundnuts, animal foods like eggs, meat and fish, green leafy vegetables, and cereals like bajra and ragi, all cooked in appetising ways; some combinations are shown in Table 15.3. Plenty of water should be drunk.

Table 15.3: Combination foods providing nutrient variety during pregnancy and lactation

Dish	*Foodstuffs used*	*Improvement possible*
	Northern Region	
Khicheri	Rice, til seed, bajra, sugar	Sprout the bajra; use Bengal gram; use vegetables, serve with curd
Stuffed paranthas	Wheat flour, potatoes, cauliflower	Add dhal powder or roasted groundnut powder to wheat flour; use cooked green leafy vegetables
Bhajis	Bengal gram flour, mixed vegetables	Sprout the Bengal gram, add boiled and roasted green leafy vegetables to the stuffing
	Southern Region	
Idli	Rice urad dhal	Use some Bengal gram powder; add a pinch of lime powder
Dosa	Broken rice, urad dhal	Use green leafy vegetables and other vegetables
Dahi vada	Rice, urad dhal, curd	Sprout the urad dhal; add a pinch of lime
Ragi puttu	Ragi	Use tuvar dhal powder or Bengal gram powder with the ragi
Sambhar rice	Rice, tuvar dhal	Add ragi of cracked wheat to rice; sprout the dhal; add a pinch of lime powder
	Eastern Region	
Ragi dosa	Ragi, wheat flour, curd	Sprout the ragi; use some sprouted tuvar dhal powder
Leto	Ragi, rice, dhal	Sprout the ragi; sprout the dhal; use mixed dhals
Puran poli	Wheat flour, Bengal gram, jaggery, coconut	Use some sprouted ragi powder; sprout the gram
	Western Region	
Dhokla	Cracked wheat masoor dhal	Use some sprouted ragi; sprout the dhal; use dhal combinations; use green leafy vegetables; add a pinch of lime powder
Debra roti	Wheat flour, dhal	—do—
Khicheri	Rice, dhal	Sprout the dhal
Sheera (savoury)	Rava, groundnuts	Use sprouted dhals, green leafy vegetables and other vegetables

GUIDELINES FOR MEAL PLANNING DURING LACTATION

By and large menu planning for lactation remains the same as for pregnancy except for consideration of the facts given below (Table 15.4 and Fig. 15.4):

Table 15.4: A balanced vegetarian diet for a nursing mother doing sedentary work

S.No.	*Food group*	*Quantity in g*
1.	Cereal and millets	330
2.	Pulses	90
3.	Milk (ml)	500
4.	Roots and tubers	100
5.	Green leafy vegetables	150
6.	Other vegetables	100
7.	Fruits	200
8.	Sugar	20
9.	Fats and oils	30

For non-veg substitute 30 g of pulse with 50 g of meat/fish/chicken/egg.

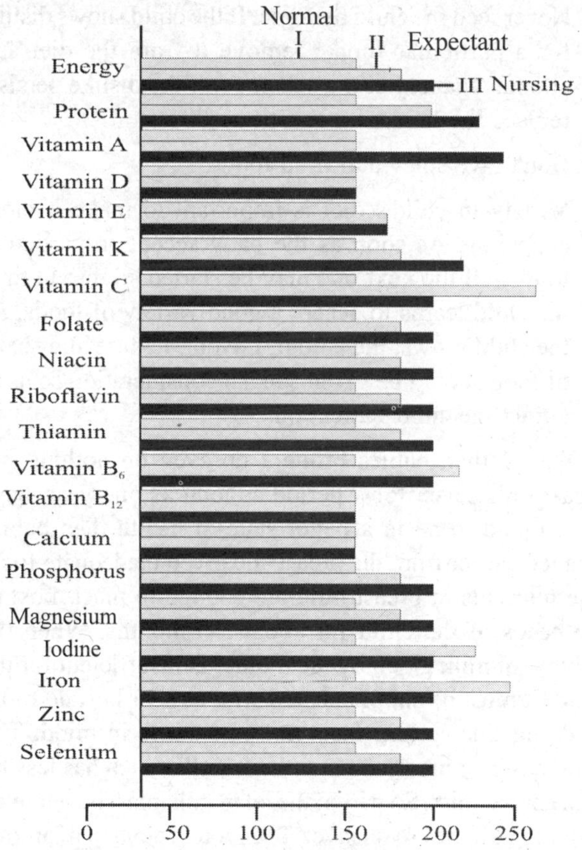

Fig. 15.4: RDA comparison of normal adult woman, expectant and nursing mothers

1. Protein requirement reaches an all time high of about 70 g per day as compared to 60 g per day in case of an expectant mother (normal adult Indian woman requires 45 g per day).
2. RDA for calories increase by 400 to 600 calories over expectant mother and 700-900 calories over normal adult woman.
3. Whereas there is no increase in calcium iron, and vitamin C requirement over expectant mother, an increase in vitamin A and B complex vitamins, especially riboflavin and niacine, as they are secreted in milk.
4. Intake of fluids (water and beverage such as juices, tea and coffee) is increased to make up for the fluids secreated in milk.

NUTRITION IN THE FIRST 6 TO 8 MONTHS

The nutrient needs of a newborn are actually higher than those for an adult when looked at in proportion to their weights. Newborns need a plentiful supply of all nutrients, and nutrients used in growth, such as vitamin D, folic acid, vitamin B_{12}, calcium, and iron are of particular importance. The newborn has one source of nutrients during the first 4 to 6 months of life: Either breast milk or formula milk. But breast milk is considered to be nutritionally superior to formula milk howsoever hard the manufactures may try to mimic human milk (Tables 15.5 to 15.8).

Table 15.5: Immunization schedule

Age	*Vaccine*
Soon after birth	BCG, Hepatitis B 1st dose, OPV 1st dose
6 weeks	Hepatitis B 2nd dose
	DPT 1st dose
	OPV 2nd dose
10 weeks	DPT 2nd dose
	OPV 2nd dose
14 weeks	DPT 3rd dose
	OPV 4th dose
6 months	OPV 5th dose
	Hepatitis B 3rd dose
9 months	Measles
15 to 18 months	MMR
18 months	DPT, OPV 1st Booster
2 years	Typhoid vaccine
5 years	DPT, OPV 2nd Booster

Table 15.6: ICMR recommended dietary allowances for infants

Nutrients	*0-6 months*	*6-12 months*
Energy (k cal)	108/kg	98/kg
Protein (gm)	2.05/kg	1.65 kg
Calcium (mg)	500	500
Vitamin A		
Retional (μg) or	350	350
B carotene (μg)	1200	1200
Thiamine (μg)	55/kg	50/kg
Riboflavin (μg)	65/kg	60/kg
Niacin (μg)	710/kg	650/kg
Pyridoxine (mg)	0.1	0.4
Ascorbic acid (mg)	25	25
Folic acid (μg)	25	25
Vitamin B_{12} (μg)	0.2	0.2

Table 15.7: ICMR recommended dietary allowance of preschool children

Nutrient	*Age (in years)*	
	1-3	4-6
Energy (k cal)	1240	1690
Protein (g)	22	30
Fat (g)	25	25
Calcium (mg)	400	400
Iron (mg)	12	18
Vitamin A		
Retional (μg) or	400	400
β carotene (μg)	1600	1600
Thiamine (mg)	0.6	0.9
Riboflavin (mg)	0.7	1.0
Niacin (mg)	8	11
Vitamin C (mg)	40	40
Pyridoxine (mg)	0.9	0.9
Folic acid (μg)	30	40
Vitamin B_{12} (μg)	0.2-1	0.2-1

Table 15.8: Balanced diet for infants (6-12 months)

S.No.	*Food groups*	*Quantity (gm)*
1.	Cereals and millets	45
2.	Pulses	15
3.	Milk (ml)	500*
4.	Roots and tubers	50
5.	Green leafy vegetables	25
6.	Other vegetables	25
7.	Fruits	100
8.	Sugar	25
9.	Fats/oils (visible)	10

* Quantity indicates milk apart from breast milk. For breast fed infants 200 ml is required.

Source: *Dietary Guidelines for Indians–A Manual,* National Institute of Nutrition, ICMR, Hyderabad, India, 1999.

In short the breast milk has following nutritional superiorities over the formula based feeding.

1. Newborn are mostly not allergic to breast milk but they often manifest symptoms of allergy to formula based diets.
2. Suckling promotes the development of the infant's jaws and teeth.
3. A close relationship, a sublime bonding develops between the mother and the child through breast feeding.
4. Breast milk develops immunity in the infant against disease.
5. It is easy to digest and assimilate.
6. It is totally hygienic.

Important in Weaning:

1. Introduce a single food at a time.
2. Begin with small quantities of food and increase the amount gradually as the child develops a liking for it.
3. Never feed the child by force. If the child shows dislike for a particular food, remove it from the diet and attempt again after a week or so. If the dislike persists replace the food by a substitute.
4. Don't give spicy and fried foods.
5. Variety in child's diet is important to make it more appealing. As soon as the baby accepts a particular food well the next one may be started so that in time the child learns to accept a good variety of foods. As the child grows, the colour, flavour, texture and shape of food should be given special consideration so as to attract the child's attention.

Thus Indian babies brought up even on nothing but breast milk, even for a period as long as one year, have been found to be in a better state of health than babies weaned earlier from the breast and given inadequate food. The nutrients in breast milk are enough to meet most of the needs of the child for about 3-6 months. When the volume of milk given by the mother is insufficient for the child, it must be supplemented with cow or buffalo milk. In doing this certain facts must be borne in mind. The child has become used to mother's milk which has less fat than animal milk. So part of the fat in milk must be removed by taking off the cream layer. The protein content of animal milk is also higher, and the sugar content lower, than in mother's milk. Hence the milk must be diluted with an equal amount of water and some sugar added to it. As the child grows older, buffalo or cow milk can gradually be given with less and less of such defatting and dilution.

A child needs plenty of boiled water. If not given adequate water, the nutrients which it gets will not be properly digested and fully utilised. In the first month of life, a child must be given as much as 200 ml of water every day (Tables 15.9 to 15.19).

Sometimes cow or buffalo milk in the quantities needed by child is suitable yet costly to buy for weaker sections. Useful milky liquids for feeding children can be made from groundnuts, coconut pieces or soyabeans. These vegetable milks resemble cow's milk in composition, and can be treated in the same way, for example by removing fat, diluting and adding sugar, when given to young babies.

While both breast milk of a well-nourished mother, and cow or buffalo milk, are all excellent foods, there are a few nutrients in which they are naturally somewhat deficient. These nutrients are all the more likely to be short in breast milk if the mother's diet is not a balanced one and itself lacks the nutrients.

The four nutrients are iron, vitamin C, vitamin A and vitamin D. For this reason, soups made from vegetables or drumstick leaves, juices of fruits, certain soft vegetables like yellow pumpkins, and shark liver oil are all very desirable foods even for a 2-3 months old baby, and should be included in the diet. Tables 15.9 and 15.10 given an account of the energy protein and foodstuff requirements of infants and children and Table 15.11 gives the sample details of an infant's feeding schedule.

Table 15.9: Energy and protein requirements for children: Birth to 6 years (per kg)

Age group	*Energy (kcal per kg)*	*Protein (grams per kg)*
0 to 6 months	108	2.0*
6 to 12 months	98	1.65*
	Daily requirements	
	Energy (kcal)	*Protein (g)*
6 months to 1 year	800-1000	13-17*
1 to 3 years	1240	22*
4 to 6 years	1690	30**

* In terms of milk protein alone.

** In terms of mixed vegetable protein of NPU (Net protein utilisation) 65 relative to egg.

Table 15.10: Energy requirement of children (by age)

Age (years)	*Boys*	*Girls*
1+	1096	1078
2+	1301	1190
3+	1463	1310
4+	1531	1458
6+	1778	1643

Table 15.11

6-9 months (weight upto 9 kg)

(a) Milk upto 450 ml a day.

(b) Porridges made from boiled rice, wheat, ragi or bajra with milk and sugar.

(c) Mashed boiled vegetables as described earlier, or boiled dhal; especially moong.

(d) Soft foods like pieces of bread, chapattis, etc.

(e) One whole egg, boiled or scrambled.

(f) Thoroughly-cooked and mashed meat and fish.

(g) Small pieces of various soft fruits.

(h) Plenty of boiled water.

9-12 months (weight upto 11 kg)

(a) Milk (400 ml a day).

(b) All the above foods in gradually increasing amounts and in more adult forms, such as small pieces of cooked vegetables or cooked meat.

(c) Hard foods to provide exercise for the new teeth and the gums, like a piece of toast, or a slice of raw carrot.

As much as 200 ml of water every day.

As the child grows slightly older, it requires a greater quantity of nutrients. Alongside, the volume of breast milk is also likely to be falling. The baby's teeth are growing and its body is beginning to manufacture the enzymes required for digestion. So a wider diversity of foods, rich in both major and minor nutrients, should be served in increasingly solid forms. Such food include mashed and cooked green leafy vegetables, ripe fruit, well-cooked eggs, meat and fish (first in the form of soups and later as small shreds), semi-solid porridges consisting of well-cooked cereals and dhals, and so on.

The change-over from mother's milk to other foods, first partly and then fully, is known as weaning. As we have seen, it should not be delayed too long lest the child's health will suffer. Nutritionally, it is a fairly crucial step. Mother's milk has a good level of nutrients. Cow or buffalo milk has even higher protein and fat level than breast milk and so the child's nutrient intake level has already gone up. In India when the changeover to solid food is made, either through animal milk or direct from the breast milk, the child quite often is just given boiled rice or wheat. This kills its hunger, but since the food is insufficient in proteins, vitamins and minerals, there is a sharp drop in the quantity of nutrients which the child is getting at a time when it is growing and needs more of them. There is need to let this not happen. Even using common ingredients like dhals, groundnut and jaggery along with rice, wheat and bajra, food of high quality can be devised. A number of low-cost weaning recipes for children 6-12 months old, suitable for use in various parts of the country, have been developed by the National Institute of Nutrition (NIN) Hyderabad. They are shown in Table 15.12.

Table 15.12: Recipes for babies 6-12 months old

Each recipe gives 500-550 calories and 15-20 grams of protein. This is half the nutritional requirement of the baby. The rest is expected to be supplied by breast milk or other milk.	
Northern Region	
1. *Chidwa kheer*	
Rice flakes 40 g	a. Soak rice flakes in water for a new minutes
Bengal gram 50 g	b. Boil Bengal gram till soft and mash
Banana 25 g	c. Mash banana and add to the dhal
Jaggery 50 g	d. Mix all the above thoroughly
2. *Meethi dhal*	
Rice 30 g	a. Roast and powder rice
Masoor dhal 60 g	b. Roast and powder masoor dhal
Palak 30 g	c. Boil palak, mash and strain through sieve
Jaggery 60 g	d. Dissolve jaggery in water and strain
	e. Mix all items to a smooth paste and boil for a few minutes
3. *Seera*	
Wheat flour 60 g	a. Roast wheat flour and cook in water
Roasted groundnuts 30 g	b. Powder roasted groundnuts
Jaggery 50 g	c. Make a paste of above with the jaggery syrup and cook for new minutes
4. *Dalia*	
Broken wheat 45 g	a. Roast wheat flour
Moong dhal 45 g	b. Roast moong dhal
Jaggery 60 g	c. Make a paste of above with the jaggery syrup and cook for a few minutes
Southern Region	
1. *Keerai pongal*	
Rice 50 g	a. Roast rice and powder
Moong dhal 50 g	b. Roast moong dhal and powder
Keerai	c. Boil keerai and strain to a pulp
(amaranth) 5 g	d. Mix all the above, add boiling water and salt and cook for a few minutes till semisolid
Oil 10 g	
Salt to taste	
Jeera to taste	e. Fry jeera in oil and add to pongal
2. *Masoor payasam*	
Masoor dhal 40 g	a. Boil masoor dhal and mash thoroughly
Wheat flour 50 g	b. Roast wheat flour
Pasalai keerai 20 g	c. Boil keerai, strain to a pulp
Jaggery 40 g	d. Dissolve jaggery in water and strain
	e. Mix all the above and break up any lumps
	f. Cook for a few minutes

Contd.

Contd.

3. *Ragi porridge* Ragi 30 g Roasted Bengal gram 50 g Keerai 30 g Jaggery 50 g	a. Malt the ragi first soak overnight in water, spread grains on a plate, and cover with a damp cloth for 2-3 days to germinate. Dry in the sun, roast to a pleasant smell, and store in an air-tight tin b. Boil keerai, strain to a pulp c. Mix ragi malt with powdered, roasted Bengal gram and keerai pulp d. Add water, cook for a short time e. Dissolve jaggery in water; strain and add to the mixture
Eastern Region	
1. *Mishti chira* Beaten rice 50 g Groundnuts 40 g Jaggery 50 g	a. Soak beaten rice in water and mash b. Roast groundnuts, powder add to the rice c. Make a jaggery syrup d. Mix powder and syrup, cook with stirring for a few minutes till semi-solid
2. *Vegetable kheer* Wheat 30 g Bengal gram 60 g Spinach (palak) 30 g Jaggery 70 g	a. Roast the wheat and powder b. Roast Bengal gram and powder c. Make a jaggery syrup d. Mix wheat and dhal powders, make a batter with the jaggery syrup e. Boil the spinach, mash and strain through cloth or sieve f. Add spinach, to the mixture, cook for a few minutes with stirring till semi-solid.
3. *Channa badma kheer* Rice 50 g Groundnut cake flour 50 g Jaggery 50 g	a. Roast the rice and powder b. Mix groundnut cake flour with rice powder, add some water and cook c. Make a jaggery syrup and add to the above d. Cook for a few minutes, stir to avoid lumps e. When semi-solid, remove from the fire.
Western Region	
1. *Bajra kheer* Bajra 50 g Masoor dhal 50 g Jaggery 50 g	a. Roast bajra and powder b. Roast dhal and powder c. Mix and cook in a little water
2. *Ragi (nachna) channa kheer* Bengal gram 50 g Ragi (nachna) flour 50 g Jaggery 50 g	a. Grind ragi flour with water and strain through a sieve b. Boil the extract c. Roast Bengal gram and powder d. Add powder to boiling extract, stir continuously and cook till semi-solid and a pleasant smell emanates e. Make and add jaggery syrup
3. *Sheng danya halwa* Wheat flour 50 g Groundnut cake four 25 g Jaggery 50 g Oil or vanaspati 5 g	a. Roast wheat flour b. Roast groundnut cake flour, mix with above c. Make a jaggery syrup, add to the above d. Cook mixture for a few minutes with stirring to avoid lumps e. Add heated oil and remove from fire

There are many baby foods in the market. The instructions given for use should be closely followed, if the best results are to be obtained. A good powdered baby food which can be made and kept at home has also been developed by NIN, Hyderabad. The method of preparation is as follows. Separately roast and separately powder the following ingredients: dehusked ragi or bajra, 60 grams; moong dhal or any other dhal, 15 grams; groundnuts, 10 gram and til seeds, 5 grams. Mix the powders with 15 grams of skim milk powder. Store in an air-tight tin or bottle. Take 3 tablespoonful, mix with a little hot water, warm and add salt or sugar. This quantity of food is enough to feed a 6-month old child three times during one day. More can be made at a time and stored. Sprouting the cereal as well as the dhal for two days, drying and then roasting to a pleasant smell, enhances greatly the quality of this home-made baby food.

Weigh the baby regularly every month, and keep a record. During the first four months, the weight should roughly double, and at the first birthday it should triple.

PREMATURE AND VERY SMALL BABIES

The premature infant is not fully developed when born. Its body weight is low, the muscles are poorly developed, there is little or no fat on the body and even the skeleton may not be fully formed. The stomach is small, so only a tiny quantity of food can be digested; this is especially true of fat. The sweat glands do not function properly and so the baby's temperature is not constant but tends to go up and down. It is therefore necessary to keep it warm and well wrapped.

Table 15.13: Balanced diet for preschool children

S.No.	*Food groups*	*Quantity (g)*	
		1-3 years	*4-6 years*
1.	Cereals and millets	120	210
2.	Pulses	30	45
3.	Milk (ml)	500	500
4.	Roots and tubers	50	100
5.	Green leafy vegetables	50	50
6.	Other vegetables	50	50
7.	Fruits	100	100
8.	Sugar	25	30
9.	Fats/oils (visible)	20	25

Source: *Dietary Guidelines for Indians–A Manual,* National Institute for Nutrition, ICMR, Hyderabad, India, 1999.

Table 15.14: ICMR recommended dietary allowance of school going children

Nutrients	*Age (in years)*		
	7-9	*10-12*	
		Boys	*Girls*
Energy (k cal)	1950	2190	1970
Protein (g)	41	54	57
Fat (g)	25	22	22
Calcium (mg)	400	600	600
Iron (mg)	26	34	19
Vitamin A			
Retional (μg) or	600	600	600
β-carotene (μg)	2400	2400	2400
Thaimine (mg)	1.0	1.1	1.0
Riboflavin (mg)	1.2	1.3	1.2
Niacin (mg)	13	15	13
Pyridoxine (mg)	1.6	1.6	1.6
Ascorbic acid (mg)	40	40	40
Folic acid (μg)	60	70	70
Vitamin B_{12} (mg)	0.2-1	0.2-1	0.2-1

Table 15.15: Composition of human milk

Nutrient	*Quantity/100 ml*
Energy (k cal)	58
Fat (g)	2.9
Calcium (mg)	31
Phosphorus (mg)	14
Iron (mg)	0.09
Protein (g)	2.7
Lactose (g)	5.3
Carotene (IU)	186
Vitamin A (IU)	296

Source: Guthrie A.H., *Introductory Nutrition*, Times, Mirror/Mosby College Publishing (International Edition)

Table 15.16: Balanced diet for school going children

S.No.	*Food groups*	*Quantity gms*		
			10-12 years	
		7-9 years	*Boys*	*Girls*
1.	Cereals and millets	270	330	270
2.	Pulses	60	60	60
3.	Milk (ml)	500	500	500
4.	Roots and tubers	100	100	100
5.	Green leafy vegetables	100	100	100
6.	Other vegetables	100	100	100
7.	Fruits	100	100	100
8.	Sugar	30	35	30
9.	Fats/oils (visible)	25	25	25

For non veg 30 g of pulse can be exchanged with 50 gm of eggs/meat/chicken/fish.

Feeding must be done with care. Suckling may be difficult, and a medicine dropper may have to be used for the first few days. Even breast milk from the mother is probably not available. The first need is to give liquids, both diluted milk and boiled water. This should be done every two hours, say about half a teaspoonful each time to start with. Gradually the quantity can be increased to one teaspoonful.

Cow or buffalo milk is too rich both in fat and in proteins to feed the child. It is essential to remove the fat as completely as possible and then to further dilute with an equal amount of boiled water. Skim milk powder can also be used. Mix 18 grams of it with 11 grams of sugar (or glucose or lactose) and add 150 ml of boiled water. If baby food is used, follow the instructions on the container. After about 3 months the premature or underweight child catches up with a normal one with weight of about 6 kg. So all the foods given to normal babies, can be started.

NUTRITION FOR 1-3 YEARS OLD CHILDREN (PRE-SCHOOLERS)

A healthy one-year old child is not yet ready for food which require to be chewed or ground, so the nutrients must be given in the form of soft foods. It has need for all nutrients and is able to take in quite a variety of foods. Of course the volume of food which it is able to eat is not large, and children are also slow eaters. In consequence it may be getting less food than it needs, and the type of food which it gets will probably be the same as that eaten by adults in the household. Yet the child's needs for calcium, and for certain vitamins (C, B_{12} and folic acid) are more than those that correspond to its food volume. A child of this age needs foods of high nutritive value to grow well.

MEAL PLANNING FOR 1-3 YEARS OLD CHILDREN

1. Offer simply prepared food and avoid any foods that are mixed together, as children need to identify what they are eating.
2. Offer at least one colourful food, such as carrot sticks.
3. Pre-schoolers like nutritious foods in all food groups with one deviation, vegetables, particularly strong-flavoured ones like onions and cabbage. Vegetables are more likely to be accepted if served raw and cut as a finger food. When serving cooked vegetables, serve them undercooked.
4. Provide at least one soft or moist food that is easy to chew at each meal. A crisp or chewy food is important too, to develop chewing skills.
5. Avoid strong-flavoured and highly salted foods because children have more taste buds than adults so these foods taste too strong to them. Use sparingly pepper and other spices, as well as acidic products such as vinegar.
6. Pre-schoolers love carbohydrate foods, including cereals, breads and crackers, as they are easy to hold and chew.
7. Smooth-textured foods such as pea soup or mashed potatoes should not have any lumps because children find this unusual.
8. Before the age of 4, at which time the skills to cut up food start to develop, food needs to be served in bite-sized pieces that are either eaten as finger foods or with a spoon or fork.
9. Serve foods warm, not hot. A child's mouth is more sensitive to hot and cold than an adult's. Also, little children need little plates, utensils and cups, as well as seats that allow them to reach to table comfortably.

The National Institute of Nutrition in Hyderabad has described palatable food preparations for 1-3 year-old children which have a high nutritive value and are made from common low-cost ingredients. These are shown in Table 15.17 and have been designed to cater to differing tastes in various parts of the country. One of these items every day can very well be given to a child aged 1 to 3 years and will take care of nearly half of his energy and protein requirements for the day. Together with his normal food, and supplemented with fresh fruits, green salads and cooked green leafy vegetables, a child will be assured of a good diet.

Likewise a meal plan has also been worked out for 3-5 years old child (Table 15.18) by NIN, Hyderabad.

As older child, about 3-5 years, can eat most adult food. An example of a balanced meal plan for this child which will provide all the nutrients, drawn up by NIN, Hyderabad, is shown in Table 15.18. This plan should be generally applicable to many areas in India since a number of alternatives are provided which cater to regional tastes.

Table 15.17: Recipes for children 1-3 years old

Each recipe gives 500-550 calories and 15-20 grams of protein. This is half the nutritional requirement of the child. The rest must come from other foods.

Ingredients	Method
Northern Region	
1. *Jowar khicheri*	
Jowar rava 50 g	a. Cook jowar rava in water
Jaggery 50 g	b. Chop up pumpkin and carrots
Moong dal 50 g	c. Mix cooked jowar, dhal and vegetables, and add jaggery syrup
Pumpkin 30 g	
Carrots 30 g	d. Warm over a slow fire for a few minutes
2. *Meethi roti*	
Wheat flour 75 g	a. Dissolve jaggery in water and strain
Groundnut cake powder 30 g	b. Mix wheat flour and groundnut cake powder with jaggery syrup and make into a dough
Jaggery 60 g	c. Roll small balls of the dough into rotis
	d. Bake the rotis on a tava using oil if desired
	e. Serve rotis with a piece of papaya and a glass of buttermilk
3. *Dhal khicheri*	
Skim milk power 30 g	a. Make milk from the skim milk powder and then set it to curds
Bengal gram 55 g	
Bajra 55 g	b. Half cook the bajra
Oil 10 g	c. Add salt to taste, hot oil and jeera
Salt, jeera to taste	d. Serve khicheri with curds
Eastern Region	
1. *Tomato soup*	
Parboiled rice 75 g	a. Boil rice and Bengal gram together till very soft
Bangal gram 50 g	
Drumstick leaves 50 g	b. Boil drumstick leaves and tomato together, strain through thin cloth or sieve
Ripe tomatoes 100 g	
Oil 10 g	c. Mix the above, add salt, cook for a few minutes, add oil
Salt to taste	
2. *Meethi khicheri*	
Puffed rice 75 g	a. Roast the dhal and powder it
Tuvar dhal 45 g	b. If puffed rice is soft, roast it and powder
Jaggery 90 g	c. Mix both powder and cook with water
Carrot 30 g	d. Add grated carrots and jaggery, cook till carrot shreds are soft
3. *Muri toffee*	
Puffed rice 60 g	a. If puffed rice is soft. Roast it and powder
Bengal gram 60 g	b. Roast Bengal gram and powder
Jaggery 60 g	c. Make a thick jaggery syrup
	d. Add rice and dhal powders to the syrup, stirring briskly to avoid formation of lumps
	e. Cook for a short time, pour into a greased plate
	f. After the mixture has set, cut into pieces
Southern Region	
1. *Jowar (cholam) upma*	
Jowar rava 60 g	a. Fry in oil the mustard, urad dhal (a little) and sliced onions
Roasted groundnuts 30 g	

Contd.

Contd.

Onion 10 g	b. Add salt and water and boil
Kothmir (dhania) leaves 10 g	c. Add jowar rava and cook till soft
Oil 10 g	d. Add powdered roasted groundnuts
Mustard, urad dhal, salt	
2. *Masala idli with chutney*	
Jowar (cholam) 50 g	a. Soak jowar and Bengal gram separately for a few hours
Urad (blackgram) dhal 25 g	
Roasted groundnuts 30 g	b. Grind separately
Carrots 30 g	c. Mix them and allow to ferment for 5-6 hours
Roasted Bengal gram 5 g	d. Add to the paste chopped-up carrots and salt
Oil 10 g	e. Prepare idlis in the usual way
(Salt, mustard)	f. Make chutney by grinding groundnuts and Bengal gram, adding salt and mustard to taste
3. *Ragi puttu*	
Ragi 60 g	a. Roast ragi and tuvar dhal separately and powder
Tuvar dhal 45 g	b. Dissolve jaggery in water and strain
Jaggery 50 g	c. Mix both powders and jaggery syrup into a paste
	d. Stream the paste till it does not stick to the sides
	e. Cool, cut into pieces
Western Region	
1. *Khaman dhokla*	
Bajra 50 g	a. Roast bajra and dhal and powder both
Masoor dhal 50 g	b. Cook in a little water
Jaggery 50 g	c. Make a jaggery syrup
	d. Add syrup to cooked mixture
2. *Ragi (nachna) chapati*	
Ragi (nachna) flour 45 g	a. Roast dhal and powder
Wheat flour 20 g	b. Mix ragi flour, wheat flour and dhal, tuvar powder and jaggery syrup and make a dough
Dhal 20 g	
Jaggery 55 g	c. Take small portion of dough, roll into rotis
	d. Fry rotis using oil on a tava
3. *Pulao with cora chutney*	
Rice 60 g	a. Chop the vegetables
Carrots 30 g	b. Cook rice, dhal and vegetables together till soft
French beans 20 g	
Pumpkin 25 g	c. Add salt to taste and heat oil remove from fire
Oil 8 g	
Tuvar dhal 30 g	
Coconut 20 g	a. Grind coconut and salt
Urad dhal 10 g	b. Season with urad dhal, chillies and mustard
Oil 25 g	
Salt to taste	c. Serve chutney with above pulao
Mustard, pinch	

Table 15.18: Meal plan for a child 3-5 years old

Time	Food	Amount
8-9 a.m.	Cooked cereal-dhal preparation	2-3 spoons
	Or	
	Idli	1-2 idlis
	Bread with butter	1-2 slices
	Or	
	Puffed whole ragi with milk	Small amount
	Soft boiled, poached or scrambled	1 egg
	Or	
	Boiled dhals	1 spoon
	Boiled milk (cow, buffalo)	½ tumbler
10.30 a.m.	Fruit juice	½ tumbler
	Or	
	Fresh seasonal fruit	One serving
12.30-1 p.m.	Cooked rice	2-4 spoons
	Or	
	Wheat or ragi chapatti	1-2 chapattis
	Boiled potato, sweet potato or tapioca (occasionally)	Small portion
	Curds or milk	½ tumbler
	Cooked green leafy or green vegetable	½ spoon
	Or	
	Raw vegetable salad three times a week in place of cooked vegetable	1½ -2 spoons
3-4 p.m.	Boiled milk (cow, buffalo)	½ tumbler
	Fish liver oil	1 teaspoon
7-8 p.m.	Cooked cereal like suji, broken wheat or ragi porridge	2-3 spoons
	Boiled dhal, fish or meat preparation	2 spoons
	Boiled milk (at bedtime)	½ tumbler

MEAL PLANNING FOR SCHOOL AGE CHILDREN

1. School-age children accept more varieties of food, but many still will not eat cooked vegetables and mixed dishes.
2. Good snack choices are important for school-age children as they do not always have the desire or the time to sit down and eat. Snacks can include fresh fruits and vegetables, juices, breads, unsweetened cereals, popcorn, biscuits, milk, yoghurt, cheese, pudding, custard, sliced meats and poultry, eggs, and peanut butter.
3. An important point that concerns children, particularly younger ones, is choking. Do not offer round foods that are easy to choke on to children who only have a few teeth. Examples are grapes, nuts, popcorn, hard candy, hot dogs and chips. These foods can easily find their way to the opening of the windpipe, and choking will result. Children should not eat while running or playing hard, which enhance the possibility of choking.
4. All children upto age 10 need to eat every 4 to 6 hours to keep their blood glucose at a desirable level; therefore, snacking is necessary between meals.
5. Snacks as well as meals should provide good sources of calcium, such as dairy foods, and iron and zinc, such as meats and legumes.
6. If a child drinks little or no milk, try adding flavorings to milk such as chocolate or strawberry, or make cocoa, milkshakes, puddings and custards.

GROWTH AND NUTRIENT NEEDS DURING ADOLESCENCE

Puberty refers to the maturation or growing up of the entire body, which starts at about 10 or 11 for females and 12 or 13 for males. In females, its peaks at age 12 and is completed by age 15. In males, its peaks at age 14 and is completed by age 19, so it starts later and lasts longer in boys. The timing of puberty and rates of growth show much individual variation. During the 5 to 7 years of pubertal development, the adolescent gains about 50 percent of adult weight. Most of the body organs double in size. Whereas the proportion of fat and muscle was similar in males and females before puberty, now males put on twice as much muscle as females, and females gain proportionately more fat. In the adolescent female, an increasing amount of fat is being stored under the skin, particularly in the abdominal area. The male also experiences a greater increase in bone mass than females. Males now need more calories, protein, iron and zinc for muscle and bone development than females; however, females, on the other hand, need increased iron due to the onset of menstruation. Due to their big appetites and calorie needs, teenage body are more likely to get sufficient nutrients than females. Females have to pack nutrients into fewer calories, which can become difficult if they decrease their food intake in an effort to lose weight or stay slender.

Table 15.19: Balanced diet for adolescents (13-18 years)

S.No.	*Food groups*	*Quantity (g)*	
		Boys	*Girls*
1.	Cereals and millets	420	300
2.	Pulses	60	60
3.	Milk (ml)	500	500
4.	Roots and tuber	200	100
5.	Green leafy vegetables	100	100
6.	Other vegetables	100	100
7.	Fruits	100	100
8.	Sugar	35	30
9.	Fats/oils (visible)	25	25

For Non-veg 30 g of pulse can be exchanged with 50 g of meat/chicken/fish/egg.

Source: *Dietary Guidelines for Indians–A Manual*, National Institute of Nutrition, ICMR, Hyderabad, India, 1999.

GUIDELINES FOR MENU PLANNING FOR ADOLESCENTS (Tables 15.19 and 15.20)

1. Adolescents need to follow the basic food group pattern more or less in the manner similar to adults.
2. The nutrients most often lacking in adolescent diets are iron, folic acid and vitamin A. Calcium may also be lacking for those who have an inadequate intake of milk and other dairy products. Significant iron sources include meats, poultry, fish, eggs, legumes and dried fruits. Vitamin C helps the iron from legumes and dried fruits to be absorbed. Leafy green vegetables are live and good sources for both vitamin A and folic acid. Vitamin A is also found in fortified milk and margarine, eggs, broccoli, and deep orange fruits and vegetables. Folic acid is present in seeds and dried beans and peas.
3. Milk, curd or other milk products as custards, ice cream, need to be offered at all meals.
4. Emphasize complex carbohydrates such as assorted breads, cereals, fruits, vegetables, potatoes, rice, and dried beans and peas. These food supply calories along with needed nutrients. Whole grain products are preferred for breads.
5. Offer well-trimmed lean meat poultry and fish. Don't think that just because these adolescents need more calories thus fatty meats are in order. Their fat calories should be less saturated.

Table 15.20: ICMR recommended dietary allowances for adolescents

Nutrients	*Boys*		*Girls*	
	13-15 years	*16-18 years*	*13-15 years*	*16-18 years*
Energy (k cal)	2450	2640	2060	2060
Protein (g)	70	78	65	63
Fat (g)	22	22	22	22
Calcium (mg)	600	500	600	500
Iron (mg)	41	50	28	30
Vitamin A				
Retinol (μg) or	600	600	600	600
β-Carotene (μg)	2400	2400	2400	2400
Thiamine (mg)	1.2	1.3	1.0	1.0

Contd.

Contd.

Riboflavin (mg)	1.5	1.6	1.2	1.2
Niacin (mg)	16	17	14	14
Pyridoxine (mg)	2.0	2.0	2.0	2.0
Vitamin C (mg)	40	40	40	40
Folic acid (µg)	100	100	100	100
Vitamin B_{12} (µg)	0.2-1.0	0.2-1.0	0.2-1.0	0.2-1.0

Table 15.21: Balanced diet for adults–Sedentary/moderate/heavy activity/(Number of portions)

Food groups	*g/ portion*	*Sedentary*		*Moderate*		*Heavy*	
		Man	*Woman*	*Man*	*Woman*	*Man*	*Woman*
Cereals and millets	30	14	10	16	12	23	16
Pulses	30	2	2	3	2.5	3	3
Milk	100 ml	3	3	3	3	3	3
Roots and tubers	100	2	1	2	1	2	2
Green leafy vegetables	100	1	1	1	1	1	1
Other vegetables	100	1	1	1	1	1	1
Fruits	100	1	1	1	1	1	1
Sugar	5	5	4	8	5	11	9
Fats and oils (visible)	5	4	4	7	6	11	8

For non-vegetarians substitute one pulse portion with one portion (50 g) of egg/meat/chicken/fish.

Source: *Dietary Guidelines for Indians–A Manual*, NIN, ICMR, Hyderabad, 1999.

Table 15.22: Sample meal plan for an adult man (Sedentary)

Meal time	*Food group*	*Raw amounts*	*Cooked*	*Servings*
Breakfast	Milk	100 ml	Milk or	½ cup
	Sugar	15 g	Tea or	2 cups
			Coffee	1 cup
	Cereals	70 g	Breakfast	
	Pulses	20 g	Item	
Lunch	Cereals	150 g	Rice	2 cups
			Phulkas	2 Nos.
	Pulses	20 g	Dhal	½ cup
	Vegetables	150 g	Veg-curry	¾ cup
	Vegetables	50 g	Veg-salad	7-8 slices
	Milk	100 ml	Curd	½ cup
Tea	Cereals	50 g	Snack	
	Milk	50 ml	Tea	1 cup
	Sugar	10 g		
Dinner	Cereals	150 g	Rice	2 cups
			Phulkas	2 Nos
	Pulses	20 g	Dhal	½ cup
	Vegetables	150 g	Veg. curry	¾ cup

Contd.

Contd.

	Milk (curd)	50 ml	Veg. raita	½ cup
	Vegetables	50 g		½ cup
	Fruit	100 g	Seasonal	1 medium

1 cup = 200 ml, Use 20 g visible fat per day.

Total cereals 1 day = 420 g pulses/day = 60 g.

Note: For non-vegetarians–Substitute one pulse portion with one portion of egg/meat/chicken/fish.

Source: *Dietary Guidelines for Indians–A Manual,* NIN, ICMR, Hyderabad, 1999.

A sample vegetarian menu for an adult woman doing sedentary work is given below:

Table 15.23: A sample vegetarian menu for an adult woman doing sedentary work

Meal	*Menu*	*Raw amounts*
Early morning	Milk/coffee/tea	Milk - 100 ml
		Sugar - 10 g
Breakfast	Upma - 11/2 cup, fruit	Cereal - 75 g
		Fruit - 50 g
Lunch	Rice - 1 cup	Cereal - 100 g
	Phulkas - 2 Nos.	
	Dhal - ½ cup	Pulse - 20 g

Contd.

Contd.

	Amaranth poriyal 1 cup	Green leafy vegetable - 100 g
	Vegetable raita	Vegetable - 50 gm
	Curd - ½ cup	Milk - 100 ml
Tea	Samosa - 2 no.	Cereal - 50 g
		Potato - 50 g
	Tea 1 cup	Milk - 100 ml
		Sugar - 10 g
Dinner	Dosa 3 nos.	Cereal - 75 g
	Sambar ½ cup	Pulse - 40 g
	Vegetable salad	Vegetable - 100 g
	Fruit	Fruit - 50 g
Bed time	Milk	Milk - 100 ml
		Sugar - 5 g

Table 15.24: Comparison of human milk with cow's and buffalo's milk

Nutrient per 100 ml	*Human milk*	*Cow's milk*	*Buffalo's milk*
Water (g)	88	87.5	81
Energy (k cal)	65	67	117
Protein (g)	1.1	3.2	4.3
Carbohydrate (g)	7.4	4.4	5
Fat (g)	3.4	4.1	6.5
Calcium (mg)	28	120	210
Phosphorus (mg)	11	90	130
Iron (mg)	—	0.2	0.2
Carotene (μg)	137	174	160
Thiamine (mg)	0.02	0.05	0.04
Riboflavin (mg)	0.02	0.19	0.1
Vitamin C (mg)	3	2	1
Caseinogen lactalbumin ratio	1:2	3:1	—

Table 15.25: Western Indian meal plan

	First day	*Second day*	*Third day*
1. On rising tea	Tea	Tea	Tea
2. Breakfast	Poha	Poha	Puri, upma Potato curry
3. Lunch	Rice, phulkas Saar, potato and palak curry, curds	Rice, phulkas, green gram chhole, bhindi masala, curds	Rice, phulkas Dhal with drum-stick, leaves, bagara Baingan, curds
4. Tea	Khaman dhoka, tea	Pakodas, tea	Boondi, tea
5. Dinner	Rice, phulkas, veg. korma with potatoes, peas and beans, dhal, curds	Rice, phulkas, palak curry, fried *tinda (koval)*, curds	Rice, phulkas, potato and tomato curry, curds

Major Dishes (Quantities in grams)

1. Saar: Red gram 10, onion 10, oil 5.
2. Dhal: Red gram 20, onion 10, oil 5.
   Dhal with palak: Red gram 50, palak 50, onion 10, oil 5.
   Dhal with drumstick leaves: Red gram 20, drumstick leaves 40, onion 10, oil 5.
3. Vegetable curry: Vegetables 40 to 60, onion 10, oil 5.

Common Dishes (Quantities in grams)

(a) Tea with milk 30, sugar 15.
(b) Rice: 75.
(c) Phulkas: Wheat flour 100.
(d) Chapattis: Wheat flour 100, oil 10.
(e) Curds: 100.

Non-Vegetarians

Substitute the vegetable curry 3 or 4 times a week with a preparation using one egg, mutton or fish 30, cooked along with some vegetables or dhal.

Fourth day	Fifth day	Sixth day	Seventh day
1. Tea	Tea	Tea	Tea
2. Thilipete (jowar roti)	Suji halwa	Bread and jam	Aloo poha
3. Rice, phulkas, cabbage and potato curry, beans, curds	Rice, phulkas, dhal with palak, bhindani khadi	Rice, chapattis, dhal, ridge gourd and methi curry, curds	Rice, phulkas, mixed vegetable, curry, dhal, palak raita
4. Besan barfi, tea	Chivda, tea	Biscuits, tea	Dahi-wada, tea
5. Rice, phulkas, dhal, cluster leaves curry, butte rmilk	Rice, phulkas, beans and tomato, curry, saar, curds	Rice, phulkas, palak curry, cauliflower and potato butte rmilk	Rice, phulkas dhal, colocasia curry (arvi)

Table 15.26: Eastern Indian meal plan

	First day	Second day	Third day
1. On rising tea	Tea	Tea	Tea
2. Breakfast	Chapatti, fried parwal	Loochi (Puri), aloo dum	Suji
3. Lunch	Rice, dhal, Fried bhindi, curds	Rice, bandha gobi, dhal, curds	Rice, fish curry dhal, butter milk
4. Tea	Tea, muri	Raw banana bhajis, tea	Seasoned dried peas, tea
5. Dinner	Phulkas, lau curry, dhal with greens (spinach), buttermilk	Phulkas, dalna (cauliflower, potato and peas), dhal with greens (drumstick leaves)	Loochi, parwal korma, amaranth curry (chaulai)

Major Dishes (Quantities in grams)

1. Dhal: Dhal 25 to 50, onion 10, oil 5.
2. Curry: Vegetables 25 to 50, onion 10, oil 5.
3. Muri/pressed rice: 25.
4. Suji halwa: Suji 75, sugar 15, oil 10.
5. Ambal: Tomato 20, tamarind 5, sugar 2. Alternatively papaya 20, tamarind 10, onion 10.

Common Dishes (Quantities in grams)

(a) Tea with milk 30, sugar 15.

(b) Wheat for chapatti/phulka or loochi: 150 for lunch and dinner, 15 for breakfast.

(c) Rice: 150-175 for full meal.

(d) Curds: 75; butter milk 100.

(e) Fish: 30.

Non-Vegetarians

Substitute meat or fish (30) or egg 3 or 4 times a week for the vegetables curry; fish is eaten by widely in Eastern India.

Fourth day	Fifth day	Sixth day	Seventh day
1. Tea	Tea	Tea	Tea
2. Chapatti, fried brinjal	Seasoned muri, tea	Loochi, fried potato	Chapatti, mixed vegetable curry
3. Rice, shukhto (mixed vegetable stew), ambal (tomato chutney), curds	Rice, fried fish, dhal with greens (drumstick leaves)	Rice, pumpkin chokha, dhal, curds	Rice, chachadi, dhal, curds
4. Muri and jaggery laddus, tea	Biscuits tea	Sandesh, tea	Seasoned pressed rice, tea
5. Rice, dhal with greens, aloo dum, buttermilk	Chapatti, papaya curry, aloo maakha	Phulkas, pakak curry, dhal	Rice, beans and tomato curry, dhal, ambal papaya chutney)

Table 15.27: Northern Indian meal plan

	First day	Second day	Third day
1. On rising tea	Tea	Tea	Tea
2. Breakfast	Puri, aloo curry, suji halwa	Rasish, chapatti, curds	Phulkas, butter, buttermilk
3. Lunch	Rice, besan khadi, aloo and palak curry, curds	Phulkas, methi and aloo curry, dhal, curds	Phulkas, rice, gobhi curry, dhal, curds
4. Tea	Chivda, tea	Besan-ka-bhujjia, tea	Aloo pakoda, tea
5. Dinner	Phulkas, sukhe matter, baingan, curds	Phulkas, beans, bhurji, tinda, curry	Phulkas, amaranth curry, curds

Major Dishes (Quantities in grams)

1. Dhal: Dhal 40, onion 10, oil 5.
2. Curry: Vegetables 50 to 75, onion 10, oil 5
3. Other dishes:

   Suji halwa: Suji 25, sugar 10, oil 5.

   Besan khadi: Bengal gram flour 30, oil 5, butter milk 50.

   Sukhe mattar: Dried peas 40, onion 5, oil 5.

   Pakoda: Bengal gram flour 25, oil 10.

   Rajmah: Rajmah 45, onion 10, oil 5.

   Sarson-ka-saag: Mustard greens 25, spinach 25, onion 5, oil 5.
4. Salad: Beans 10, carrots 30, tomato 10, onion 10.

Common Dishes (Quantities in grams)

(a) Tea with milk 30, sugar 15.

(b) Wheat phulkas: Wheat flour 175 for lunch, 150 for dinner.

Wheat chapatti: Wheat flour 75.

Wheat puri: Wheat flour 50, oil 10.

(c) Rice: 150 for full meal.

(d) Curds: 75.

(e) Butter milk: 100.

Non-Vegetarians

Substitute meat or fish or egg (30), 3 or 4 times a week for vegetable curry.

Fourth day	Fifth day	Sixth day	Seventh day
1. Tea	Tea	Tea	Tea
2. Besan pura, butter milk	Namkeen paratha, tea	Aloo paratha, curds	Missi roti, curds
3. Phulkas, ridgegourd curry, spinach	Phulkas, rice, dhal, carrot and beans, curry	Phulkas, bhindi masala, palakvali dhal, curds	Chapatti, rice, bharka gobhi, dhal, curds
4. Gulab jamun, tea	Samosas, tea	Sev, tea	Gobi pakodas, tea
5. Rice, rajmah, vegetable salad, butter milk	Makki-ki-roti, sarson-ka-saag, butter milk	Phulkas, kabuli channa, calabash-cucumber curry, butter milk	Phulkas, aloo mattar, butter milk

Table 15.28: Southern Indian meal plan

	First day	Second day	Third day
1. On rising tea	Coffee	Coffee	Coffee
2. Breakfast	Wheat chapatti, brinjal curry, coffee	Rava upma, coffee,	Idli, sambar, coffee
3. Lunch	Rice, onion sambar, French beans curry, butter milk	Rice, dhal, avial, butter milk	Rice, dhal with brinjal, carrot and cabbage curry, curds
4. Tea	Onion pakoda, coffee	Raw banana bhajis, coffee	Roasted groundnuts, coffee
5. Dinner	Rice, dhal with keerai, tomato rasam, curds	Pulkas and rice, palak curry, dhal, Plain, butter milk	Wheat dosa, coconut chutney, butter milk

Major Dishes (Quantities in grams)

1. Sambar with onions: Red gram dal 20, onion 30, oil 5.

   Sambar with lady's fingers: Dal 25 onion 10, oil 5, lady's fingers 50.

   Sambar with drumsticks: Dal 15, onion 10, oil 5, drumsticks 50.

2. Dhal, plain: Red gram dhal 25, onion 10, oil 5.

   Dhal with keerai: Green gram 20, onion 10, oil 5 keerai 50.

   Dhal with brinjal: Red gram dhal 20, onion 10, oil 5, brinjal 25.

   Keerai (amaranth), or ridge gourd: Vegetables 50, onions 10, oil 5.

3. Others dishes:

Avial: Potato/brinjal 25, drumsticks/raw banana 15, French beans/fresh coconut 10, coconut oil 3, curds 25.

Vegetable korma: Peas/beans/potato/onion 10, carrot 15, oil 5, curds 25.

Carrot and cabbage curry: Carrot 100, cabbage 25, onion 10, oil 5.

Drumsticks leaves fry: Drumstick leaves 50, onion 10, oil 5.

Colocasia leaves fry: Colocasia leaves 50, oil 5.

Salad: Tomato/onion/carrot/French beans 20.

Common Dishes (Quantities in grams)

(a) Coffee with milk 50, sugar 15.

(b) Wheat phulkas: Wheat flour 100.
    Wheat chapatti: Wheat flour 75, oil 10.
    Wheat puris: Wheat flour 75, oil 10.

(c) Rice: 200 for one meal.
    Rice: 100 for second meal.
    Rice: When combined with wheat at same meal, rice 50 plus, wheat 100.

Fourth day	Fifth day	Sixth day	Seventh day
1. Coffee	Coffee	Coffee	Coffee
2. Puri, potato curry, coffee	Vermicelli upma, coffee	Dosa, coconut chutney, coffee	Idli, sambar, chutney, coffee
3. Rice, dhal with palak, French beans, curry, curds	Rice, sambar with lady's fingers, drumstick	Rice, vegetable korma, keerai curry, curds	Rice, keerai curry, fried colocasia leaves, curds
4. Sundal, coffee	Fried pressed rice, coffee	Banana, coffee	Idli, upma, coffee
5. Rice, dhal salad, butter milk	Rice, dhal cluster, beans, curry, curds	Phulkas and rice, plain thick dhal, ridgegourd curry, butter milk	Phulkas and rice, drumstick sambar, mint chutney, butter milk

Non-Vegetarians

Substitute the vegetables curry shown above 3 or 4 times a week with a preparation using an egg, mutton 30 or fish 30, cooked with some vegetables.

Table 15.29: Energy requirement (Kcal/24 hrs) of male and female 60 years and above with different body weights

Sex	*Body weight kg*	*Energy requirement for sedentary activity Kcal*
Males	60	1976
	65	2072
	70	2176
	75	2280
Females	60	1864
	65	1944
	70	2024

(Nutrient requirement and recommended dietary allowance for Indians, ICMR, 2002).

Table 15.30: Balanced diet for an elderly person for a day

Foodstuff	*Quantity (raw) g*	
	Males	*Females*
Cereals	350	225
Pulses	50	40
Vegetables	200	150
Green leafy vegetables	50	50
Roots and tubers	100	100
Fruits	200	200
Milk and milk products	300	300
Sugar	20	20
Fats and oils	25	20

(**Source:** *"Dietary Tips for Elderly"*, NIN, ICMR, Hyderabad, 2000).

TIPS ON MEAL PLANNING FOR VEGETARIANS (Tables 15.21 to 15.30)

1. Do not include many foods that offer only plenty of calories, like fat and sugar. In order to ingest adequate nutrients, vegetarians need a well-balanced, varied diet with a minimum of empty calories.
2. Include an animal source of protein at each meal, such as milk, curd and cheese.
3. For adequate protein, and also vitamins and minerals, use a variety of plant protein sources: Legumes, grain products, nuts and seeds, and/or vegetables at each meal.
4. Nuts and seeds are commonly used as snacks in roasted vegetables diet. Some are toasted lightly to bring out flavours. Nuts and seeds play a minor role in menu planning for vegetarians as compared to legumes, grains and vegetables, probably in part due to their high fat content (about 50 percent) and their relatively high cost.
5. A wide variety of vegetables should be used when planning vegetarian diets. Steaming or microwave cooking vegetables is a preferred method of preparation as it best retains flavours, nutrients and colour.
6. Vegetarian need to be concerned about iron consumption; therefore, offer good source of iron: Legumes, tofu (a soybean product), dark green vegetables, watermelon, whole grain and fortified cereal grain products and dried fruits. Iron that is present in animal products absorbed more readily into the body than iron from plant sources, and a factor that aids in absorbing iron is vitamin C. Therefore, be sure to offer at all meals vitamin C-rich foods such as citrus fruits and juices, tomatoes, broccoli, melons, potatoes and peppers.

7. Vitamin B_{12} is generally found only in foods of animal origin. Tempeh (cultured soybean cake) contains vitamin B_{12}, however, most part of it may not be bio-available to the body. Because the liver can store a year's worth of vitamin B_{12}, some time may pass before a deficiency becomes apparent. If adequate B_{12} is not available, a supplement may be needed.
8. Dairy products contribute most of the calcium. Vegetables and legumes provide calcium, though unfortunately not enough to meet daily needs. Vitamin D can be made by the body in the skin when ultraviolet light from the sun beams falls down directly on the skin. Vegans may need vitamin D supplements if they are not getting enough sun, which could be the case in colder climates or due to customs like veil system for ladies prevalent in rural India.
9. Vegetarians also have to remain particular about zinc nutrition as plant food components such as phytate and certain types of fiber inhibit zinc absorption. Important sources of zinc such as legumes nuts and seeds (especially peanut butter), soybean products (such as tofu), whole grains and cereals need to be included in vegetarian menus.

BENEFITS OF GOOD NUTRITION AND HEALTH HABITS FOR BODY FUNCTIONING

Usefulness of a good nourishing diet lie in meeting our needs for protein, calories and other essential nutrients. It also helps in preventing:

- Birth defects and low birth weight in pregnancy.
- Poor growth and poor resistance to disease in infancy and childhood.
- Poor resistance to disease in adult years.
- Deficiency diseases, such as cretinism (lack of the mineral iodide), scurvy (lack of vitamin C), and anemia (lack of the mineral iron, vitamin folate, or other nutrients). Meeting our needs for the mineral calcium helps prevent: Some adult bone loss.
- Obtaining small intake of the mineral fluoride and minimizing sugar intake helps prevent: Dental caries (decay). However, fluoride at more than 1-2 ppm is injurious to health.
- Eating enough dietary fiber helps prevent: Digestive problems, such as constipation, and possibly some forms of cancer like colon cancer.
- Eating enough vitamin A and beta-carotene (plants produced precursor of vitamin A) may help reduce: Susceptibility to some cancers, especially in smokers. Moderation in caloric intake helps prevent: Obesity and related diseases, such as diabetes mellitus, hypertension, cancer and coronary heart disease.
- Limiting intake of the mineral sodium helps prevent hypertension and related diseases of the heart and kidney in susceptible people.
- Avoiding intake of saturated fat helps prevent: Premature heart disease.
- Moderation in intake of essential nutrients by using vitamin and mineral supplements wisely, if at all supplement intake becomes inevitable.
- It prevents: Most chances for nutrient toxicities.

Exercise

Adequate, regular exercise helps prevent:

- Obesity.
- Non-insulin dependent (adult-onset) diabetes mellitus.
- Coronary heart disease.
- Some adult bone loss.
- Loss of muscle tone.

Lifestyle

Minimizing alcohol intake helps prevent:

- Liver disease.
- Foetal alcohol syndrome.
- Accidents.

In addition, not smoking, minimal use of medications, no illicit drug use, adequate sleep, and limiting stress provides a more complete approach to good nutrition and health.

TIPS FOR HEALTHY NUTRITION IN GENERAL

1. Eat a variety of foods.
2. Maintain healthy weight.
3. Choose a diet low in fat, saturated fat and cholesterol.
4. Choose a diet with plenty of vegetables, fruits and grain products.
5. Use sugars only in moderation.
6. Use salt and sodium only in moderation.
7. Drink plenty of water (around 2.5 liters for an adult) less at meals and more between meals.

STUDY QUESTIONS

1. Enumerate the important points that prove, valuable while planning meals for vegetarians.
2. How do you proceed to plan menus for expectant and nursing mothers?
3. Give 'To the point tips' on meals planning for infant and toddlers, pre-schoolers, schoolers and adolescents.
4. What are the benefits of good nutrition and health habits and how one can maintain healthy nutrition?
5. Explain the importance of nutrition of pre-schoolers and adolescents.

CHAPTER 16

Meal Planning in Indian Context

> ***Chapter Outlines***
> - Indian scenario
> - Balanced diet
> - Five basic food groups
> - Tips for using daily food guide
> - Study questions

INDIAN SCENARIO

Diet has acquired a new meaning today as a result of health consciousness exercised by a reasonably good proportion of the literate population. Calories are counted before they are consumed and a healthy balance is maintained between caloric intake and expenditure. Though many of them are still the victims of sedentary lifestyle, faulty eating habits and obesity; some people have started realising the importance of nutritious foods–complex carbohydrates, fruits and vegetables. They are also understanding, though slowly, the ills of over consuming saturated fat and cholesterol rich foods.

However, majority of our population is poor, illiterate and still subsists on the diet that is both qualitatively and quantitatively far from satisfactory. Ironically, the people who need more nutritious and calorie rich food–farmers, labourers and other manual workers–are seen facing the onslaughts of malnutrition. At one end of the nutrition spectrum is this undernourished majority struggling to earn two square meals a day and at the other end are the prosperous over weight individuals indulging in faulty eating habits and over consumption sans exercise. The one causative factor of both under nutrition and over nutrition is by ignorance, the other being availability of food, or the lack of it. It is the lack of knowledge of what comprises a healthful diet that goes in significant way to contribute towards the malnourishment of either kind.

BALANCED DIET

The concept of balanced diet was perhaps the first lesson in nutrition we should learn in life as early as possible. We should learn that a judicious mix of all essential nutrients–proteins, carbohydrates, fats, minerals, vitamins and water–as required by our body, comprises a healthful diet. Infact, there are two basic functions which a healthful diet should perform. First, it should minimize the risk of all nutrition related deficiency diseases. Secondly, it should minimize the risk of diseases associated with over consumption. For a nutritionist, a major challenge arises when he is asked to recommend a balanced diet which on one hard should provide all essential nutrients and on the other should be inexpensive, easy to make, tasty and acceptable to all. This is a daunting task particularly in a country like India, where a sizeable segment of the population is poverty stricken.

Added to this, to further compound the matter, is a wide variety of dietary habits of Indians which are largely governed by different cultures, geographic locations, climatic conditions and cropping patterns. Also, the growing affluence of the middle class is gradually posing yet another problem–faulty eating habits leading to excessive consumption of undesirable food resulting in overweight with its deleterious effects on health. Finally, the dietary recommendations need to be presented in ways that are easily understandable, more feasible to be accepted and that can be put into practice by people in order to have a favourable impact on their dietary practices. To cope with this list of challenges is no mean task for any nutritionist and meal planner.

An ideal diet cannot be defined. Hence one must not be very specific while advocating for a particular diet or be very general in the dietary counseling. One must understand that the concept of healthful diet differs from one person to the other. Infants, young children and adolescents need nutritionally rich diets to meet the demands of their growing bodies. Likewise, physiological status, such as pregnancy and lactation also puts mothers under stress, raising their daily nutritional requirements. Men require higher amounts of all nutrients as compared to women. Old age calls for a simple, bland but nutritious diet. Physical work activity determines one's nutritional requirements as demand for nutrients differs from person to person carrying out sedentary, moderate or heavy type of physical work.

All this lead us to the concept of recommended dietary allowances (RDAs). On the basis of height of an Indian adult, body weight of 60 kg and 50 kg for reference man and reference women should be used in arriving at RDAs. The notion behind the concept of RDA is that individuals of similar age, sex and physical activity levels may have different nutrient needs. Both genetic and environmental factors are, presumably, involved. The needs of an individual are rarely known. Thus, if an adequate intake of nutrient is to be assured for all individuals, the nutrient standard should be established at the upper end of the range of requirements of the group. These standards most often are actually above the need of most individuals. Hence, sometimes it becomes difficult to achieve. It is seen that those groups with relatively low energy intakes–teenage girls, adult women and the elderly persons–are usually those finding most difficulty in partaking the recommended levels of intake. Also the "problem nutrients"–calcium, iron, vitamin B-complex, magnesium, zinc, folic acid are generally not consumed in recommended amounts by these groups. The obvious reason for this is limited amount and variety of food available for consumption by the majority population.

Nutrients intake by those with low purchasing capacity, living in both urban and rural areas is far below RDA. One of the most reasonable remedies for this would be food fortification and consumption of supplements. One must also keep in mind the practical difficulties which crop up in this process. Identification of a suitable food for fortification is a major hurdle in India. Food choices vary widely amongst different population groups. The second available alternative of consuming supplements to ensure adequate intake of these problem nutrients, is also a distant dream, due to reasons like cost of the supplement, low purchasing power, ignorance, resistance to change, etc.

Against like dismal scenario, prescription of healthful diet, to serve the purpose of majority population groups of the country is a real challenge. It is practically impossible for anyone to weigh the nutrients as recommended and formulate the diets accordingly. RDAs more importantly serve as reference points for us to consume nutritionally adequate diets. We need not include any new food item or change to any new dietary pattern in order to consume a healthful diet. What we need presently is to bring about slight modifications in the existing diets of our people. Quality more or less remaining unchanged, a little increase in the quantities and nutritionally compatible combinations of the food items normally consumed will take care of the nutrient needs of people to a greater extent.

Overconsumption leads to number of health complications. Obesity, atherosclerosis coronary heart disease, some cancers, hypertension, diabetes and dental caries are a few problems which can be linked to overconsumption.

A diet that provides adequate quantities of essential nutrients without providing a surplus of calories is absolutely essential for maintenance of health. It is also known that in order to be healthy our daily energy intake should match the amount of energy spent during daily physical activity. And to get the required energy, protein, fat and carbohydrates are recommended to be included in the diet in the following—protein may range from 10% to 15% of calories, fat from 20% to 30% and carbohydrate from 55% to 70%—all provided through a variety of sources.

A nutritious diet that provides adequate quantities of all essential nutrients and sources of energy from a variety of foods in amounts needed to achieve and maintain desirable body weight is necessary for good health and for vigorous defence mechanisms against diseases.

The RDAs are not intended for use by consumers, not are the goals for individual dietary intakes. Rather, they are standards against which nutrient intakes can be compared. They are used to evaluate the nutrient content of population food supplies, of foods provided in government-sponsored or other feeding programs, and for related purposes. In fact consumers need a more accessible and easy-to-use guide to menu planning. Several consumer-oriented assessment systems have been designed to fill specific needs.

Because food composition table and RDAs (appendix) are too complex to use by the average consumer, several simplified tools have been developed. Among these are the basic food groupings and exchange lists.

Depending on the major nutrients present in them, Indian foods have been grouped into five basic food groups. For a convenient and nutrionally effective meal planning, various every day foods from the basic food groups are included in the diet in specific amounts and kinds. Hence usage of food group system makes it conventient for a meal manager to plan meals in accordance with the daily dietary requirements of family or any other target group. Food group system lays emphasis on consuming a wide variety of food through judicious selection of foods from each group. A rational approach of choosing foods daily from each group in moderate number and amount (servings) so that all foods groups find representation in meal plan to make it balanced in terms of nutrients and in keeping with dietary requirements.

FIVE BASIC FOOD GROUPS (Table 16.1)

As per the 'Food Guide', the group are given hereunder:

1. Milk-pulse-egg-meat-fish group of protein foods.
2. Primary protective vegetable and fruit group.
3. Secondary protective vegetable and fruit group.
4. Cereal and millet or grain group.
5. Oil, fats and sugar group.

1. Protein Food Group

This group includes milk, pulses, legumes, nuts, eggs, meat, fish and poultry. Basically, it is a protein providing food group which supplies protein inputs for growth and maintenance. Foods included in this group also supply some B-Vitamins such as thiamine, niacin and riboflavin. Besides being protein suppliers, eggs, milk and liver are also good sources of iron. Milk, especially is a rich source of calcium. Each serving of this group supplies 4-6 gm of protein.

Given hereunder are salient features of foods belonging to this group:

1. Among pulses and legumes there are tur, masur, moong, cholas and dry whole grains, beans, peas etc. providing variety and freedom for making various combination to a meal planner. Among nuts and oil seeds also there are many that are in common like groundnut and seasame.
2. Included in the milk category are, apart from milk, curd and other preparations containing whole milk. The food item 'egg' included in human diet pertains to hens' egg and one egg weighing 40-60 gm is taken as one serving.

2. Primary Protective Vegetable and Fruit Group

The group is made up of two sub groups, namely (a) Yellow orange fruit and vegetable and green leafy vegetables (b) Vitamin C rich vegetable and fruits.

The first sub group (a) further comprises two types: (i) Yellow orange fruits and vegetable and (ii) Green leafy and light green leafy vegetable such as cabbage and onion tops.

Food belonging to the type (i) are rich sources of beta-carotene, and type (ii) apart from including green leafy vegetables, such as spinach, fenugreek, coriander, amaranth and radish tops, also encompasses light green leafy vegetables, such as cabbage and onion tops.

The second sub-group includes papaya, apricots, mango, carrots, orange, cantaloup, goose berries etc.

A single serving from this group meets half the daily requirements of vitamin A by supplying its precursor, the β-carotenes.

Second sub group (b) is constituted by vitamin C rich vegetables and fruit comprising, pineapple, tomato, strawberries, citrus fruits (oranges, sweetlime, grape fruits etc.) amla (Indian gooseberry), guava, drumstick and cabbage. These foods are high in dietary fiber and vitamin C.

3. Secondary Protective Fruit and Vegetable Group

Foods belonging to this group supply minerals, vitamins, besides being the largest source of dietary fiber.

The individual foods include ladyfinger, pumpkin cucumber and brinjal; bitter gourd, all ash-gourd, namely bottle, snake, ridge gourds; all immature beans and peas, beetroot, radish, potatoes, sweet potatoes and fruits like banana, melon, grapes, berries etc.

4. Cereal and Millet or Grain Group

The group provides proteins and calories as carbohydrates. The foods in this group supply more than half of the day's requirements for proteins and calories. The group includes jowar, bajra, maize, ragi, rice, wheat and their products such as rice flakes, vermicelli (senvaya) samoline (suji) and fine wheat flour (maida).

Table 16.1: Food guide with five basic food groups

	Sub group I	*Sub group II*	*Sub group III*
(1) Protein food group	Nuts, legumes pulses	Milk and assorted products, eggs	Meat, fish, poultry
(i) Individual foods in each sub group	Groundnut, walnut almonds legumes and their dahls, moong, masur etc.	Milk, skim dry and condensed curd, cheese yoghurt and butter	Organ (liver) and muscle meat chicken, drumstick and breast milk, eggs meat and fish.
(ii) Nutrients present	Protein, thiamine, iron in pulses and legumes Protein, fat vitamin, riboflavin and niacin in nuts	Calcium, riboflavin phosphorus, lactose thiamine and vitamin D, whole milk supplies vitamin A too	Iron (mostly hemo iron), thiamine, niacin, phosphorous liver meat rich in B_{12}, egg yolk rich in cholesterol.
(iii) Serving size (one serving)	25 gm (one tea cup of dahl or legume of medium consistency)	150 gm (one cup milk, one cup curd, one egg)	30 gm meat chicken or fish fillet (without bone) piece
(iv) Number of servings normally required per day	-------------------------	4-6----------------------	
(2) Primary protective vegetable and fruit group	Yellow orange fruits and vegetables, green leafy vegetables	Vitamin C rich vegetables and fruits	
(i) Individual foods in each sub group	Carrot, orange, papaya, mango; all green leafy vegetables, e.g., spinach, cabbage mustard etc.	All citrus fruits gooseberry, guava tomato	
(ii) Nutrients present	β-carotene and other carotenoids (precursors of vitamin A) dietary fiber and to smaller extent other vitamins and minerals	Vitamin C, dietary fiber. To a lesser extent other vitamins and minerals	
(iii) Serving size	50-75 gm (A cup half full of cooked vegetables, half cup shredded carrot	50-75 gm, one small orange or a sweet lime or a medium size tomato	
(iv) Number of servings	------------------------- 2 or more -------------------------		
(3) Secondary protective fruit and vegetable group			
(i) Individual foods in the group	All other vegetable and fruits like sweet potato, ladyfinger bitter gourd, potato, brinjal and all gourds		
(ii) Nutrients present	Abundant source of dietary fiber, vitamins and minerals		
(iii) Serving size	50-70 gm. Half a cup cooked vegetable or one fruit		
(iv) Number of servings	------------------------- 2 or more -------------------------		
(4) Cereal and millet or grain group			
(i) Individual foods in the group	Rice, wheat and their preparations, jowar, bajra, maize, ragi		
(ii) Nutrients present	Carbohydrates, proteins, thiamine and iron		
(iii) Serving size	25 gm. One medium chapatti, half a cup cooked rice, one slice of bread		
(iv) Number of servings	------------------------- 6 to 12 -------------------------		
(5) Oil, fat and sugar group			
(i) Individual foods in the group	Oils, fats, sugars, jaggery		
(ii) Nutrients present	Fats and sugars		
(iii) Serving size	25 gm (one spoonful of oil), 25 gm of sugar or jaggery		
(iv) Number of servings	------------------------- Minimum one -------------------------		

Legumes include dried beans, peas and lentils. They are all seeds of leguminous plants, and they either have been allowed to dry in their pods before being picked or have been dried after being shelled. Green beans and green peas are also legumes, but are picked in their immature state, and are not as rich nutritionally as legumes. Legumes are good sources of some B vitamins and iron and average 22 percent protein by weight (except for the soyabean, which is 40 percent protein). They contain no cholesterol, and most are low in fat, except for soyabeans, which contain fat but considerably less (and less saturated) than meats.

Legumes can be stored for long periods of time and are economical to use. However, they are not without a couple of concerns. Whole beans and peas (not split peas or lentils) must first be hydrated before cooking, a slow process during which water enters through the hilum, the point at which each bean or pea was attached to its pod, because the skin is impermeable to water. Soaking can be accomplished faster by boiling the legumes in water for a few minutes, and then setting them aside to soak, or by pressure cooking for added time. An alternative to rehydrating legumes is to buy them canned, if available. Whether canned or soaked, beans and peas have a tendency to produce flatulence or gas in people who do not eat them very often. This effect is due to non-digestible carbohydrates in beans and peas that intestinal bacteria break down for food and produce gas as a by-product. This problem can be reduced by making sure the legume is cooked thoroughly (because uncooked starch is harder to digest) and also by disposing of the soaking water.

Cereal grains are the fruits or seeds of cultivate grasses and include wheat, corn, rice, rye, barley, oats, millet and sorghum. Buckwheat, although not a true cereal grain because it is not a member of the grass family, is considered to be one because of its grasslike structure. Cereal grains, such as rice and oats, are cooked in water until they become hydrated, which softens the grain, makes it more digestible, and improves the flavour. During cooking, gelatinization takes place, which means that the starches in the grain absorb water and swell tremendously, causing a thickening of the mixture. From cereal grains are made both hot and cold breakfast cereals, flours used in baking starches used in thickening foods such as puddings and grayish and dried pastes used to make pastas such as macroni, spaghetti, and egg noodles.

Cereal grains are good source of iron and B vitamins, particularly thiamin, riboflavin and niacin. Whole grains that have not been milled or refined are also good sources of fiber and minerals.

Since proteins of cereals are not of very good quality and to take care of this limitation two or more cereals are eaten along with pulse and legume combinations so as to improve the protein quantity by mutual supplementation of amino acids. As a matter of fact, cereal (grain) proteins when eaten together with pulses or legumes make the missing essential amino acids mutually available. For example grains (cereals) are deficient in the essential amino acid lysine and legumes are deficient in methionine, but from grain and legumes together the body receives complete protein, that is, all the eight essential amino acids.

5. Oil, Fat and Sugar Group

This group also known as the fuel group mainly yields energy. Whereas fats and oils are condensed forms of energy, the sugars, are quickly available sources of energy. Jaggery is a crude unrefined sugarcane juice in concentrated form which contains, in addition to sugar sucrose, certain minerals like iron.

Simple single (glucose, fructose) and double (sucrose) sugars are used to sweeten our daily foods and beverages. Indians, as somebody has very aptly said, have a sweet tooth and hence sugar (sucrose) occupies an important place in their diets, although it is not a nutritional necessity. Oils and fats enhance the palatability of foods and are used for seasoning and dressing of foods. In addition, they also impart qualities like texture and flavour to foods and increase their satiety values. Fats and oils also become sources of fat soluble vitamins namely, vitamin A,D,E and K. Naturally, saturated fats like butter and ghee are rich natural sources of vitamin A. Hydrogenated fats such as vanaspati are fortified with vitamin A. Also oils and fats are needed to supply essential fatty acids to human body.

Whereas main edible oils are all of vegetable origin obtained from groundnut, sesame, coconut and mustard; the fats include butter, ghee, margarine and vanaspati.

A minimum level of fat (20-30 gm) thus is always necessary in diet. However, a high fat diet is deleterious to health and plays no less role in the genesis of obesity, atherosclerosis and a host of other diseases.

Apart from foods listed and discussed in five basic food groups, there are certain others that, though in alienable part of Indian diet, are not included in the food groups. These include pickles, spices and condiments. Table salt

(Sodium chloride) is another such case. Although most of these are taste flavour and aroma imparting, some of them like iodized salt (source of iodine) and lime smeared betel leaf (source of calcium), also provide certain nutrients in sizable amounts.

TIPS FOR USING DAILY FOOD GUIDE

1. First step is to know the RDA for different age groups.
2. The next step is to prepare a food list i.e., a list of quantities of various food groups to be included in the diet so that it is balanced and can meet the RDA. This can be done by:
   i. Selecting foods from all the five food groups.
   ii. Deciding the quantities of the selected foods as multiples of portion sizes.
3. Include at least the minimum number of servings as recommended for each food group in the food guide.
4. Include atleast one food from protein food group (group 1) in each meal.
5. Grain group (group 4) should supply not more than 65-70% of total energy needed.
6. Cereals and pulses combinations are consumed in such a way that the former supplies 4 to 5 times more proteins than the latter (Cereals 7: Pulses 1).
7. Oil, fat and sugar group (group 5) should not contribute more than 20% of the total energy. Table sugar (sucrose) and jaggery should not contribute more than ¼th of the recommended caloric contributions (20%) of this group.

By following the basic tenets of five food groups systems, one cannot only plan one's meal well but also can undertake the nutritional evaluation of one's dietary intake.

Thus a convenient, quick and fairly accurate nutritional evaluation of the diet can be made by using 'the exchange lists'. The technique in addition, also enables the dietition, housewife or any other meal manager to plan the diets with one or more nutrients in restricted amounts by an easier to follow method.

Exchange List of Foods

One defines an exchange list as a table which contains a group of foods in specified amounts with approximately equal carbohydrate, protein and fat levels. This does not mean that the values of two foods within the group are identical. It is but natural that there would be some differences in the values but these tend to nullify each other owing to the variety of foods that are selected by the subject from within the group on day to day basis.

Food Groups and Food Exchange System

Various food items that are commonly consumed in our country which are the main source of nutrients in our diet were discussed. Normally these foods are used in formulating nutritionally adequate diets for various categories of people to meet their needs as per nutritional standards (RDA) and also for formulating special diets for therapeutic purposes. In order to do this conveniently 'food group system' and food exchange system are widely followed.

The food group system converts quantitative nutrient data into food related information that can be used both by consumer and health professionals in diet planning to achieve nutritional adequacy.

The five group plan allows a person to plan his/her diet to achieve the nutritional adequacy as per Recommended Dietary Allowances. Information on foods which are rich sources of nutrients are given in Table 16.1.

The five food group system can be used by health professionals for the following purposes:

1. **Tool for nutritional assessment and screening:** A brief dietary history system can disclose inadequacies of nutrient from any of the five groups. This information can be the first clue for the possibility of the subject may be at the risk of developing nutritional deficiency.
2. **Tool for nutritional counselling:** The dietary history based on the five food group system allows a health team to counsel or teach a patient about nutrition.
3. **Explaining therapeutic diets to a patient:** Therapeutic diets are scientifically based on nutrient composition and food groups which can be used in menu planning.
4. **Food labelling and surveillance system:** Food groups can be used for food labelling and for nutrition surveillance system.

The Food Exchange System

Food exchange system allows one to choose a variety of foods with adequate nutrients. The food exchange system is important in planning a nutritious diet. Essentially the food exchange system can be used to select foods in familiar measures that are adequate in nutrient content and satisfy the requirement of a given individual.

Menu Planning

The five food group plan permits an individual to plan a menu to achieve nutrient intakes as specified by RDA. The food exchange system is important in this planning of a nutritious diet. The two components, namely, nutrient density and balance are achieved when these guidelines are used. The food exchange system can be used to select a variety of foods that are adequate in nutrient content and satisfies requirement.

STUDY QUESTIONS

1. What is the concept of balanced diet that you must bear in mind while planning meals for a common Indian?
2. Explain the 'Five food group' and 'Food exchange' systems that make the cornerstones of meal planning in Indian context.
3. What are the main points that you must consider while using daily food guide for meal planning?

CHAPTER 17

Food Exchange List: An Introduction

Chapter Outlines

- Salient features of the food exchange list
- Use of the food exchange list for meal planning
- Detailed versions of food exchange list
- Study questions

SALIENT FEATURES OF THE FOOD EXCHANGE LIST

Food exchange list includes the foods commonly used being grouped into 7 main groups on the basis of similarities in nutrient composition. The exchange list system intends to make diet planning easier, practical and meaningful. As a matter of fact, the exchange list of any food group includes specified amounts of various foods in that group with approximately equal carbohydrate, protein, fat, vitamin and mineral content (fruits and vegetables being exceptions).

Any food within a given list can be replaced with any other in the list as it provides more or less the same nutritive value. With the use of this system, nutritionally balanced and varied diets can be easily planned by choosing adequate number of exchanges from each group. When energy and protein requirements are fulfilled at the first place, all other nutrient requirements too are likely to be met. Only vitamin A and C become exceptions and fulfilling their requirements need suitable selection of foods from the vegetable and fruit exchange lists. Similarly, selection of iron rich foods helps ensure adequacy of iron.

The seven main food groups in the food exchange system are milk, meat and pulse, vegetables A and B, fruit, cereal, fat and sugar and one exchange of each normally represents commonly measured/procured units of food or its multiple.

Source: Nutritive Value of Commonly used Foods. Adapted from Department of Foods and Nutrition, Lady Irwin College, New Delhi which has been modified from; Handbook of Diet Therapy. Dorothea Turner. The University of Chicago Press, 1959. With due acknowledgment to both the sources.

The salient features of each of the 7 food groups (Tables 17.1 and 17.2) of the food exchange list are as follows:

1. **Milk:** One cup whole milk (cow's) forms the basis of this exchange providing 8 g protein and 170 Kcal per 250 ml. Other milk products can by substituted for 1 cup cow's milk in amounts that provide 8 g protein. In case skimmed milk is used in a normal diet, 2 additional fat exchanges may be added, because of the negligible fat content of the milk.
2. **Meat and Pulse Exchange:** These two exchanges are interchangeable and are characterized by high protein content. One exchange of meat or pulse is that amount which provides 7 g protein.

   Meat Exchange: This includes meat, fish, poultry, egg, paneer, cheese, proteinex etc. One exchange of meat approximately equals 30-40 g of edible portion of flesh food, which is less than 1 serving.

   Pulse Exchange: Pulses, soyabean and its products are included in this exchange and 1 exchange approximately equals 30 g, which is one serving, with the exception of soyabean.
3. **Vegetables A and B:** Vegetables are divided into those that contain negligible or ≤ 3.5 g % carbohydrate, i.e.,

Table 17.1: Comprehensive food exchange list

Sl. No.	Food exchange	Wt. of raw food (g) (approx.)	Measure of raw food (approx.)	Calories	Protein (g)	Carbohydrate (g)	Fat (g)
1.	Milk	250	1 cup	170	8	12	10
2. a.	Meat	40	1 egg	70	7	Nil	5
b.	Pulse	30	3 tbsp	100	7	17	Nil
3. a.	Vegetable A	100	½ cup	20	1	<3.5	Nil
b.	Vegetable B	100-150	½ cup	40	2	7	Nil
4.	Fruit	80-100	1 portion	40	Nil	10	Nil
5.	Cereal	20	3 tbsp	70	2	15	Nil
6.	Fat	5	1 tbsp	45	-	-	5
7.	Sugar	5	1tbsp	20	-	5	-

Table 17.2: Food plan

Sl. No.	Food exchange	No. of exchange	Approximate amount (g)	Energy (Kcal)	Protein (g)	Carbohydrate (g)	Fat (g)
1.	Milk	2	500	340	16	24	20
2. a.	Meat	1	40	70	7	Nil	5
b.	Pulse	2	60	200	14	34	Nil
3. a.	Vegetable A	2	200	40	2	7	Nil
b.	Vegetable B	2	200-300	80	4	14	Nil
4.	Fruit	1	80-100	40	—	10	Nil
5.	Cereal	9	180	630	18	135	Nil
6.	Fat	7	35	315	—	—	35
7.	Sugar	5	25	100	—	25	—
				1815	61	244	60

vegetable A and those with 7% carbohydrate, i.e., vegetable B. Vegetable A provides negligible amount of carbohydrate unless 2 or more than 2 exchanges are used, and in such cases, 2 exchanges of vegetable A are considered equivalent to 1 exchange of vegetable B. Some vegetables like root vegetables which have approximately 20% carbohydrate are included in the cereal exchange.

4. **Fruit:** One exchange is that amount of fruit that would provide 10 g carbohydrate and this amount is represented by majority of the fruit in one serving portion. Some fruits however, like banana, mango do not represent average serving sizes per exchange due to their higher carbohydrate content, as also canned fruit and dried fruit. The amount per exchange of these fruit is therefore less as compared to the average of the exchange.

5. **Cereal:** This includes cereals, bread products, pastas and some high carbohydrate vegetables like potato, colocasia and yam. One cereal exchange provides 15 g carbohydrate which is equivalent to approximately 20 g dry cereals, 30 g bread and 50-60 g potatoes and other root vegetables included in this group.

6. **Fat:** This group includes fats, ghee, oil, butter, cream, nuts and oilseeds containing 5 g of fat. One exchange provides 45 Kcal and equals 5 g (1 tsp) in the case of fats and oils. Nuts provide some protein also besides energy.

7. **Sugar:** This may be added to the diet to fulfill the energy requirements and for increasing palatability. One teaspoon or approximately 5 g sugar provides 5 g carbohydrates and 20 Kcal and may be considered as one sugar exchange.

Food adjuncts: Miscellaneous items like tea, coffee, spices and vinegar lend interest to the diet but have insignificant nutrient content in the amounts commonly used these may thus be included in the diet plans without calculations.

Detailed exchange lists follow the comprehensive food exchange list.

Food Plan

The prepared food plan can then be translated into menu/ menus by dividing the daily food allowance into a meal pattern, suitable for the individual.

USE OF THE FOOD EXCHANGE LIST FOR MEAL PLANNING

Meal Pattern: Distribution of exchange between different meals: (Tables 17.3 and 17.4)

- The first step in meal planning using the food exchange list is to prepare the food plan for the day. The food plan consists of the total numbers of exchanges of each of the seven food groups, constituting the food exchange system, which fulfills the given nutritional requirements.
- Preparation of the food plan includes assessing the approximate amounts of milk, meat and pulse that a person can afford, depending on the socio-economic status and preferences, which will provide most of the protein requirements and part of the energy requirements.
- Sufficient amounts of vegetable and fruit are also included based on economic status and preferences, to ensure adequacy of vitamin A and C in the diet.
- The energy and protein values provided by milk, meat, pulse, vegetables and fruit are calculated.
- The remaining energy requirement is then provided by the cereal exchange, fat exchange and sugar. The cereal exchange also provides the remaining required protein.
- The food exchanges in the food plan should, as far as possible, is used in whole numbers.
- The second step in meal planning is the preparation of the meal pattern. This involves distributing the food exchanges from the total food plan, as evenly as possible, between the various meals. This ensures balance of nutrients between the meals and nutritional adequacy of each meal.

Table 17.3

Food group	*Meal and No. of exchanges per meal*				*Total No. of exchanges*
	B	*L*	*L*	*D*	
Milk	¾	½	¼	½	2
Meat	1	-	-	-	1
Pulse	-	1	-	1	2
Vegetable A	-	1	-	1	2
Vegetable B	-	1	-	1	2
Fruit	-	-	1	-	1
Cereal	2	3	1	3	9
Fat	2	2	1	2	7
Sugar	2	-	1	2	5

- The third step is the translation of the food allowances in the meal pattern into a menu plan suitable for the individual. Several menus can be made based on the same meal pattern.
- This method of meal planning can be used for low, medium or high cost diets by (a) adjusting the amount of different food exchanges used, but providing the same nutrient content and (b) by selecting suitable foods within an exchange.
- The detailed exchange list of each food group permits easy substitution of foods, thus adding flexibility, interest, variety and ease in meal planning.
- Occasionally, exchanges may be carried from one meal to another without exceeding the total. While planning a day's balanced diet with its detailed nutrient composition, it is advisable to calculate the nutrient intake of each meal besides the total day's nutrient intake.
- Suppose a diet providing 2000 kcal and 60 g protein approximately, has to be planned for an adult belonging to the middle income group. Using the steps listed a food plan is first drawn up based on the socio-economic status.

  Based on the meal pattern, one or several menus (menu plan) may be planned. The approximate amounts of various foodstuffs which may be used under each exchange can be determined from the detailed food exchange lists should be rounded off to the nearest practical whole number. For example, 27 g may be taken as 30 g.
- Variations in the menu can easily be introduced within the same meal pattern. For example, at breakfast, instead of porridge, milk and two toasts may be planned or two parathas and curd.

Table 17.4: Menu plan

	Menu	*Ingredients*	*Exchange group*	*No. of exchange*	*Approx. amount*
Breakfast	1. Porridge	Milk	Milk (cow)	¾	185
		Broken	Cereal	1	120
		Wheat	Sugar	2	10
	2. Toast	Sugar	Cereal	1	30
		Bread	Fat	1	6
	3. Fried egg	Butter	Meat	1	50
		Egg	Fat	1	5
Lunch	1. Chapatti/	Fat	Cereal	3	60
	rice	Atta/rice	Pulse	1	30
	2. Bengal	Bengal gram	Veg A	½	50
	gram with	bottle gourd	Fat	1	5
	bottle gourd		Veg B	½	80
			Fat	1	5
	3. Capiscum	Capiscum	Milk (cow)	½	125
	veg	Fat	Veg A	½	50
	4. Curd	Curd	Veg B	¼	50
	5. Salad	Cucumber	Milk (cow)	¼	65
		Tomato	Sugar	1	5
Tea time	1. Tea	Milk	Cereal	1	20
		Sugar	Fat	1	5
	2. Mathri	Maida	Fruit	1	60
		Fat	Cereal	2	40
	3. Fruit	Mango	Veg B	1/3	20
Dinner	1. Vegetable rice	Rice	Veg B	1/3	15
	with sprouts	Carrot	Veg B	1/3	15
		Peas	Pulse	1	30
		Onion	Fat	1	5
		Green gram	Milk (cow)	½	125
		Whole	Veg A	½	50
		Fat	Veg A	½	50
	2. Spinach	Curd	Cereal	1	20
	raita	Spinach	Sugar	2	10
		Cucumber	Far	1	5
	3. Salad	Vermicelli			
	4. Sweet	Sugar			
	vermicelli	Fat			

Given hereunder are the detailed versions of the Food Exchange List.

DETAILED VERSIONS OF THE FOOD EXCHANGE LIST

MILK EXCHANGE

Protein: 8 g, Carbohydrate: 12 g, Fat: 10 g, Energy: 170 Kcal

Foodstuff	*Amount (g)*	*Protein (g)*	*Carbohydrate (g)*	*Fat (g)*	*Energy (Kcal)*
Cow's milk	250	8	11.0	10.3	168
Buffalo's milk	185	8	9.3	12.0	216
** Skim milk (liquid)	320	8	14.7	Nil	93
Whole milk powder	31	8	11.8	8	154
Curd	258	8	7.7	10.3	155
Skim milk (powder)	21	8	10.7	Nil	75
Channa from cow's milk	44	8	0.5	9.2	117
Channa from buffalo's milk	60	8	4.7	13.8	175
Cheese	33	8	2.1	8.3	115
Khoa from buffalo's milk	55	8	11.3	17.2	231
Khoa from cow's milk	40	8	0.0	10.4	165
Khoa from skim buffalo's milk	36	8	9.3	0.6	72

Need to add two fat exchanges as the 'milk types' are without fat.

MEAT EXCHANGE

Protein: 7 g, Fat: 5 g, Traces of Carbohydrate, Energy: 70 Kcals

Foodstuff	*Weight (g)*	*Protein (g)*	*Fat (g)*	*Energy (Kcal)*
Egg yolk	39	7	11.3	13.8
Egg	53	7	7.0	81
Egg white	58	7	-	26
Fowl	27	7	0.2	29
Goat meat	32	7	1.2	38
Goat liver	35	7	1.1	38
Sheep liver	35	7	2.6	53
Mutton, muscle	38	7	5.1	73
Pork	37	7	1.7	43
Crab	63	7	6.1	106
Hilsa	32	7	6.2	87
Katla	35	7	0.8	39
Pomfret	41	7	0.5	33
Prawn	37	7	0.4	32
Singhara	34	7	1.0	53
Channa	38	7	7.9	101
Cheese	29	7	7.3	101
Channa, buffalo	52	7	1.2	162
Proteinex	12.5	7	-	28
Sausages	80	7	23	273

PULSE EXCHANGE

Protein: 7 g, Negligible fat, Carbohydrate 17 g, Energy: 100 Kcals

Foodstuff	*Weight (g)*	*Protein (g)*	*Fat (g)*	*Carbohydrate (g)*	*Energy (Kcal)*
Bengal gram whole	41	7	2.2	25	148
Bengal gram dal	34	7	1.8	20	125
Black gram dal	29	7	0.4	17	101
Cow pea	29	7	0.3	16	94
Green gram whole	29	7	0.4	16	97
Green gram dal	28	7	0.3	17	101
Lentil	29	7	0.2	16	96
Bean, dry	35	7	0.4	20	105
Rajma	30	7	0.5	18	105
Redgram dal	31	7	0.5	18	104
Soyabean	16	7	3.2	3.4	70
Nutrinuggets	14	7	0.1	4.2	48

100 g soaked and sprouted green gram provides approximately 0.63 mg thiamine, 0.6 mg riboflavin, 4.1 mg niacin and 82 mg vitamin C.

- At lunch/dinner, different vegetables and pulses can be planned. Instead of curd, a milk based dessert could be given or paneer. Noodles with vegetables could be given instead of rice/chapatti and vegetables. Pulse could be given in the form of soup or sprout salad. Cereal pulse and vegetables could be combined to make dosa and sambhar.
- At tea time, various snacks could be given such as samosa, sandwich, cutlet, poha, upma, biscuits or other similar items.
- In a normal diet planned, the energy provided by the diet may be equal to the RDA or approximately ± 50 Kcal. In a vegetarian cereal based diet, the protein intake usually exceeds the RDA. Energy and protein intake should be as near the RDA as possible in the case of therapeutic diets.
- To plan a meal for a family consisting of individuals of different ages and sex, the total energy requirement may be calculated using the 'Consumption Units' given by (Nutritive Value of Indian Foods, 1999) for individuals of various ages, in relation to the adult sedentary male. The same proportions may be used as a rough estimate of the total protein requirement and the serving portions for each family member.
- Finally a note of caution. Do not start meal planning with a preconceived menu or a particular dish. This results in losing the advantage of flexibility, variety and time economy introduced by the use of the food exchange list method.

VEGETABLE -A EXCHANGE

Carbohydrate: 3.5 g, Protein: 1 g and Negligible fat

2 exchange of vegetable A can be considered equivalent to

1 exchange of vegetable B

Foodstuff	*Carbohydrate %*
Bathua leaves	2.9
Bottle gourd	2.5
Cucumber	2.5
Ghosalas	2.9
Lettuce	2.5
Mustard leaves	3.2
Parwar	2.2
Radish leaves	2.4
Radish white	3.4
Ridge gourd	3.4
Snake gourd	3.3
Spinach	2.9
Tinda	3.4

VEGETABLE-B EXCHANGE

Carbohydrate: 7 g, Protein: 2 g, Negligible Fat, Energy: 40 Kcal

Foodstuff	*Weight (g)*	*Carbohydrate (g)*	*Protein (g)*	*Energy (Kcal)*
Amaranth	115	7	4.6	52
Beetroot	80	7	1.4	34
Bitter gourd	167	7	2.7	42
Brinjal	175	7	2.5	42
Broad beans	97	7	4.4	47
Cabbage	152	7	2.7	41
Capsicum	166	7	2.1	39
Carrot	66	7	0.6	32
Cauliflower	175	7	4.5	53
Colocasia leaves	103	7	4.0	58
Drumstick	192	7	4.8	50
Coriander leaves	111	7	3.7	49
Fenugreek leaves	117	7	5.1	57
French beans	165	7	2.6	41
Jack fruit tender	75	7	1.9	38
Knolkhol	184	7	2.0	39
Ladies finger	109	7	2.0	38
Mushroom	163	7	2.3	47
Mint leaves	121	7	5.8	58
Onion small	56	7	1.0	33
Peas	44	7	3.2	41
Pumpkin	152	7	2.1	38
Tomato	194	7	1.7	39
Turnip	113	7	0.6	33

FRUIT EXCHANGE

Carbohydrate: 10 g, Negligible Protein and Fat, Energy: 40 Kcal

Foodstuff	*Weight (g)*	*Carbohydrate (g)*	*Energy (Kcal)*
Amla	74	10	42
Apricot	86	10	46
Apple	75	10	44
Banana	40	10	42
Cherries	72	10	46
Dates, fresh	30	10	43
Grape fruit	143	10	46
Grapes	61	10	41
Guava	80	10	45

Contd.

Contd.

Lemon sweet (nimbu)	92	10	54
Lichi	73	10	44
Lime sweet (malta)	128	10	46
Lime sweet (mausami)	107	10	46
Loquat	104	10	44
Mango, ripe	59	10	44
Melon, musk	286	10	49
Orange	92	10	44
Papaya	139	10	44
Pear	84	10	44
Pineapple	93	10	43
Plums	90	10	47
Pomegranate	69	10	44
Raspberry	86	10	48
Raisins	13	10	41
Sapota	47	10	46
Water melon	303	10	49

CEREAL EXCHANGE

Carbohydrate: 15 g, Protein: 2 g, Negligible Fat, Energy: 70 Kcal

Foodstuff	*Weight (g)*	*Carbohydrate (g)*	*Protein (g)*	*Energy (Kcal)*
Bajra	22	15	2.6	79
Barley	22	15	2.5	72
Bread, white	29	15	2.3	69
Bread, brown	31	15	2.7	76
Biscuits, salty	28	15	1.8	150
Biscuits, sweet	21	15	1.3	96
Cake, plain	31	15	1.0	88
Cake, sponge	25	15	1.5	67
Cornflakes	18	15	1.4	72
Jowar	21	1	2.1	73
Maize, dry	23	15	2.5	79
Noodles, macroni, spaghetti	20	15	2.3	70
Oatmeal	24	15	3.3	90
Ragi	21	15	1.5	69
Rice	19	15	1.3	66
Rice flakes	20	15	1.3	65
Rice, puffed	20	15	2.1	66
Semolina	20	15	2.1	70

Contd.

Contd.

Wheat, flour	22	15	2.7	75
Wheat, flour (refined)	21	15	2.3	73
Vermicelli	19	15	1.7	67
Colocasia	71	15	2.1	69
Lotus stem (dry)	29	15	1.7	63
Potato	66	15	1.0	64
Potato sweet	53	15	0.6	64
Yam	58	15	0.8	64

FAT EXCHANGE

Fat: 5 g, Negligible Carbohydrate and Protein, Energy: 45 Kcal

Foodstuff	*Weight (g)*	*Protein (g)*	*Fat (g)*	*Energy (Kcal)*
Butter	6	0	5	45
Ghee	5	0	5	45
Hydrogenated oil	5	0	5	45
Almonds	8	1.7	5	53
Cooking oil	5	0	5	45
Cashew nuts	11	2.3	5	66
Coconuts, dry	8	0.3	5	53
Coconuts, fresh	12	0.5	5	53
Gingerly seeds	12	2.2	5	58
Groundnuts, roasted	13	3.4	5	74
Walnuts	8	1.3	5	55
Bacon	10	3.5	5	60
Cream, light 20%	25	Nil	5	45
Cream 40 %	15	Nil	5	45
Mayonnaise	6	Nil	5	45

Source: Nutritive Value of Commonly Used Foods, Department of Foods and Nutrition, Lady Irwin College, New Delhi (With due acknowledgment).

STUDY QUESTIONS

1. Discuss the purposefulness of the food exchange list system.
2. Explain the salient features of each of the food system of the 7 food group of the food exchange list.

CHAPTER 18

Protein Quality and Its Evaluation

Chapter Outlines

- Protein quality
- In vitro evaluation of protein quality
- In vivo evaluation of protein quality
- Index of nutritional quality
- Study questions

PROTEIN QUALITY

Animal experimentation in rats, during the early part of the twentieth century, revealed that milk protein promoted optimal growth, as evidenced by a far higher weight gain on casein feeding as compared to wheat protein. Zein, a corn protein, didn't support growth at all, as the rats digesting it, as a protein source, were seen to lose weight. A more intensive research into the cause effect aspect of such outcomes led to the conclusion that differences in growth supporting abilities of these proteins are due to their varying amino acid compositions. Years of experimentation have made it clear that quality of a various proteins depends upon its essential amino acid content. Human body needs amino acids in different amounts. Therefore, a good quality protein is the one that supplies different essential amino acids in the proportion in which they are needed by the body for the synthesis of tissue protein for their growth and maintenance. They are also referred to as complete proteins. Proteins of animal origin, such as those present in milk, meat, fish, egg and poultry are capable of promoting optimum growth and maintenance and are good quality or complete proteins as compared to plant proteins.

A poor quality protein, on the other hand, either completely lacks or has a slow content of an essential amino acid. Such an amino acid is termed as limiting amino acid as it bears the cross of limiting the nutritive quality or completeness of that protein. Proteins of plant origin, namely those from cereals, pulses, legumes, nuts, seeds or vegetables are incomplete proteins.

To ensure optimum dietary protein levels, it becomes imperative to evaluate the quality of proteins in different foodstuffs. Towards this end, a number of indices of protein quality, obtainable either by laboratory (*in vitro*) or biological (*in vivo*) methods, have been devised by nutritionists. Whereas comparison of the amino acid composition of the test protein with that of a high quality protein (milk or egg protein), or with a reference amino acid pattern devised by world health organization, is the hallmark of *in vitro* evaluation; *in vivo* assessment is based upon the ability of the test protein to support growth and maintenance in a living subject by promoting cellular synthesis and thereby causing the retention of the ingested protein nitrogen in the body.

Since conversion of dietary proteins into free amino acids by the process of gastrointestinal digestion is essential prerequisite for the absorption and utilization of proteins therefore, proteins that are easily digestible, e.g., egg proteins and milk proteins, are utilized in an optimum or near optimum manner as compared to the proteins of wheat and other cereals, that are partially digested due to the presence of :

(i) Protease husks of incompletely hydrolyzable polysaccharides around protein rich portions of the grains.

(ii) Protease inhibitors such as trypsin inhibitors in soyabeans.

An index of digestibility of a protein, termed as Digestibility Coefficient (D.C) is thus defined as the percentage of dietary nitrogen consumed that finds its way into the blood circulation after the completion of digestive process. 'Digestibility Coefficient' is calculated from the following formula:

$$\text{Digestibility Coefficient} = DC$$

$$\frac{\text{Dietary N - (Total N in feces - Endogenous N in feces)}}{\text{Dietary N}} \quad 100$$

Where 'endogenous N in feces' is the nitrogen present in the feces of the subject on a protein free diet.

IN VITRO EVALUATION OF PROTEIN QUALITY

Chemical Score or Amino Acid Score

A complete protein is the one that contains all the amino acids essential for human beings in proportions in which they are required by the human body. The assigning of chemical score or amino acid score to a protein involves comparing the content of each essential amino acid of the test protein with that of the same amino acid present in the standard reference protein (like egg protein) or a reference amino acid pattern devised by FAO/WHO (Table 18.1).

Table 18.1: Reference amino acid pattern devised by FAO/WHO

Amino acids	*Requisite level in mg per g of protein*
Isoleucine	40
Leucine	70
Lysine	55
Methionine + Cystine	35
Pheynylalanine +Tyrosine	60
Threonine	40
Tryptophan	10
Valine	50
Total	360

Such a comparison, based upon the following formula, yields a value for each essential amino acid.

$$\text{Amino acid score} \quad \frac{\text{mg of amino acid present in 1 g of the test protein}}{\text{mg of amino acid in 1 g of reference protein}}$$

Essential amino acid of the test protein that scores the lowest value is called the limiting amino acid of that protein. And the amino acid score or chemical score of the test protein is the lowest score obtained by one of the essential (limiting) amino acid. For instance, soyabean protein has chemical score of 75 as sulphur containing amino acids methionine and cysteine of soyabean protein constitute 75 percent of the same amino acids (methionine and cysteine) present in the reference protein. If soyabean protein is fed as a protein source to human subjects about 75 percent of its each essential amino acid will be utilized for protein synthesis in body tissues (due to the constraint imposed by the limiting amino acids on their complete utilization). Consequently, 75 percent of its nitrogen is retained in the body and the rest excreted in the urine causing wastage.

Generally lysine, threonine, sulphur containing amino acids (methionine and cysteine) and tryptophan are the limiting amino acids in proteins. In practice, therefore, amino acid scores are determined for these amino acids only.

Chemical or amino acids score, though a crude approximation of protein quality, yet gives values obtained as protein quality index that agree well with those obtained by biological methods.

Other advantages of this method lie in its simplicity and convenience. The principle underlying the amino acids score evaluation can also be used to determine the nutritive quality of a mixture of proteins purely by theoretical calculation based upon the amino acid composition of the individual proteins constituting the protein mixture.

Another *in vitro* method of protein quality assessment, the pepsin digest index, which also evaluates the digestibility of the given test protein by the gastric enzyme pepsin, is not commonly used for protein quality evaluation owing to the cumbersome nature of the procedure involved.

However, protein quality, or the nutritional value of a protein, is meaningful only in terms of usefulness of a protein for specific vital purposes such as growth, replacement of metabolic losses and damaged tissues, reproduction, lactation, and general well-being. The usefulness of a protein may differ for several of these functions. Further, a measure of usefulness of a protein based on chemical analysis of its amino acid makeup is complicated by a number of factors. These include accuracy of the analytical method under conditions that can preclude the detection of one or another amino acid or cause its destruction, availability and digestibility of the protein from foods that many not be readily broken down by digestive enzymes or absorbed through the intestine, and factors contributing to unpalatability of the protein-containing food. Yet another factor that has a bearing on the accuracy of results is amino acid imbalance. It is possible to have an excess of one or more amino acids relative to other in a protein. This can have a negative effect on growth etc.

These objections to chemical analysis of amino acid content to determine protein quality are not encountered when a biological method, such as an animal feeding study, is used. However, in this case a different set of obstacles is encountered. One of the most obvious is how closely results obtained with laboratory animals apply to humans. Even where questions of digestibility and vital response are ruled out, the palatability differences between species must be considered in arriving at a valid measure of the nutritional usefulness of a protein source. Notwithstanding these difficulties, research has shown that results obtained with young rats generally are applicable to humans, and feeding tests under controlled conditions are far more easily carried out on rate than with humans. Such tests may be run under a variety of experimental conditions which then influence the interpretations that may be given for the nutritional findings.

In brief, it can be said that, *in vivo* protein quality determination or the biological methods of protein quality assessment are the methods of choice due to their being the closer estimates of the protein utilization in human biological systems.

IN VIVO EVALUATION OF PROTEIN QUALITY

Among the various methods of *in vivo* protein quality estimation, the biological value is the most prevalent one.

Biological Value

This method of protein quality appraisal is most favoured one. It measures the extent of protein nitrogen retention for growth or maintenance in the experimental animals and the nitrogen retained is expressed as the percentage of the total nitrogen that has been absorbed by the intestinal tract and is calculated using the following equation:

$$\text{Biological Value} \quad \frac{\text{N retained}}{\text{N absorbed}} \quad 100$$

$$\text{B.V.} = 100 \times \frac{\text{Dietary N - (Total N in feces - Endogenous N in feces) - (Total urinary N - Endogenous N in urine)}}{\text{Dietary N - (Total N in feces - Endogenous N in feces)}}$$

In order to evaluate the biological value of a given protein food, it becomes imperative to feed it to the experimental animals (mostly rat) as an exclusive protein source during the test period and the nitrogen content of the diet, urine and feces determined. Also the content of the urine and feces is determined for the same animal experimental model by keeping on protein free diet in order to assess the endogenous nitrogen in feces and urine.

Highest biological values are found in the egg protein (90 to 98) and cow's milk casein (85-90). Plant proteins like those of rice and soybean, on the other hand have biological values around 75. Among animal proteins only gelatin has the lowest biological value owing to the complete absence of the essential amino acid tryptophan. Generally, protein with biological values of more than 70 provide adequate nutrition in terms of growth support provided the caloric intake is adequate.

Net Protein Utilization (NPU)

Apart from its essential amino acid composition, the other factor that contributes to the quality of a protein is its digestibility. NPU is one such index that also takes into account the relative digestibility of the protein.

Infact, NPU is BV multiplied by digestibility and gauges both digestibility of food protein and the biological value of the amino acid content that gets absorbed after the food protein digestion. NPU value of a protein expresses the proportion of the food nitrogen that is retained by the body for tissue building and maintenance, whereas BV represents the proportion of the absorbed nitrogen retained by the body.

$$\text{NPU} = \frac{\text{Dietary N - (Total N in feces - Endogenous N in feces) - (Total urinary N - Endogenous N in urine)}}{\text{Dietary N}} \quad 100$$

In terms of biological value:

NPU = BV × digestbility coefficient.

Generally, proteins of animal origin are rapidly and easily digested. Thus in most animal proteins NPU is almost equal to BV. In proteins of plant origin, many a time, the NPU values do not approximate biological values:

Nitrogen Balance Index (NBI)

Nitrogen balance is defined as the slope of the line in the nitrogen balance VS absorbed nitrogen graph. Alternatively, it can be calculated by the following equation:

$$\text{NBI} = \frac{\text{N Balance at a given N intake - N Balance on N free diet}}{\text{Absorbed N}}$$

Since basically NBI and BV represent the same index of the protein quality and that is why NBI determinations is not much in vogue.

Net Dietary Protein Value ND_pV:

This index is an improvement over NPU as it takes into account in addition, the quality (percentage of protein in the diet) aspect as well.

$ND_pV = NPU_{op} \times$ percentage of protein in the diet

NPU_{op} means that net protein utilization of the test protein is determined at a given level of protein in the diet, i.e., at operational conditions.

Protein Efficiency Ratio

BV, NPU and NBI are the biological indices of protein quality that are based on nitrogen balance studies. In an alternative procedure that obviates the difficult steps of N estimation in faecal and urinary matter in studies based on N balance, the protein quality appraisal is made by measuring the weight gain in growing animals rats per gram pf protein intake when the protein under test is the exclusive source of protein in the diet. Thus PER is defined as the change in body weight, i.e., growth, relative to the amount of protein eaten. Generally growing rats (3-4 weeks old) are fed the test protein over a period of 4 weeks as an exclusive protein source in an otherwise standard diet at a level cy 9.09% of its total daily energy intake.

While egg has a PER value of 3.5, the tryptophan deficient protein geltin has a PER of 1.2. In certain countries there is a practice to mention the PER values on the food labels in order to indicate the nutritional value of the protein present in the food. Figure 18.1 and Table 18.2 depicts the PER values of 'Common Proteins'.

Table 18.2: Nutritive quality (Biological) of certain proteins

Protein source	*BV*	*NPU*	*PER*
Egg	96	96	3.5
Milk	90	85	2.7
Meat	80	76	3.2
Fish	80	74	3.5
Rice	80	77	1.7
Maize	60	50	1.0
Food yeast	32	30	2.4
Whole wheat	66	61	1.1
Potato	68	63	1.9
Bengal gram	74	61	1.1

Though PER value of a protein is less precise index vis-à-vis BV and NDP, it is the convenience in its determination that, makes it a widely practised method.

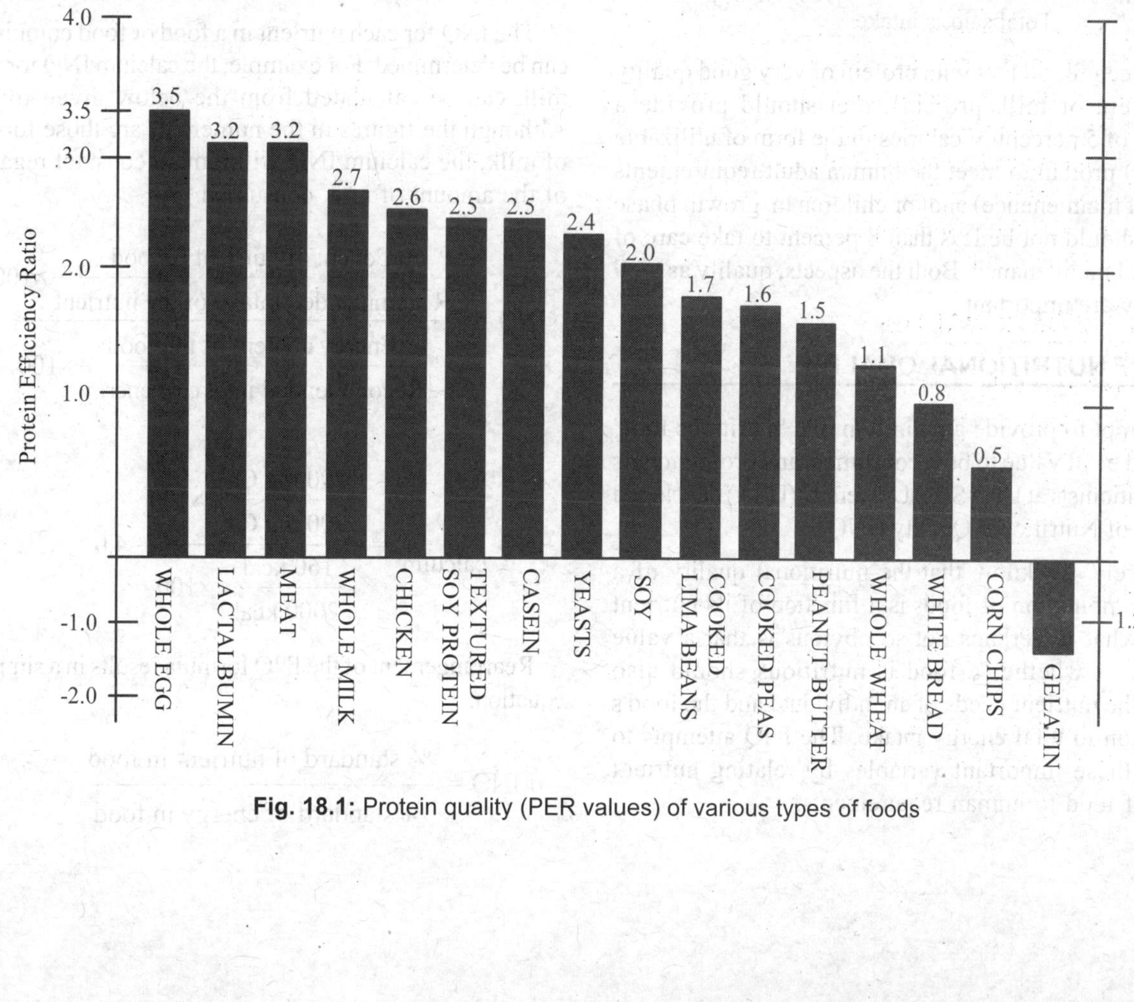

Fig. 18.1: Protein quality (PER values) of various types of foods

Generally PER values are expressed relative to the PER value of a diet that contains 10 percent casein, whose PER is taken as 2.5.

Net Protein Ratio

NPR is an improvement over PER in a way, as consideration is also made of the role of protein in maintenance even in growing animals by having one more group of animals being fed on protein free diet. The weight loss by rats on protein free diet is assumed to be equivalent to the amount of protein required for tissue maintenance.

$$\text{NPR} = \frac{\text{Wt. gain on diet containing test protein + Wt. loss on protein free diet}}{\text{Total protein intake with test protein as the protein source}}$$

Net Dietary Protein Calories Percent (NDP cal %)

Conventionally protein content of the diet is expressed as percent of the total weight of the diet. However the knowledge of protein content as a percentage of total caloric intake is also essential in various types of dietary plannings and nutritional interventions.

$$\text{NDP Cal \%} = \frac{\text{Protein calories}}{\text{Total caloric intake}} \times 100 \times \text{NPU}_{op}$$

It has been found that with protein of very good quality (egg protein or milk protein), diet should provide a minimum of 5 percent of calories in the form of utilizable (available) protein to meet the human adult requirements (largely of maintenance) and for children in growth phase the level should not be less than 8 percent to take care of growth and maintenance. Both the aspects, quality as well as quantity are important.

INDEX OF NUTRITIONAL QUALITY

In an attempt to provide a definition of a 'nutritious food' that would be of value to both consumers and professionals alike, nutritionists at Utah State University (USA) developed the Index of Nutritional Quality (INQ).

Intuitively, we know that the nutritional quality of a food or combination of foods is a function of its nutrient content; what is perhaps not so obvious is that a value judgment of whether a food is nutritious should also consider the nutrient needs of an individual and the food's contribution to total energy intake. The INQ attempts to consider these important variables by relating nutrient content of food to human requirements.

When individual food choices are limited either in quantity or variety, perhaps for health or economic reasons, it becomes increasingly important to select foods that provide an adequate intake of essential nutrients. The INQ was developed to identity foods that have a beneficial nutrient: energy ratio, relative to a standard. When originally introduced, the standard used was the RDA, but refinement of the INQ concept has led the research group to prefer a standard energy level (1,000 or 2000 kcal) as the energy reference point. The INQ is defined as follows:

Table 18.3: Standards used for INQ determination

2,000 kcal	16 mg iron
50 g protein	3,000 mg sodium
4,000 IU vitamin A	5,000 mg potassium
60 mg vitamin C	350 mg cholesterol
1.2 mg riboflavin	78 g total fat
900 mg calcium	

Source: R.G. Hansen and B.W. Wyse, Using the INQ to Evaluate Foods, Nutrition News 42(1) :2, 1979. Courtesy National Dairy Council.

The reference values for adults currently used for certain nutrients are listed in Table 18.3. However, this need to be modified in respect of Indian context.

The INQ for each nutrient in a food or food combination can be determined. For example, the calcium INQ for whole milk can be calculated from the below given formula. Although the figures in the numerator are those for 1 cup of milk, the calcium INQ will remain constant regardless of the amount of milk consumed.

$$\text{INQ} = \frac{\dfrac{\text{Concn. of nutrient in food}}{\text{Recommended intake of the nutrient}} \times 100}{\dfrac{\text{Energy content of the food}}{\text{Recommended intake of energy}} \times 100}$$

$$\text{INQ}_{\text{calcuim}} = \frac{\dfrac{290 \text{ mg Ca}}{900 \text{ mg Ca}} \times 100}{\dfrac{160 \text{ kcal}}{2000 \text{ kcal}} \times 100} = 4.0$$

Rearrangement of the INQ formula results in a simplified equation:

$$\alpha \text{ INQ} = \frac{\text{\% standard of nutrient in food}}{\text{\% standard of energy in food}}$$

$$INQ_{calcuim} = \frac{290 \text{ mg calcium}/900 \text{ mg calcium}}{160 \text{ kcal}/2{,}000 \text{ kcal}}$$

$$= \frac{0.32}{0.08} = 4.0$$

Stated in this way, it becomes apparent that 1 cup of milk provided 32 percent of the calcium allowance and 8 percent of the energy allowance; based on total adult requirements, therefore, milk supplies four times as much calcium as energy. An INQ equal to 1.0 or more for any nutrient indicates that the food has a beneficial nutrient : energy ratio for that particular nutrient.

The previous example shows that milk is a good source of calcium relative to energy. An examination of Table 18.4 reveals that milk has several nutrient INQs greater than 1.0 and also provides more than 30 percent of the dietary standard for the two nutrients.

Table 18.4: INQ of milk

	Milk	
	INQ	*% Standard*
Energy	1.00	08.0
Protein	2.00	16.0
Calcium	4.00	32.0
Iron	0.09	00.75
Vitamin A	0.95	07.6
Thiamin	1.16	09.3
Riboflavin	4.10	32.9
Vitamin C	0.48	03.8

Source: Adapted from R.G. Hansen and B.W. Wyse. Using the INQ to Evaluate Foods, Nutrition News 42(1):c, 1976. Courtesy National Dairy Council.

The two parameters–INQ and the percent standard–provide useful information in selecting nutritious foods. Individuals who wish to reduce their energy intake while maintaining an adequate nutrient intake should plan their meals to meet their desired level of energy consumption and choose foods with most or all of the nutrient INQs equal to or greater than 1.0.

STUDY QUESTIONS

1. How do you explain the concept of protein quality and apply it to design a low cost, protein nourishing diets.
2. Give a detailed description of 'Amino acid score' as an apt index of *in vitro* protein quality evolution.
3. Explain the two most common *in vivo* indices of protein quality evaluation, namely 'Biological Value' (BV) and 'Net Protein Utilization' (NPU). What additional feature(s) does NPU have, that makes it a better index vis-à-vis BV?
4. Write short notes on:

   (i) Protein Efficiency Ratio (PER).

   (ii) Net Protein Ratio (NPR).
5. Explain the terms Net Dietary Protein Calorie Percent (NDP Cal%) and Index of Nutritional Quality (INQ) and their relevance to evaluate the nutritional quality of diet.

CHAPTER 19

Malnutrition and Its Assessment

Chapter Outlines

- Protein malnutrition
- Starvation
- Protein energy malnutrition in (PEM)
- Biochemical changes in protein energy malnutrition
- Calcification of protein energy malnutrition
- Predicting the duration of malnutrition
- Overnutrition
- Body mass index (BMI) as a yardstick of under nutrition and overnutrition
- Poverty-malnutrition-underdevelopment and again poverty: The vicious circle
- Study questions

Malnutrition is a term used to refer to a disease condition resulting from an absolute or relative deficiency or excess of one or more nutrients. It can be overt or covert, either manifesting clinically or occurring latently, detectable by routine clinical examination or sensitive laboratory—biochemical tests of nutritional status respectively. Malnutrition can occur in five forms, namely, undernutrition, starvation, specific deficiency, imbalance and overnutrition. Opinions on what constitutes malnutrition, and recommendations for avoiding the problem, have been refined over time. Early studies considered 'lack of protein alone' or lack of both protein and calories, i.e., an overall decrease in food intake, to be the most troubling deficiencies in the diets of underfed children, especially in the developing countries.

Ingested protein is broken down into amino acids, which are then recycled to build the specific proteins needed by the individual at any given time. Proteins, as we all know, form many structural elements of the body and carry out most cellular processes. Likewise, when faced with a lack of calories, the body breaks down amino acids for energy instead of using them to make new proteins.

With prosperity and affluence coming to selected sections of our society, the tendency for overnourishment has become prevalent leading to the other kind of malnutrition, the overnutrition. Here we shall briefly discuss these three forms of malnutrition only.

PROTEIN MALNUTRITION

It is the most important and widespread nutritional problem among young children of developing countries, including India, today. The clinical syndrome, called kwashiorkor, occurs mainly in children 1 to 3 years of age and is precipitated by weaning an infant from breast milk onto a starchy, protein poor diet. This name originated in Ghana meaning "the sickness of the older child when the next one is born". It is a consequence of feeding the child a diet adequate in calories but deficient in proteins. It may become clinically, manifest when protein requirements are increased by infection, for example gastroenteritis, malaria or worm infestations. The syndrome is characterized by poor growth, low plasma protein levels, muscle wasting, edema, diarrhea, and increased susceptibility to infection. The presence of subcutaneous fat clearly differentiates it from caloric starvation. The maintenance of fat stores is due to the fairly good carbohydrate intake that results in high blood insulin level. As a matter of fact, the high insulin levels interfere with the adaptations undertaken in starvation.

Specifically, fat is not mobilized as an energy source and consequently ketogenesis does not take place, and there is no transfer of amino acids from the skeletal muscle to liver. The lack of dietary amino acids results in diminished protein synthesis in all tissues. The liver becomes enlarged and infiltrated with fat, reflecting the need for hepatic protein synthesis for the formation and release of lipoproteins from this tissue. In addition, protein malnutrition impairs the function of the gut, resulting in malabsorption of calories, protein, and vitamins, which accelerates the disease. The consequences of the disease include a permanent stunting of physical growth and poor intellectual and psychological development.

STARVATION

Starvation, or an overall deficit in food intake, including both calories and protein, leads to the development of a syndrome known as nutritional marasmus. Marasmus is a word of Greek origin meaning "to waste". Although not restricted to any age group, it is most common in children under 1 year of age. In developing countries early weaning of infants from breast milk is a common cause of marasmus. This may result from pregnancies in rapid succession, the desire of the mother to return to work, or switching from breast feeding to infant diets, especially when economically deprived tend to dilute it with water to make it last longer. This practice leads to insufficient intake of calories. Likewise, diarrhea and malabsorption can develop if safe water and sterile procedures are not used.

In contrast to kwashiorkor; subcutaneous fat, hepatomegaly, and fatty liver are absent in marasmus because fat is mobilized as an energy source and muscle provides adequate amino acids to the liver for the synthesis of glucose and hepatic proteins. Low insulin levels allow the liver to oxidize fatty acids and to produce ketone bodies for other tissues. Ultimately, energy and proteins reserves are exhausted, and the child starves to death.

PROTEIN ENERGY MALNUTRITON (PEM)

The most common form of malnutrition in the world today is protein energy malnutrition (PEM). In the developing countries inadequate intake of protein and energy is all too common, and it is usually the infants and young children who suffer the most. While the actual symptoms of protein energy insufficiency vary widely from case to case, it is common to classify all cases as either marasmus or kwashiorkor. Marasmus is usually defined as inadequate intake of both protein and energy and kwashiorkor as inadequate intake of protein in the presence of adequate energy intake. More often than not, the diets associated with marasmus and kwashiorkor may be similar with the kwashiorkor being precipitated by conditions of increased energy demand. The marasmic infant will have a thin, wasted appearance and will be small for its age. If the PEM continues long enough the child will be permanently stunted in both physical and mental development. In kwashiorkor, on the other hand, the child will often have a deceptively plump appearance due to edema. Other tell-tale symptoms associated with kwashiorkor are dry, brittle hair, diarrhea, dermatitis of various forms, and retarded growth. Perhaps the most devastating result of the marasmus and kwashiorkor is reduced ability of the afflicted individuals to fight off infection. They have a reduced number of T lymphocytes (and thus diminished cell-mediated immune response) as well as defects in the generation of phagocyte cells and production of immunoglobulins, interferon, and other components of the immune system. Many of these individuals die from secondary infections, rather than from the starvation itself. With the process of development catching on, classical marasmus and kwashiorkor are on the decline, but milder forms of protein energy malnutrition often prevail.

BIOCHEMICAL CHANGES IN PEM

Marasmic child is endocrinologically adapted to the low energy supply. He is able to maintain his blood sugar and plasma protein at normal levels at the cost of muscle and fat tissue. This endocrinological adaptation comes from the fact that blood insulin levels are low and levels of gluconeogenic hormones are fairly good.

The child with kwashiorkor doesn't adapt well from endocrinological point of view owing to normal blood insulin levels and consequently plasma protein levels fall. This results in edema of face and feet as plasma proteins play significant part in maintaining the normal osmotic pressure and fluid exchange levels in the tissues. If the kwashiorkor condition persists for a long time, the child's liver also gets infiltrated with abnormal quantities of fat. A quick comparison of the salient features of two contrasting forms of malnutrition is given in Table 19.1.

Table 19.1: Contrast between marasmus and kwashiorkor

Characteristic	*Marasmus*	*Kwashiorkor*
Appearance	Thin and emaciated	Cheek area full wasting present
Age	6 months to 2 years (generally)	1-3 years (generally)
Edema (face and feet swelling)	Absent	Present
Mentation	Hungry	Anorexic (Apathetic)
Endocronologic adaptation	Present	Absent
Serum albumin	Normal	Low

CLASSIFICATION OF PROTEIN ENERGY MALNUTRITION

PEM can be classified according to different schemes. These schemes are based on weight for age, height for age and nutrition deprivation.

Weight for Age Based Classification

A. Wellcome Classification

Expected standard weight is in the 50th centile of Harward standard	*Without edema*	*With edema (swelling of face and feet)*
60-80% of expected std. wt.	Undernourishment	Kwashiorkor
Less than 60% of expected std. wt.	Marasmus	Marasmic kwashiorkor

B. Gomez Classification

% of Standard wt. (50th Centile of Harvard or NCHC Std.)

≤ 60%	III Grade Malnutrition
61-75%	II Grade Malnutrition
76-90%	I Grade Malnutrition
> 90%	Normal

C. Indian Academy of Paediatrics Classification

≤ 50%	IV Grade	Severe
51-60%	III Grade	Severe
61-70%	II Grade	Moderate
71-80%	I Grade	Mild
> 80%	Normal	Normal

Height for Age Based Classification

A. Mclarn's Classsification

< 80 % of the std.	Dwarf
80 - 93%	Short
93-105%	Normal

B. Vishveshwara Rao's Classification

< 80% of the std.	Poor (Stunted)
80 - 90%	Mild retardation
91-100%	Normal

C. Waterlow's Classsification

< 85% expected height for age	Severe Malnutrition (Stunted)
85 - 90%	Moderate
90 - 95%	Marginal
> 95%	Normal

Nutrition Deprivation Based Classification

A. Seone and Latham's Classification

Group	*Weight to height ratio*	*Conclusions*
A. Normal	Normal height to weight ratio	Normal nutrition
B. Undernourished but not height retarded	Height normal for age, weight for height low	Acute malnutrition
C. Undernourished and height retarded	Height and weight is less for age, weight for height low	Acute or chronic malnutrition
D. Height retarded but not undernourished	Height for age low, weight for height is normal	Chronic malnutrition

B. Weight to Height

> 75%	Severe Malnutrition
75 - 84%	Moderate Malnutrition
85 - 90%	Marginal Malnutrition
> 90%	Normal Malnutrition

C. Waterlow's Qualitative Classification Based on Height for Age and Weight for Height

Normal	Weight for Height	≥ 80% Standard
	Height for Age	≥ 90% Standard
Stunted	Weight for Height	≥ 80% Standard
	Height for Age	< 90% Standard
Wasted	Weight for Height	< 80% Standard
	Height for Age	≥ 90% Standard
Wasted and Stunted	Weight for Height	< 80% Standard
	Height for Age	< 90% Standard

Children with grade III and IV or severe forms of malnutrition (Indian Academy of Pediatrics Classification) comprise 10 per cent of the child population of India and are at maximum risk of dying from PEM. Since prevalence of infection is very high in such children, they require urgent medical attention.

PREDICTING THE DURATION OF MALNUTRITION

The index weight for height gives little information on chronic malnutrition which is sometimes, accompanied by normal weight for height. In other words, children with poor linear growth but adequate weight for height would be classified as perfectly normal by weight for height alone which actually would not be true. These children can, however, be identified if height for age is also taken into consideration along with weight for height. The extent of height deficit in relation to age may be regarded as a measure of the duration of malnutrition. This concept has been proposed by Seone and Latham (1971) and a classification based on weight for height, weight for age and height for age has been suggested by them. The advantage of this classification (indicating below) is that it helps to find out the type and duration of malnutrition.

While evaluating the usefulness of anthropometric measurements such as height, weight, arm circumference, Sastry and Vijayaraghavan (1973) found that Seone and Latham classification was better as compared to others.

Wasting and Stunting

Waterlow (1972) has recommended use of only weight for height and height for age. In this classification children with low weight for height are considered as 'wasted' those with height deficit are considered as 'stunted'. Accordingly, the following classification was suggested.

Differentiation of Wasting and Slanting

The interpretation guidelines for judging wasting and stunting are given in Table 19.2.

Waterlow does not regard children who are not wasted but only stunted as malnourished through their weight for age is low "because increasing their food intake may simply cause obesity". Beaudry-Darisme and Latham (1973) also made similar observations. However, Rao and Naidu (1977) observed that nutritional dwarfs gained as much weight and height as did normal children on nutritional supplementation over a 14-month period. Thus, longer periods of nutritional rehabilitation would make a nutritional dwarf gain both height and weight proportionately making him less of a dwarf after nutritional rehabilitation and he can move towards normalcy.

Table 19.2: Interpretation guidelines for judging wasting and stunting

Nutritional status	*Height for age*	*Weight for age*	*Weight for height*
Normal	Normal	Normal	Normal
Past chronic malnutrition (nutritional dwarf)	Low	Low	Normal
Current short duration malnutrition	Normal	Low	Low
Current long duration malnutrition	Low	Low	Low

Nutritional status	*Weight for height*	*Height for age*
Normal	Normal	Normal
Wasted but not stunted (acute malnutrition)	Low	Normal
Stunted but not wasted (nutritional dwarfs)	Normal	Low
Wasted and stunted (acute over chronic malnutrition)	Low	Low

Classification by Standard Deviations

Preschool children are classified according to standard deviation classification as Median -1 SD, Median -1 SD to -2 SD, Median -2 SD to 3 SD, Median -3 SD, Median + 1 SD to - 2 SD, Median + 2 SD to -3 SD and Median + 3 SD.

It is necessary to give the whole distribution of Z-scores to relate the measurements to the reference population. For most group of population comparisons, where uniformity is important, the standard cut-off points of ± 2 SD from the mean are used.

Severe acute malnutrition (SAM) or severe wasting is defined by very low weight-for-height (below -3 Z-scores of the median WHO child growth standards), a mid-upper arm circumference < 115 mm, or by the presence of nutritional edema. SAM remains one of the major killers of children under five; it contributes to approximately 1 million child deaths every year. Globally, it is estimated that 26 million children under five years are severely acutely malnourished, most of whom live in South Asia and in sub-Saharan Africa. India alone is home to 8,105,000 children with SAM (31.2% of the world's severely wasted children).

Majority of our children with grade I or II PEM, thought not at risk of immediate death, yet vulnerable to illness and erosion of nutritional status to a higher grade (severe) of malnutrition. Lacking in vitality, stamina, strength and predominantly, they are not normal. They are the lesser amongst equals, in whom genetic potential has not been given full expression.

In fact the prevalence of malnutrition is a global phenomenon. Globally, nearly 195 million children younger than five years are undernourished and the problem is most obvious in developing countries. In India alone we have above 75 million malnourished children below the age of 5 years, the largest number in the world. Malnutrition triggers an array of health problems in children, many of which can become chronic. As we have observed that criteria laid out for classifying malnutrition are based upon changes in the height-weight values form those expected for a particular age group, it can be said for sure that malnutrition leads to weight loss, stunted growth, weakened resistance to infection hindered mental development and disrupted cognition by producing structure damage to brain, and in the worst cases, early death. The effect are particularly devastating in the first few years of life because:

i. Children grow rapidly and thus the need for protein and energy is greatest of all phases in life.
ii. They are more active and hence need more energy per unit weight.
iii. Their immune system is not fully developed and thus predisposes them to infection.
iv. They are dependent on adults for nutrition.

And since malnutrition prevails the most in the underdeveloped countries, the basic reason is traced to poverty's. That's why poverty is most appropriately defined as the inability to purchase minimum food for dfaily caloric needs. Malnutrition alters educational preparedness and, later, work force productivity, making it an unacceptable risk for its victims as well as for nations strength and competitiveness. Hence prevention of malnutrition among young children should remain the best policy not only on moral grounds but on economic one's as well. The immediate expense on nutrition programmes and interventions should be considered a critical investment for the future.

OVERNUTRITION

Perhaps another serious nutritional problem in this country is excessive energy consumption. In fact, obesity is the most frequent nutritional disorder of the affluent sections of the society. It is worthwhile to consider some of the metabolic consequences of obesity. One striking clinical feature of overweight individuals is a marked elevation of serum free fatty acids, cholesterol, and triacylglycerols irrespective of the dietary intake of fat. Obesity is obviously associated with an increased number and/or size of adipose calls resulting from long time high energy intake. Furthermore, these cells contain fewer insulin receptors and thus respond poorly to insulin, resulting in increased activity of the hormone-sensitive lipase. The increased lipase activity along with the increased mass of adipose tissue is probably sufficient to explain the increase in circulating free fatty acids. These excess fatty acids are, of course, carried to the liver, where they are broken down to acetyl CoA, which is a precursor for both triacylglycerol and cholesterol synthesis. The excess triacylglycerol and cholesterol are released as very low density lipoprotein particles, leading to higher circulating levels of both triacylglycerol and cholesterol and resultant atherosclerosis.

A second striking finding in obese individuals is higher fasting blood sugar levels and decreased glucose tolerance. About 80% of adult onset diabetics are overweight. Again the culprit appears to be the decrease in insulin receptors, since many adult onset diabetics have higher than normal insulin levels. Because of these metabolic changes, obesity is one of the primary risk factors in coronary heart disease, hypertension and diabetes. This is nutritionally significant because all of these metabolic changes are reversible. Quite often reduction in ideal weight is the single most important mode of nutritional therapy. Furthermore, when the individual is at its ideal body weight, the composition of the diet becomes a less important consideration in maintaining normal serum lipid and glucose levels. Any one who is more than 10% above the 'standard' weight for people of the same age, sex, height, race and body frame is termed overweight and the one having more than 20% of this weight is called obese.

Overwight is thus defined as body weight between 10 to 20 percent over desirable weight. Obesity is 20 percent or more over desirable weight. It is classified into three categories: mild, moderate and severe. Mild obesity is 20 to 40 percent, moderate obesity is 40 to 100 percent, and severe obesity is 100 percent or more over desirable weight. Over 90 percent of obese fall into mild category, which can be treated with diet exercise and behaviour modification. Body Mass Index (BMI), Weight/(Height)^2 values also reflect a person's status with respect to obesity and overweight. BMI values of 22.7 and 22.4 denote ideal weight for men and women respectively. Similarly BMI values of 26.9 (men) and 27.2 (women) and 31.4 (men) and 31.8 (women) for men and women denote 20 percent and 40 percent overweight respectively. An obese individual, as we all know, is at an increased risk of hypertension, high blood cholesterol levels, diabetes and coronary heat disease. A few tips to stay healthy and to avoid the twin maladies of overweight and obesity, and to live longer are given hereunder:

i. Eat plenty of fiber, which is present in substantial amounts in unrefined wheat flour (atta) fruits with their skin, sprouts, corn and raw vegetables.

ii. Avoid fast foods—it's high in cholesterol and low in fiber.

iii. Eat fresh foods—storage leads to loss of vitamin B, and more importantly, vitamin C—the natural antioxidants.

iv. Eat only lean meat—have it grilled, backed or roasted.

v. Don't eat while you are reading, cooking or talking on telephone.

vi. Stay off salted and fried snacks as much as possible and use cucumber, radish and carrots as salads as much as possible

vii. Chew your food slowly and take small mouth fulls. Avoid late meals.

viii. Your visible fat (oil and ghee) intake should not be more than 20 gm per day, half oil and half ghee.

ix. Take plenty of water, not less than 2.5 liters per day.

Body Mass Index (BMI) as a Yardstick of Under and Overnutrition

Many formulae have been proposed to describe the way in which weight varies with height during growth. Rao and Singh (1970) found that Quetlet's Index—Weight/Height^2 was independent of age in preschool children. Malnourished children have lower values of weight/height^2. Dugdale (1971) showed that weight/height$^{1.6}$ is age independent after one year and can be used to grade nutritional status of children.

In general, these indices, essentially, provide the same information as weight for height. The one disadvantage of using weight for height or any index based on weight and height singly is that even when nutritional intervention over a period of time brings about significant improvement in height and weight, there may not be perceivable change in distribution of weight for height values as compared to the baseline data, since both weight and height increase, as happens during normal growth. Any index in which both the parameters increase with age, one as the numerator and the other as denominator, fails to show a significant increase (Naidu and Rao, 1979).

BMI in Adults: After the cessation of linear growth around 21 years, weight for height indicates muscle-fat mass in the adult body. The ratio of Weight (in kg)/Height (m) is referred to as Body Mass Index (BMI). It provides a reasonable indication of the nutritional status of adults. The BMI has good correlation with fatness. It may also be used as indicator of health risk. The following classification has been suggested by James *et al.* (1988) and Luizz *et al.* (1992).

BMI class A	*BMI class B*	*Presumptive diagnosis*
< 18.5	< 18.5	Thin
18.5-24.9	18.5-22.9	Normal
25-29.9	23-24.9	Pre obese, overweight, with marginal risk
30.0-34.9	25.0-29.9	Class I obese, with moderate risk
35.0-39.9	30.0-34.5	Class II obese, with severe risk
> 40.0	> 35.0	Class III morbid obese, with very severe risk

BMI class A is for Caucasian (European), BMI class B is for Asian/Indian.

Mid-Upper Arm Circumference for Age

The arm circumference (AC), as an absolute measurement, varies little between the ages of one and four years. It correlates well with weight and weight for height. In view of its simplicity, and that it does not require expensive equipment, arm circumference has been suggested as an index to assess the nutritional status of children.

POVERTY-MALNUTRITION-UNDERDEVELOP MENT AND AGAIN, POVERTY: THE VICIOUS CIRCLE

We have seen that hunger, both manifest (lack of adequate quantity of food to completely fill the bellys) and hidden (lack of balanced diet), affect physical and mental development leading to an unloading sequence of 'malnutrition ill health-in efficiency-malnutrition'. Table 19.3 incorporates a few terms related to this phenomenon that besets the underdeveloped countries including India.

Eating Disorders

Fasting and feeding are not always imposed upon people by nature. More often than not, human psyche or circumstances make them impose these conditions upon themselves. An *eating disorder* is to eat, or avoid eating, which negatively affects both, one's physical and mental health. It is marked by extremes. It is present when a person experiences a feeling of either too much or too little urge to eat.

Anorexia nervosa is an eating disorder that involves a psychological loss of appetite and self starvation, resulting from a distorted body image. Various social pressures associated with adolescence/puberty, also known as the age of innocent rebellions, seem to become the causative agents in this disorder which prevails mostly in females. **Bulimia nervosa**, on the other hand, is an eating disorder in which large quantities of food are taken at one time (binging) and then purged from the body by vomiting, use of laxatives, diuretics and other means. Like anorexia nervosa, bulimia also afflicts female adolescents and youth. However, the frequency of affliction of males with bulimia is sizeable as compared to anorexia nervosa. The starvation diet in anorexia nervosa takes a toll causing deterioration into the health of adolescents and youth. It can lower the heart and breathing rates, blood pressure and body temperature. It can cause osteoporosis, constipation, stunting and cessation of menstruation in the female, who incidentally are its major victims. Bulimia nervosa too creates health problems. For instance, repeated vomiting tendency damages teeth and gums and even doesn't leave esophageous and stomach unscathed. A number of bulimics have consistent heart burn and sore throats. Repeated loss of fluids either due to frequent vomiting or laxative usage causes electrolyte imbalance in the body. This goes a long way to tell upon the state of heart leading to irregular heart beats and associated problems. Apart from anorexic nervosa and bulimia nervosa there are other eating disorders generalized as: Eating Disorder not Otherwise Specified (EDNOS). These disorders combine characteristics of anorexia nervosa and bulimia along with attendant psycho-social-neural aberrations. There are no simple causes or solutions to the eating disorders as they are rooted in biological, psychological and social facets of human persona.

In the present materialistic era, of cut throat competitions, conflicts and costly life styles; the urge and yearning for pleasure, physical appearance and popularity makes one tread the path of faulty eatings. Eating disorders are also a manifestation of an *ostrich like* behaviour where the person makes eating as the scapegoat for hiding problems whose answers have become elusive for him/her. A girl or woman, or occasionally a boy or adult, use self starvation or bringing as a means of exercising some control direction over his/her environment in a bid to deal with the problem of self image and inadequacy. In this age of literacy and enlightenment, it is important to gain awareness about these disorders so as to stear either clear without falling prey to them or to drive them out taking them as stumbling blocks in the pursuit of real accomplishment, progress and actualization.

To prevent eating disorders, parents, peers and professionals should counsel the adolescents and youth focusing on following points:

- On discouraging and restricting dieting, meal skipping and fasting.

Table 19.3: Certain terms associated with the vicious circle of 'poverty-undernutrition-disease-inefficiency-underdevelopment-poverty'

Poverty: It is the inability to purchase minimum food for daily caloric needs.

Absolute poverty: The income level below which a minimally nutritionally adequate diet plus essential non-food requirements are not affordable.

Anemia: A condition in which the hemoglobin concentration (the number of red blood cells) is lower than normal as a result of a deficiency of one or more essential nutrients, such as iron, or due to disease.

Daily calorie requirement: The average number of calories needed to sustain normal levels of activity and health, taking into account age, sex, body weight and climate.

Famine: A situation of extreme scarcity of food, potentially leading to widespread starvation.

Food security: Assumed access for every person, primarily in production or purchase, to enough nutritious food to sustain productive human life.

Foreign exchange: currency acceptable for use in international trade, such as US dollars. The value of one currency in terms of another is the *exchange rate*.

Gross domestic product (GDP): The value of all goods and services produced within a nation during a specified period, usually a year.

Gross national product (GNP): The value of all goods and services produced by a country's citizens, wherever they are located.

Hunger: A condition in which people lack the basic food intake to provide them with the energy and nutrients for fully productive, active and healthy lives.

Infant mortality rate (IMR): The annuál number of deaths of infants under one year of age per one thousand live births.

Inflation: An increase in overall prices, which leads to a decrease in purchasing power.

International Monetary Fund (IMF): An inter-governmental agency which advances loan to countries that have foreign exchange and monetary problems. These loans are conditioned upon the willingness of the borrowing country to adopt economic policies designed by IMF.

Low birth weight infants: Babies born weighing 2,500 grams (5 pounds, 8 ounces) or less who are especially vulnerable to illness and death during the first month of life.

Malnutrition: Failure to achieve nutrient requirements, which can impair physical and/or mental health. Malnutrition may result from consuming too little food or a shortage or imbalance of key nutrients, e.g., refined sugar and fat.

Poverty line: An official measure of poverty defined by national governments. In the United States, for example, it is based on ability to afford USA's Thrifty Food Plan.

Recession:A period in which a country's GDP declines in two or more consecutive three-month periods.

Structural adjustment: Economic policy changes, often imposed upon an indebted country by its lenders as a condition for future loans, intended to stimulate economic growth. These generally involve reducing the role of government in the economy and increasing exports.

Stunting: Failure to grow to normal height caused by chronic undernutrition during the formative years of childhood.

Sustainability: Society's capacity to shape its economic and social systems so as to maintain both natural resources and human life.

World Bank: An inter-governmental agency which makes long-term loans to the governments of developing nations.

Under five mortality rate: The annual number of deaths of children under five years of age per one thousand live births.

Underemployment: A situation where a large portion of the population is not fully employed round the year.

Undernutrition: A form of mild, chronic, or acute malnutrition which is characterized by inadequate intake of food energy (measured by calories), usually due to eating too little. Stunting, wasting and being underweight are common forms of undernutrition.

Underweight: A condition to which a person is seriously below normal weight for her/his age. The term can apply to any age group, but is most often used as a measurement of undernutrition in children under five years of age.

Vulnerability to hunger: Individuals, households, communities, or nations who have enough to eat most of the time, but whose poverty makes them especially susceptible to changes in the economy, climate, or political conditions.

Wasting: A condition in which a person is seriously below the normal weight for his height due to acute undernutrition.

- On informing the adolescents and the youth about the changes that occur during puberty, reassuring them that they all are normal and natural
- On eradicating misconceptions about nutrition, normal body weight and approaches to weight loss.
- On emphasizing positive nutrition and healthful food properties free form obsessions and hypocracies.

To make adolescents and youth reach their potential, the society has to groom them positively giving them right direction, impetus and momentum. The concept of 'care' enunciated by UNICEF for children and other member of the household, applies to the adolescents, and youth as well. Care is the provision in the household and community of time, attention and support to meet the physical, mental and social needs and adjustments of growing child and other household members in the different age group. Evidently, the concept of care refers to the behaviours performed by care givers that effect nutritional intake, health and psychosocial development. The society owes this to the incoming generation to ensure their hassle free growth and development for making them apt for an efficient takeover of the societal reins.

STUDY QUESTIONS

1. Explain the term 'Malnutrition'. Discuss 'Starvation', 'Protein malnutrition' and 'Protein energy malnutrition' in the context of malnutrition.
2. Giving a brief description of biochemical changes that occur in PEM, discuss the classification of PEM based on various schemes.
3. What do you understand by the terms 'Overweight' and 'Obesity'? What tips would you give to the people to stay fit and avoid overweight and obesity?
4. How can you use 'Body Mass Index' (BMI) as a yardstick to assess over and undernutrition?
5. Explain the term 'Eating Disorders' and give their different types.

CHAPTER 20

Setting Nutritional Requirements

Chapter Outlines

- General principles of deriving RDA
- RDA recommendations by Nutrition Expert Groups
- Energy
- Protein
- Fat
- Minerals
- Vitamins
- Study questions

Human beings need a wide range of nutrients to lead a healthy and active life and these are derived through the diet they consume daily. The components of their diets must be chosen judiciously to provide all the nutrients they need in adequate amounts and in proper proportions. The amount of each nutrient that is required by a person depends upon his age and physiological status. Adults need nutrients for maintaining constant body weight and ensuring proper body function. Infants and young children who are growing rapidly require nutrients not only for maintenance but also for growth. They require relatively more nutrients (2-3 times) per kg body weight than adults. In special physiological conditions like pregnancy and lactation, adult woman needs additional nutrients to meet the extra demand for foetal growth and maternal tissue expansion in pregnancy and milk secretion during lactation. These extra intake of nutrients are essential for the normal growth of the embryo and of the infant in the early postnatal life.

There are certain general guiding principles in arriving at dietary allowances for various groups. The nutritional requirement of an individual and the dietary allowances for a group or a population are distinctly different. The former depends upon the age, body weight and the physiological and metabolic status of the individual. The latter must also take into consideration individual variation within the group, the quality of the diet, the effect of cooking and processing and the bioavailability of nutrients from the diet.

GENERAL PRINCIPLES OF DERIVING RDA

A number of approaches have been used in arriving at the nutritional requirements of an individual and the RDA for a population. The general principles are:

i. **Dietary intakes:** This approach has been used in arriving at the energy requirements of children. Energy intakes of normally growing healthy children are made use of for recommending energy intakes.

ii. **Growth:** The level of any particular nutrient in the breast milk intake, sufficient for satisfactory growth has been utilized for defining requirements in an early infancy.

iii. **Nutrient balance:** The minimum intake of nutrient for equilibrium (intake = output) in adults, and nutrient retention consistent with satisfactory growth in children, have been used widely for arriving at the protein requirements.

iv. **Obligatory loss of nutrients:** The minimal loss of any nutrient or of its metabolic product (viz., nitrogenous end products in the case of proteins) through normal routes of elimination, viz., urine, faeces and sweat is determined on a diet devoid of or very low in the nutrient (for example, a protein free diet). This information is used to determine the amount of nutrient to be consumed daily through the diet to replace the obligatory loss. In infants and children, growth requirements are added to the above maintenance requirement.

v. **Factorial approach:** In this approach, the requirements for different functions are assessed separately, and added up to arrive at the total daily requirement. This is the basis of arriving at energy requirements. Earlier, this was the approach employed for assessing the protein requirement.

vi. **Nutrient turnover:** Data from turnover of nutrients in healthy persons, using isotopically labelled nutrients have been employed in arriving at requirements of certain nutrients. Requirements of vitamin A, vitamin C, iron and vitamin B_{12} have been determined on this basis. Earlier, radioisotopic labelled compounds were utilized and currently compounds labelled with a stable isotope are being increasingly used to determine the turnover of nutrients in the body. Stable isotopes are particularly useful in infants, children and in women during pregnancy and lactation where radioisotopes are counter indicated.

vii. **Depletion and repletion studies:** This approach has been employed in arriving at the requirement of water-soluble vitamins. The levels of vitamin or its coenzyme in serum or tissue (erythrocytes, leucocytes) are used as a biochemical marker of the vitamin status. Requirements of ascorbic acid, thiamine, riboflavin, niacin and pyridoxine have been established employing this approach. The subjects are first fed a diet very low in the nutrient under study till the biochemical parameters reach a low level after which response to feeding graded dose of the nutrient is determined. The level at which response increases rapidly is an indication of requirement.

Further, RDA is derived from a knowledge of the average requirement of nutrients for each physiological group. Based on the nutrient requirements arrived at by one or more of the approaches described above, the RDA is computed after taking into consideration the individual variability and nutrient bioavailability from the diet. In defining the RDA for a specific nutrient, it is assumed that the requirement of all the other nutrients are adequately met. The concept of RDA is tenable only under this condition. In addition, RDA is applicable only to a healthy normal population living under normal conditions.

As a matter of fact, the RDA takes into account the variation that exists between individuals and a level of intake is chosen which includes an allowance for this variation. It thus aims at meeting the requirement of nearly all individuals in a population. In practice a level of intake corresponding to the mean plus 2 standard deviation, which covers the requirements of 97.5% of population, is chosen to define RDA. This had been termed as safe level of intake and the chance of finding this level inadequate is not more than 2.5%. This safe level approach is not used in the case of energy, since excess energy intake is as undesirable as inadequate intake, only the average requirement of energy is defined as RDA. Energy balance is also reported to be homeostatically regulated.

Thus RDAs are taken to be the estimates of intakes of nutrients which individuals in a population group need to consume to ensure that the physiological needs of all subjects in that population are met. But it needs to be recognised that RDAs are not meant to be used as standards to determine whether or not a given individual's requirement has been met. As mentioned earlier, RDA for all nutrients, except for energy is the mean requirement value to which, an alloance corresponding to 2SD, that is 25% of the mean, has been added. While this clearly implies that an individual who has an intake at the RDA level will run very little risk of inadequacy, it does not imply that an individual who has an intake below the RDA is necessarily at risk, since there will be several individuals in a population whose requirements will be well below the RDA. This point must be kept in mind while applying RDA at the individual level. For this purpose, the probability approach may have to be used.

Another important consideration in arriving at RDA is the bioavailability of the nutrients from the diet. Bioavailability depends both upon the nutritive value of the particular nutrient and on the quality and components of the whole diet. For certain nutrients, bioavailability from the diet is a critical factor, viz., iron, protein, Ca, vitamin B_{12}, β-carotene. For proteins, the essential amino acid composition, i.e., the quality of the dietary protein is also important. In a normal mixed diet from which protein is derived from several sources like cereals, legumes, milk, flesh foods and so on, there is a mutual supplementation effect, and the quality of the protein tends to be higher than the protein from any of its individual constituents like cereals or pulses. For iron, absorption from food becomes a critical factor, since it is influenced both by absorption promoters (ascorbic acid, meat, etc.) and absorption inhibitors (phytate, tannin, oxalate etc.) present in the diet. The diets habitually consumed in India which are based predominantly on cereals and other plant foods, are high in inhibitors and low in promoters, and hence, iron absorption from such diets is only 2 to 5 per cent.

In case of certain nutrients like vitamin A and niacin, provitamins are present in foods which can be converted into the respective vitamins in the body. For example, β–carotene can give rise to vitamin A and tryptophan can yield nicotinic acid or niacin. The extent of absorption of β–carotene depends on its source in the diet, and the amount of tryptophan available for conversion depends on the quality of protein in the diet. These factors need to be taken into account in defining the RDA for vitamin A and nicotinic acid.

RDA RECOMMENDATIONS BY NUTRITION EXPERT GROUPS

The Nutrition Advisory Committee of the Indian Research Fund Association, now called the Indian Council of Medical Research, recommended for the first time in 1944 dietary allowances for Indians in respect of energy, proteins, iron, calcium, vitamin A, thiamine, ascorbic acid and vitamin D. These recommendations were revised in 1958 in respect of energy and protein. The Nutrition Expert Group of the Indian Council of Medical Research in 1968 revised the earlier recommendations of nutrient allowances for Indians in respect of all nutrients, except energy. This group also considered the desirable levels of intake of additional nutrients like folic acid, vitamin B_{12}, vitamin D and fat. In making these recommendations, the group was guided both by the safe allowances of various nutrients suggested by expert groups of the Food and Agricultural Organization and the World Health Organisation, as well as by data on the nutrients requirement of Indians. These recommendations were again revised in 1978 by an Expert Group of the ICMR and allowances were updated and revised in respect of several nutrients.

In April 1988, nutrient allowances for Indians were again examined in detail by an Expert Committee of the ICMR and detailed recommendations are now made with respect to safe levels of intake of many nutrients. The basis of these recommendations is discussed in detail in this report in 1988. These recommended intakes are not summarised along with some guidelines for their use.

ENERGY

Assessment of Energy Requirements

Currently, it is recommended that energy requirement must be assessed in terms of energy expenditure rather than in terms of energy intakes. Energy intake may vary from day-to-day, on some days it may be above the energy expended and on others below it. Body energy reserves (viz., fat) help to maintain normal energy expenditure over short periods even when the daily intake is below requirement. Over a long period of time, however, people tend to maintain energy balance and constant body weight.

The principle of using energy expenditure to arrive at estimates of energy requirements cannot be over-emphasised. An analysis of the energy intake data is unhelpful since it is possible to have a grossly inadequate intake by individuals who in the face of maintaining normal energy expenditure respond by weight loss so that they become substantially underweight. This is particularly so, among population in developing countries like India. Such population may be able to maintain their low body weights by reducing metabolic activity of their body tissues in an attempt to adjust to the low intakes. Recommended dietary intake of energy is not intended for this type of population, but to healthy and active population. The assessment of energy expenditure is therefore a more logical approach where one can specify the energy requirements in terms of energy output for productive work and leisure activity. This does imply that there is a need to specify the appropriate weight of the individual and the quantum of physical activity that is considered 'desirable' for the same individual. Energy intake far above the actual requirement is harmful, leading to hazards of obesity and its deleterious consequences. On the other hand, energy intakes far below the requirement leads to undernutrition and loss of body weight. Hence, in contrast to many other nutrients, no safe allowance is made in the case of energy and only the average requirements are defined.

Reference Man and Reference Woman

Taking into account the body weights of well-nourished Indian adults who had satisfactory growth during childhood, the reference man and woman have been redefined as having body weights of 60 kg and 50 kg respectively. These body weights corrrespond to desirable weights for their current heights.

Factorial Approach for Estimating Energy Requirements

The Committee has adopted the procedures used by the FAO/WHO/UNU Expert Consultation for deriving the estimates of energy requirements of adult Indians, both for men and non-pregnant, non-lactating women (Tables 20.1 to 20.7).

Table 20.1: Energy requirements (Kcal/24 hr) of adult males and females aged 18-30 years with different body weights

	Male				*Female*			
	Activity				*Activity*			
Body Wt. (kg)	*BMR*	*Sedentary*	*Moderate*	*Heavy*	*BMR*	*Sedentary*	*Moderate*	*Heavy*
35					960	1536	1824	2400
40	1225	1960	2328	3063	1030	1648	1957	2575
45	1300	2080	2470	3250	1100	1760	2090	2750
50	1370	2192	2603	3425	1170	1872	2223	2925
55	1445	2312	2746	3612	1240	1984	2356	3100
60	1515	2424	2882	3788	1310	2096	2489	3275
65	1590	2544	3021	3975	1380	2208	2622	3450
70	1660	2656	3154	4150	1450	2330	2755	3625
75	1755	2806	3335	4388				

Table 20.2: Energy requirement (Kcal/24 hr) at different ages of adult males and females with different body weights

		Age 31 to 60 + yrs				*Age above 60 yrs*	
		Activity				*Activity*	
Gender	*Body Wt. (kg)*	*BMR*	*Sedentary*	*Moderate*	*Heavy*	*BMR*	*Sedentary*
Males	45	1325	2120	2518	3313	1040	1664
	50	1380	2208	2622	3450	1105	1768
	55	1435	2296	2727	3588	1170	1872
	60	1485	2376	2822	3713	1235	1976
	65	1540	2464	2926	3850	1295	2072
	70	1695	2552	3031	2988	1360	2176
	75	1650	2640	3135	4125	1425	2280
Females	40	1120	1792	2128	2800	965	1544
	45	1160	2856	2204	2900	1015	1624
	50	1200	1920	2280	3000	1065	1704
	55	1240	1984	2356	3100	1115	1784
	60	1285	2056	2442	3213	1165	1864
	65	1325	2120	2518	3313	1215	1944
	70	1365	2184	2594	3413	1265	2024

Table 20.3: Balanced diet for adults

S.No.	*Food group*	Activity					
		Sedentary		*Moderate*		*Heavy*	
		Man	*Woman*	*Man*	*Woman*	*Man*	*Woman*
1.	Cereals and millets (g)	420	300	480	360	690	480
2.	Pulses (g)	60	60	90	75	90	90
3.	Milk (ml)	300	300	300	300	300	300
4.	Roots and tubers (g)	200	100	200	100	200	200
5.	Green leafy vegetables (g)	100	100	100	100	100	100
6.	Other vegetables (g)	100	100	100	100	100	100
7.	Fruits (g)	100	100	100	100	100	100
8.	Sugar (g)	25	20	40	25	55	45
9.	Fats/oils (visible) (g)	20	20	35	30	55	40

For Non Veg. 30 g of pulse can be substituted with 50 g of Meat/Chicken/Fish/Egg.

Source: *Dietary Guidelines for Indians–A Manual*, NIN, ICMR, 1999.

Table 20.4: ICMR recommended dietary allowances for adults

Sex	*Activity*	*Energy* *Kcal*	*Protein* *g*	*Fat* *g*	*Calcium* *mg*	*Iron* *mg*	Vitamin A *Retinol* *μg*	Vitamin A *β carotene* *μg*	*Thiamine* *mg*	*Riboflavin* *mg*	*Niacin* *mg*	*Pyridoxin* *mg*	*Vit.C* *mg*	*Vit.* B_{12} *μg*
Males	Sedentary	2425	60	20	400	28	600	2400	1.2	1.4	16	2.0	40	1
	Moderate	2845	60	20	400	28	600	2400	1.4	1.6	18	2.0	40	1
	Heavy	3800	60	20	400	28	600	2400	1.6	1.9	21	2.0	40	1
Females	Sedentary	1875	50	20	400	30	600	2400	0.9	1.1	12	2.0	40	1
	Moderate	2225	50	20	400	30	600	2400	1.1	1.3	14	2.0	40	1
	Heavy	2925	50	20	400	30	600	2400	1.2	1.5	16	2.0	40	1

Table 20.5: ICMR Recommended dietary allowances for an expectant mother

Nutrient	*Normal adult woman*	*Pregnant woman*
Energy (Kcal)		
Sedentary	1875	2175
Moderate	2225	2525
Heavy	2925	3225
Protein (g)	50	65
Fat (g)	20	30
Calcium (mg)	400	1000
Iron (mg)	30	38
Vitamin A		
Retinol (μg)	600	600
(or)		
β carotene (μg)	2400	2400

Contd.

Contd.

Thiamine (mg)		
Sedentary	0.9	1.1
Moderate	1.1	1.3
Heavy	1.2	1.4
Riboflavin (mg)		
Sedentary	1.1	1.3
Moderate	1.3	1.5
Heavy	1.5	1.7
Niacin (mg)		
Sedentary	12	14
Moderate	14	16
Heavy	16	18
Pyridoxine (mg)	2.0	2.5
Ascorbic acid (mg)	40	40
Folic acid (μg)	100	400
Vitamin B_{12} (μg)	1	1

Table 20.6: ICMR recommended dietary allowances of a nursing mother

Nutrient	Period of Lactation					
	0-6 months			6-12 months		
	Sedentary activity	Moderate activity	Heavy activity	Sedentary activity	Moderate activity	Heavy activity
Energy (kcal)	1875 +550	2225 +550	2925 +550	1875 +400	2225 +400	2925 +400
Protein (g)	75	75	75	68	68	68
Fat (g)	45	45	45	45	45	45
Calcium (mg)	1000	1000	1000	1000	1000	1000
Iron (mg)	30	30	30	30	30	30
Vitamin A						
Retinol (μg) or	950	950	950	950	950	950
β-carotene (μg)	3800	3800	3800	3800	3800	3800
Thiamine (mg)	0.9 +0.3	1.1 +0.3	1.2 +0.3	0.9 +0.2	1.1 +0.2	1.2 +0.2
Riboflavin (mg)	1.1 +0.3	1.3 +0.3	1.5 +0.3	1.1 +0.2	1.3 +0.2	1.5 +0.2
Niacin (mg)	12 +4	14 +4	16 +4	12 +3	14 +3	16 +3
Pyridoxine (mg)	2.5	2.5	2.5	2.5	2.5	2.5
Ascorbic acid (mg)	80	80	80	80	80	80
Folic acid (μg)	150	150	150	150	150	150
Vitamin B_{12} (μg)	1.5	1.5	1.5	1.5	1.5	1.5

Table 20.7: Composition of mother's milk

Nutrient	Quantity / 100 ml
Energy	65 kcal
Protein	1.1 g
Carbohydrate	7.4 g
Fat	3.4 g
Calcium	28 mg
Iron	Negligible
Vitamin A (Retinol)	137 IU
Thiamine	0.02 g
Riboflavin	0.02 g
Vitamin C	3 mg

Source: Gopalan C., Ramasastri B.V. and Balasubramanian S.C. (2000). *Nutritive Value of Indian Foods*, NIN, ICMR, Hyderabad, India.

Energy requirements are best determined by measurement of energy expenditure. Energy expenditure, from physiological point of view, is made up of three major components:

i. Basal Metabolic Rate (BMR).

ii. Regulatory thermogenesis, which is categorised into obligatory and facultative components and includes the metabolic response to food ingested, i.e., the use of energy in digesting, absorbing, storing and disposing of ingested nutrients as also the response of the body to stimuli such as cold, stimulants and drugs.

iii. Physical activity, which includes both the cost and quantum of the activity as well as the type of activity viz., (a) essential economic or occupational activities, and (b) discretionary activities, which include household tasks, socially desirable activities and activities aimed at maintenance of physical fitness.

For all practical purposes, the components of energy expenditure related to regulatory energy output or thermogenesis are known to merge into measurements related to the cost of physical activity. Consequently the new simplified approach has only two principal components of energy expenditure : BMR and physical activity. Assessment of energy requirements is thus based on specifying the needs for the basal metabolic rate and then considering all physical activity costs as effectively occurring in the fed state (i.e., inclusive of the energy costs of thermogenesis).

Energy Requirement During Pregnancy and Lactation

Pregnancy

During pregnancy additional energy is needed to support the growth of the foetus, placenta and maternal tissues as well as to meet the increased basal metabolic rate (BMR). Since BMR increases by about 5% during the first and second trimester and by about 12% during the third trimester.

As per FAO/WHO expert group the total energy cost of pregnancy for a woman weighing 55 kg, has been estimated to be 80,000 kcals. Of this, about 36,000 kcals is deposited as fat which is utilized subsequently during lactation. Based on these estimates the FAO/WHO Expert Group recommended an extra daily allowance of 150 kcals during the first trimester and 350 kcals during the rest of pregnancy. For a reference Indian woman, whose body weight is 50 kg, the total energy cost of pregnancy has been estimated to be approximately 73,000 kcals and the energy expenditure during normal pregnancy would be 23,000 kcals. The additional daily requirement to meet the increased energy expenditure alone would thus be about 120 kcals during the second and third trimester of pregnancy. This level however, would not allow for the deposition of fat, which is used during lactation to meet the additional energy needs for mild secretion. On the basis of such evidences, the 1978 ICMR committee felt that extra energy intake is desirable not only for the growth of foetus and maternal tissue, but also for the deposition of fat which can be utilized for meeting the increased energy demands during lactation and therefore, recommended an additional intake of 300 kcal/day during the second and third trimesters of pregnancy.

Lactation

Additional energy required during lactation computed from the volume of milk secreted, its energy content and the efficiency of conversion of food energy into milk energy.

Estimates of additional energy needs during lactation by the FAO/WHO Expert Group in 1973 is based on optimal milk output of 850 ml and efficiency of conversion of 80 per cent. On the basis of this computation the additional intake of energy recommended during the first 6 months of lactation is 550 kcal/day. In this computation the contribution of fat deposited during pregnancy is all taken into account. On the same lines, the ICMR, expert committee (1978) also recommended an additional energy allowance of 550 kcal/day for the first 6 months of lactation. Since Indian women continue to lactate beyond 6 months, albeit with reduced milk output, upto one year, an extra allowance of 400 kcal/day was recommended for periods from 6 months to 1 year.

The present committee recommends that the earlier RDA for energy for these two groups be retained as there has been no additional evidence to justify a change.

Infants and Children

Infants: Energy requirement of infants as recommended by the FAO/WHO/UNU is adopted for Indian infants also. The values for different ages during infancy are given in Table 20.8.

Table 20.8 : Energy requirements of infants

Age	*Kcal/Kg*	
0-3 months	116	Average during the first year = 103 kcal/Kg
3-6 months	99	
6-9 months	95	
9-12 months	101	

Children: Following the suggestion of the 1985 FAO/WHO/UNU Expert Consultation, the energy needs of children of 1-10 years are computed. These computations for boys and girls are given in Tables 20.9 and 20.10. The energy requirements for different age ranges are shown in Table 20.9. These values are not substantially different from those recommended in 1978.

Table 20.9: Energy requirements of children (kcal/d)

Age group	*Body*	*Girls*
1-3 years	1287	1193
4-6 years	1752	1630
7-9 years	2075	1833
10-12 years	2194	1965
13-15 years	2447	2056
16-18 years	2642	2064

Table 20.10: Energy requirements of children (kcal/d)

Age (Yrs)	*Boys*	*Girls*
1 +	1096	1078
2 +	1301	1190
3 +	1463	1310
4 +	1531	1458
5 +	1778	1643
6 +	1948	1790
7 +	2030	1858
8 +	2034	1872
9 +	2160	1892
10+	2140	1907
11+	2193	1956
12+	2248	2032
13+	2340	2037
14+	2468	2066
15+	2534	2065
16+	2586	2070
17+	2662	2061
18+	2677	2061

The energy requirements suggested for preschool children that have been given in the Table 20.9, correspond closely to the values (Table 20.11) observed in well-to-do preschool children of Hyderabad, which were determined over a period of one year on 6 occasions and the values representing the average of these observations were tabulated.

Table 20.11: Observed energy intakes of well nourished Indian preschool children

Age (yrs)	Energy intake (kcal)	
	Per day*	kcal/kg
2-3	1223 ± 24	107
3-4	1467 ± 367	93
4-5	1530 ± 370	92
5-6	1500 ± 378	98

* Mean ± S.D.

Guidelines for the Use of Recommended Dietary Allowances of Energy

1. Energy allowances represent only the average requirement and no allowance is to be made for any safety margin, in contrast to other nutrients (such as protein), since excess intake of energy has undesirable consequences.
2. Energy requirement for adults are given in terms of a Reference Man and Woman. Energy requirement of other individuals of different body weights and age have to be calculated as suggested. In computing average energy requirement of a population also, weighed averages will have to be used.
3. Energy requirement of adults should be related to energy expenditure rather than to intake. In case of children below 10 years of age, however, energy requirements are related to intakes for satisfactory growth.
4. For malnourished children, the recommended intakes for the actual age should be used and no adjustments for actual body weights should be made.

Variability in Energy Requirements and Their Implications for Assessing Energy Deficiency

Energy requirement of an adult varies over a wide range depending upon the gender, age, body, size and weight and the degree of physical activity. Based on the daily variation in energy intakes, it has been suggested that the energy requirement of an individual also varies over a wide range with a coefficient of variation of over + 12.5% on a body weight basis. This variation is said to include both intra and inter-individual variations.

A critical analysis of the available data in the literature indicates that within individual variability in 24 hours energy expenditure or BMR of an individual on different level of intakes varies within a coefficient of variation of +5%. These conclusions are based on carefully conducted studies on 24 hours, energy expenditure in a whole body calorimeter over several times.

PROTEIN

Dietary proteins provide amino acids for the synthesis of body proteins and other biologically important nitrogenous compounds in the body. Adequate protein intake is essential during growth when new tissue proteins are being synthesised. However, in the adult, dietary protein is essential to synthesise only those new proteins that will replace those which are constantly being broken down. During pregnancy and lactation additional proteins are required for the synthesis of foetal tissue proteins and milk proteins respectively. Dietary proteins should supply the eight essential amino acids (EAA) in the proper proportions needed by the body. The other twelve amino acids present are not considered essential since the body can synthesise them from other carbon and nitrogen sources. Since most of the body N is derived from proteins, the terms 'protein' and 'N' requirements are used interchangeably.

Protein requirements have been determined by several methods like (a) N balance (b) obligatory N loss and (c) factorial method. Although the factorial method was used earlier, greater reliance is currently placed on the balance method which reflects physiological reality and provides a true estimate of requirements of body proteins. The 1985 recommendations of the FAO/WHO/UNU have been based largely on N balance data.

In India considerable experimental data exist on the protein requirements of adults. In recent years too, there have been some systematic studies to determine the protein requirements of Indian preschool children through N balance experiments on their habitual diets.

Protein Quality

An important factor in relation to defining protein needs is the quality of protein, since the efficiency of utilisation of a dietary protein depends upon its ability to supply the required amounts of essential amino acids (EAA). Animal proteins in general are of higher quality since they contain

EAA, an important determinant of protein quality, in right proportions. Egg protein in particular is used as reference against which the quality of other proteins are compared. Vegetable proteins are generally of poorer quality than animal proteins, not only because of lower digestibility but also because of their deficiency in one or the other of the essential amino acids, like lysine, methionine, etc. The relative biological quality of the mixture of vegetable proteins which are present in Indian diets that are based on cereals and pulses is only about 65 compared to the 100 of egg proteins.

Taking into consideration the available data on protein requirements in relation to the 1978 ICMR recommendations and the 1985 FAO/WHO/UNU recommendations, the 1988 ICMR Expert Group has adopted the following principles in fixing the protein requirements of Indians:

1. Nitrogen balance data (both short term and long term) obtained under appropriate conditions should form the basis for arriving at minimum maintenance nitrogen requirements.
2. Daily protein requirements in different age groups should be expressed on a g/kg body weight basis. The safe level of requirement is given by the Mean + 2SD of the mean requirements.
3. Requirements for proteins should be derived by a two-step process. First, the level of requirement according to age has to be chosen and next the actual amount has to be calculated by multiplying with the standard body weight for that age (Tables 20.12 to 20.16). Only during adolescent and adult periods have requirements to be indicated according to gender.
4. The coefficient of variation of 12.5% which was used by the 1985 FAO/WHO/UNU Committee should be used for all groups. This figure covers both intra-individual and inter-individual variation.
5. Nitrogen values of 8 mg/kg body weight for adults and 10 mg/kg for children as suggested by the 1985 FAO/WHO/UNU Expert Consultation are accepted for miscellaneous endogenous losses.
6. The requirement for protein should be given in terms of the average quality of the Indian diet, proteins from which are considered to have a NPU of 65%.
7. In computing the protein requirements of children the body weight standards are to be used as the reference values of weight for age.
8. The deliberations of the FAO/WHO/UNU Expert Group brings out the fact that the theoretical growth requirements based on factorial gains in nitrogen for children below 10 years of age have to be increased by a factor of 50% to obtain the physiological growth requirements. Similarly, during second half of pregnancy, the actual nitrogen retentions are 50% higher than the computed accretions of tissue nitrogen, though the FAO/WHO/UNU group disregarded this fact and recommended only the additional requirement of 925 g protein during pregnancy obtained by the factorial method. If 50% additions are used in calculating the growth requirement of children, a similar correction seems logical in arriving at the protein requirements for foetal growth in pregnancy.
9. For adults, 0.5 g per kg body weight of (milk) protein is adequate. For other groups the minimum protein requirements as suggested by the FAO/WHO/UNU consultation are accepted. The following are the recommendations of the committee for dietary protein allowances for different groups.

Adults

The average daily protein requirement of an Indian adult, in terms of a high quality protein like milk/egg at the physiological level is estimated to be 0.5 g/kg. This requirement figure has been based on an obligatory loss of urinary and faecal nitrogen of 45 mg, per kg and miscellaneous N loss through sweat etc. of 8 mg/kg. The factorial value thus obtained has been increased by 50% to obtain the requirement at the physiological level. Assuming a coefficient of variation of 12.5% the safe level of intake (M + 2SD) for an adult will be 0.625 g of protein per kg in terms of a high quality protein. When adjusted for the lower quality of dietary proteins with 65 NPU, the safe level of intake in terms of dietary protein will be 1.0 g/kg/day. A number of N balance studies in Indian adults indicate that the minimum intake of dietary protein for N equilibrium in Indian adults ranges from 0.5-0.66 g/kg with a mean of 00.58 g per kg which after allowing for the sweat loss of N, works out to 0.7 g/kg. The corresponding safe level of intake (M + 2SD) will be 0.88 g/kg which is close to the RDA derived from the factorial method. The RDA for adults is given in Table 20.12.

Table 20.12: Protein requirements of adults

Grou	*Body weight*	*Requirement g*	
	kg	*Per kg*	*Per day*
Men	60	1.0	60
Women	50	1.0	50

Pregnancy and Lactation

Protein requirement during pregnancy and lactation have also been assessed by the factorial method. Protein requirement during pregnancy has been computed on the basis of N accretion for foetal growth and expansion of maternal tissue. Based on the body weight gain of 12 kg in a normal, healthy and well nourished pregnant woman, the daily N deposited during the three trimesters is estimated to be 0.1, 0.5 and 0.9 g respectively. After increasing by 50% to convert the factorial value into physiological value for N accretion, and 25% for individual variation (i.e., M + 2SD), the safe level of intake in terms of a high quality protein during the three trimesters will be 1.2, 6.0 and 10.5 g respecitvely. After adjusting for the dietary protein quality of NPU 65 the safe additional intake during the later half of pregnancy recommended by the committee is 15 g/day.

During lactation, protein requirement has been computed on the basis of secretion in milk of 9.4 g protein per day during 0-6 months and 6.6 g during 6-24 months, which correspond to 820 ml and 600 ml of milk respectively with protein content of 1.15 g/100 ml. Assuming a 70% efficiency of conversion of dietary protein into milk protein and a 25% for individual variation (i.e., M + 2SD) the safe additional daily intake will be 16.8 g and 12.8 g during the first six months and during 6-12 months respectively. In terms of dietary protein of NPU 65, safe daily intake would be 26 g and 18.5 g respectively. The committee has recommended, during lactation, an additional daily intake of 25 g during the first six months and 18 g during 6-12 months of lactation.

Protein allowances during pregnancy and lactation are shown is Table 20.13.

Table 20.13: Protein requirement during pregnancy and lactation

Group	*Daily additional requirement g*	*Total daily requirement g*
Pregnant women	15	65
Lactating women:		
0-6 months	25	75
6-12 months	18	68

Infants

Infant protein requirement at various periods during the first year of life are derived from the breast milk intake of normally growing infants as has been done by the 1985 FAO/WHO/UNU consultation. These figures are given in Table 20.14.

Table 20.14: Protein requirement g/kg of infants

Age (months)	*Daily requirement*
0-3	23.00
3-6	01.85
6-9	01.65
9-12	01.50

Children

The requirements of children of various age groups are also computed by the factorial method employing the procedure adopted by the 1985 FAO/WHO/UNU consultation. In these computations, the maintenance N requirements of children as given by the 1985 FAO/WHO/UNU Expert Group and the N content of body weight increment of normally growing children have been used. The factorial value is increased by 50% to obtain the physiological requirement for growth. A safe allowance of 25% (M + 2SD) has been used to arrive at the safe intake. Safe intakes in terms of dietary protein have been arrived at using an NPU value of 65 for dietary proteins. In computing the total daily allowance of proteins for children at different ages, the body weight standards of well to do Indian children have been used. A comparison of the estimated safe allowance of proteins by the modified factorial method with those actually determined by long term N balance among 3-5 years old children, that is 1.75 g/kg, provides ample support to the present recommendations of protein for children. The recommended daily allowances of protein for children are given in Table 20.15.

Table 20.15: Protein requirements of boys and girls

	Boys			*Girls*		
Age (yrs)	*Body wt (kg)*	*Requirement per kg (g)*	*Total daily requirement (g)*	*Body wt (kg)*	*Requirement per kg (g)*	*Total daily requirement (g)*
1-2	10.54	1.81	19.1	9.98	1.81	18.1
2-3	12.51	1.67	20.9	11.67	1.67	19.5
3-4	14.78	1.61	23.8	13.79	1.61	22.2
4-6	19.20	1.52	29.2	18.69	1.52	28.4
7-9	27.00	1.48	40.0	26.75	1.48	39.6
10-12	35.54	1.46	51.9	37.91	1.45	55.0
13-15	47.88	1.40	67.0	46.66	1.33	62.1
16-18	57.28	1.31	75.1	49.92	1.21	60.4

Protein Quality

In arriving at the RDA for protein in terms of the proteins actually present in Indian dietaries, a value of 65 NPU that has been found in several experimental studies has been used.

Protein Calorie Ratio of Diets

It is useful to consider together the protein and energy requirement on habitual Indian diets. The protoein requirement can be expressed as the ratio of protein calories to total dietary calories (PE%). A comparison of this PE% value with the protein energy % of the diet will indicate whether diets can fulfil protein needs if an adequate quantity of the diet is eaten to meet the energy requirement. This concept is useful because in many population groups enough diet is not consumed to meet energy needs, resulting in energy deficits. The ratio of protein requirement, expressed as the ratio of protein calories to the energy requirements is given in Table 20.16 for various population categories. It will be seen that a PE% between 8 and 12 would meet the protein requirement of any group provided its energy needs are met.

Table 20.16: Protein energy ratios

Group		*Recommended protein intake g/day*	*Recommended energy intake kcal/day*	*Protein energy ratio (%)*
Reference adult (Moderate activity)				
Man		60	2900	8.3
Woman		50	2200	9.1
Pregnant woman		65	2500	10.4
Lactating woman (0-6 m)		75	2750	10.9
Preschool children:				
1-3 years		21	1240	6.8
4-6 years		29	1690	6.9
7-9 years		40	1950	8.2
Adolescents:				
13-15 years	Boys	67	2450	10.9
	Girls	62	2060	12.0
16-18 years	Boys	75	2640	11.4
	Girls	60	2060	11.7

FAT

Fat is a major nutrient and has several functions. Fat is a concentrated source of energy and increases the energy density of the diet. Fat in the diet also helps in the absorption of beta-carotene and other fat soluble vitamins. Dietary fat must also provide essential fatty acids (EFA) which are the functional components of membrane lipids and have other important metabolic functions. Fat may have other functions which are as yet unclear. While a minimum amount of fat has to be present in the diet to meet the minimum essential requirement of the two unsaturated EFAs, excess of fat in the diet is considered harmful. Hence the minimum level, the desirable level and the safe upper limit of fat intake have to be considered.

Fat Intake in India

Diet surveys by the National Nutrition Monitoring Bureau (NNMB) in 10 States of India show that daily intake of visible fats vary from 3 g to 20 g/day per consumption unit in rural India; in many states as much as quarter of population may not have any visible fat at all in their diets. In urban areas middle and upper income groups have daily intakes of visible fat that range from 20-42 g. Thus the average intakes of urban dwellers are much higher than those in rural areas. These low intakes of fat reflect both the low availability of edible oils and fat in the country and the low purchasing power. Based on current production of edible oils and fats in the country, per capita availability works out to only 15-17 g/day, made up of about 10-12 g vegetable oils, 3 g of vanaspati and 2-5 g of ghee. The nature of the edible oil used varies from one part of the country to the other; groundnut oil in the West and South, coconut oil in Kerala, rape/mustard oil from Punjab to West Bengal along the Gangetic plain and safflower oil in parts of North Karnataka and Southern Maharashtra.

Invisible Fats and Their Significance in Indian Dietaries

Some fat is present in most food. This fat content has been usually expressed as crude ether extracts. The invisible fat thus determined was considered earlier as of not much consequence in contributing to the dietary intake of fat. However, in recent years, the use of more vigorous methods which extract both bound and free fat have shown that significant quantities of invisible fat are present in common dietary items like cereals, pulses, condiments, fresh coconuts, nuts and oilseeds. The total quantity of invisible fat therefore depends on the kind of diet eaten. The diets of even poor people which consist predominantly of cereals and have little or no visible fat contain significant quantities of invisible fat. The invisible fat from cereals and pulses alone contribute as much as 6 en % or 16 g of invisible fat in adult diet that provide 2400 kcal. In average Indian diets in many parts of the country. The total visible plus invisible fat contributes about 15% of the dietary energy, though in the diets of poor income groups, this reduces to about 10.5% of dietary energy. Continuous intake of daily diets providing an average of about 15% of energy from fat does not lead to any fat deficiency. A daily Indian diet which provides 2400 kcal will thus carry about 40 g of fat a day, out of which 25 g will be invisible fat and 15 g visible fat. The upper income groups in urban areas tend to consume daily about 50 g of visible fat. Besides this they consume high amounts of milk and fat rich foods the invisible fat content of which can contribute another 30-50 g fat a day. This group forms only a very small per cent of our population and may have a fat intake in excess of 30 per cent of dietary energy.

Quality of Fat

Besides being a concentrated source of energy, fats are also a source of essential fatty acids (EFA). Fats are made up of fatty acids which include saturated fatty acids like palmitic and stearic, monounsaturated fatty acids like oleic and polyunsaturated fatty acids like linoleic (lin) and linolenic (len). The latter two cannot be synthesised in the body and have to be supplied through dietary fat. Dietary fat with an equal proportion of saturated, monounsaturated and poly-unsaturated fatty acids components have been considered as desirable.

Linoleic and linolenic fatty acids are further metabolised in the body into other fatty acids of greater chain length and unsaturation which have important biological functions. Some of them form part of cell structures and others have a specific role in vision and in the function of the central nervous system. Also linoleic and linolenic acids are converted into prostaglandins, thromboxanes and prostacyclines which have extremely important functions in such areas as regulating blood pressure, blood viscosity, muscle contraction, pain relief, male fertility and female conception and normal delivery.

Fats like ghee, hydrogenated fats and coconut oil are comparatively saturated and are poor source of EFA. Other edible oils are better source of EFA, their levels ranging from 10% in palmolein to 25% in grouindnut oil, 50% to 70% in cottonseed, corn, sunflower, soyabean and safflower oils. Linolenic acid content is found to be high in mustard/rapeseed (13%) and soyabean (5%). Essential fatty acid composition (lin and len) of commonly consumed edible oils and fats are given in Table 20.17.

EFA Requirements

The desirable amount of linoleic acid to be consumed by a normal adult person has been placed at 3 en%. The requirements of linoleic acid during pregnancy and lactation are higher, i.e., 4.5 and 5.7 en% respectively. The EFA requirement of children is placed at 3 en% (Table 20.17).

Table 20.17: Linoleic (Lin), Linolenic (Len) acid content of edible oils (g/100 g)

Oil	*Lin*	*Len*	*Total EFA*
Ghee	1.6	0.5	2.1
Coconut	2.2	-	2.2
Vanaspati	3.4	-	3.4
Palmolein	12.0	0.3	12.3
Rape/Mustard	13.0	9.0	22.0
Groundnut	28.0	0.3	28.3
Rice bran	33.0	1.6	34.6
Sesame	40.0	0.5	40.5
Cotton seed	50.3	0.4	50.7
Corn oil	50.0	2.0	52.0
Sun flower	52.0	Trace	52.0
Soyabean	52.0	5.0	57.0
Safflower	74.0	0.5	74.5

The invisible fats present in many Indian food materials have a high linoleic acid content (rice 50%, wheat 55%, Bengalgram 65% and linolenic acid contents of about 3%). The invisible fat in spices have a particularly high content of linolenic acid (5.4%). As a result, average Indian diet predominantly based on cereals and some pulses including the diets of poor income groups carry sufficient linoleic acid levels and a proportion of linolenic acid as well. A study of such populations indicate that the EFA status as reflected in the fatty acid components present in their blood is satisfactory. Although their diet may contain very low amount of visible fat, the quantity of EFA and the levels of invisible fats compensate for the lack.

Fat Requirement of Indians

Considering the EFA requirement of different groups (Table 20.18) and knowing that the total invisible fat (bound and free) in a cereal based diet can meet more than half the linoleic acid requirement of an adult, the following recommendation on minimal intakes of fat is made. The visible fat should preferably be in the form of an oil containing at least 20% linoleic acid. Apart from providing the essential fatty acids, visible fat in the diet has other desirable functions such as improving the palatability and increasing the calorie density of the diet. A higher calorie density in the diet is essential for feeding young children so as to provide the needed calories.

Adult

Taking into account the linoleic acid content of invisible fat, a 5 energy (en %) of visible fat derived from oils having at least 20% lin would meet the adult need. Another 10 energy % would come from invisible fat with an average EFA content of 20% contributed by cereals and pulses, spices, condiments, nuts and oilseeds and other components in habitual Indian diets. The visible fat intake on the basis of 5 en% would be about 12 g/day. Although a minimal intake of 12 g visible fat can meet the EFA requirement, a higher level of intake of 20 g/day is desirable to provide energy density and palatability to the diet.

Children and Adolescents

The linoleic acid requirement of older children is also 3 en%. As with adults, their minimum visible fat intake would also be 5 en% and since their daily energy needs are also about 2400 kcal, the minimum quantity of visible fat intake also would be 12 g/day. As suggested for adults, the desirable level of visible fat intake in the case of older children and adolescents is also 20 g/day.

Young Children

The linoleic acid requirement of young children has been placed at 3 en% which can be satisfied by minimal intake of 10 g/day of visible fat. However, more fat is needed in their bulky cereal based diets to provide enough calories to meet their energy needs. It is suggested that their daily visible fat intake could be 25 g/day.

Pregnancy

The linoleic acid requirement during pregnancy is 4.5 en%. Taking into account the contribution from the invisible fat, 12.5 en% visible fat would meet the EFA requirement. The corresponding visible fat intake will be 30 g/day. This level of fat intake would also provide the necessary calorie density to their diets.

Table 20.18: Fat requirement of Indians

Group	*EFA requirement*	*Invisible fat*[a]	*Minimum visible*[b] *fat*		*Suggested desirable visible fat intake*	
	en %	*en %*	*en %*	*g/day*	*g/day*	*en %*
Adults[c]	3	10	5	12[c]	20[c]	9
Older children[c]	3	10	5	12	22	9
Young children	3	10	5	8	25	15
Pregnant woman	4.5	10	12.5	30	30	12.5
Lactating woman	5.7	10	17.8	45	45	17.5

a. Contains 20% EFA, about 6% from cereals and pulses and rest from milk, nuts, spices, etc.

b. EFA at least 20%.

c. Average for males and females.

Lactation

The linoleic acid requirement during lactation has been placed at about 6 en%. After taking into account the contribution from invisible fat, the visible fat requirement of lactating women can be placed at 17.5 en% so as to supply the high level of EFA needed. This would correspond to a daily intake of 45 g of visible fat. This level of fat in the diet would provide adequate energy to enable a nursing woman to meet her higher energy needs.

Infants

Adequately breast fed infants receive nearly 30 g fat per day, of which about 10% is linoleic acid and 1% linolenic acid. Breast milk would thus meet the EFA needs of infants, which is about 6 en%. The superiority of breast milk over the cow and buffalo milk must be emphasised, since the former contains longer chain n-6 and n-3 PUFA which are biologically more potent.

Infants who have been weaned completely or partially should be given enough vegetable oil with high linoleate content so as to provide 6 en% as linoleic acid.

Upper Limit of Fat

Although a minimum amount of fat is essential to provide EFA, fat intake above a certain level is also undesirable, being associated with health hazards like cardiovascular diseases and obesity. Fat intake should not exceed 30% of total caloric intake, out of which 10% each should be saturated, monounsaturated and polycusaturated fats. Since 10-15% of the fat intake comes from invisible fats, the visible fat intake should be below 20%, i.e., below 40-50 g per day.

MINERALS

Important minerals are calcium, phosphorus, magnesium and the electrolytes, sodium and potassium.

Calcium and Phosphorus

Because of their close relationship these nutrients are taken together. The desirable ratio of Ca: P is 1:1.5 for infants and 1:1 for all other groups (Table 20.19).

Table 20.19: Suggested intakes of calcium and phosphorus (mg/d)

Group	*Calcium*	*Phosphorus*
Adult:		
Men	1000	400
Women	1000	400
Pregnancy and lactation	1600	1000
Infants	500	750
Children:		
1-9 years	400	400
10-15 years	600	600
16-18 years	500	500

Magnesium is a component of cells and is essential for various metabolic reactions. Magnesium concentrates in the bone and it is important for maintaining electrical potential in nerves and muscle membranes. Mg deficiency leads to neuromuscular dysfunction. Mg occurs widely in foods and plant foods are particularly rich in it. Dietary deficiency of Mg is therefore, unlikely to occur in the Indian population. No specific recommendations are made with regard to dietary intake of Mg.

Sodium and Potassium

Since sodium intake is high in India and a high intake is associated with hypertension, there is a need for fixing limits of intake of sodium. There is no information available on the body turnover of Na and K in tropical country like India where Na and K can be lost significantly in sweat. In the absence of such data no specific recommendations for Na and K are made.

Trace Elements

At present, fifteen trace elements are believed to be essential for the mammalian species, of which eight elements are known to be required by man (Tables 20.20 to 20.23). These are Iron (Fe), Zinc (Zn), Copper (Cu),

Table 20.20: Suggested daily intake of trace elements by an Indian adult

Chromium	67 μg
Copper	2.2 mg
Manganese	5.5 mg
Zinc	15.5 mg

Table 20.21: Iron requirement in pregnancy

Loci of additional requirement	*Gross loss*	*Iron requirement during entire pregnancy (mg)*
Foetus	240 mg	240
Expansion of maternal red cell mass	400 mg	400
Obligatory loss	14 μg/kg	170
Total		180

Chromium (Cr), Cobalt (Co). Iodine (I), Manganese (Mn), Molybdenum (Mo) and Selenium (Se). However, only the deficiency of a few of these elements is observed in man. Iron and iodine deficiencies are widespread, while deficiencies of Cu, Zn, Cr and Se have been reported in recent years. So far the requirement of these trace elements could not be defined for two important reasons: (a) data on their content in foods are not available, hence intake could not be established, and (b) their requirement (but for Fe and I) have not been experimentally studied.

Iron

Iron requirements are derived by using the factorial approach which takes into account the basal loss in case of men, basal loss + menstrual loss in case of women and basal loss + growth requirement in case of children. Dietary iron requirements are prescribed at a level of absorption of 3% in adult men from habitual diets based on mixed cereals.

Iron Requirement for Women

Based on the available data for Indian and Western women, the following additional requirement can be taken into consideration for assessing iron requirement during pregnancy for Indian women of 50 kg body weight.

The mean requirement during the first trimester is not increased. It is similar to the normal requirement of 0.70 mg, while during the second and third trimester, the daily requirement is 3.3 mg and 5 mg respectively.

Lactation

Iron requirement during lactation is the sum of the requirement of the mother and that required to make up the iron lost in breast milk. Since there is amenorrhoea during lactation, the basal requirement will be the same as in adult man, i.e., 14 mg/kg. For lactation, the requirement is about 1 mg/day, or 16 μg/kg, as the total requirement turns out to be the same as for a normal woman, namely 30 μg/kg.

Dietary Requirement of Iron

The recommendations are based on systematic computation of the daily requirement of adults and also of children and adolescents of different age groups.

Based on these considerations of the iron requirement in different groups, the requirement of absorbed iron per kg body weight shown in Table 20.22 are drawn up. Taking into account the absorbed iron requirement for different physiological groups and the iron absorption of 3% for the habitual diets based on mixed cereals, the total dietary iron requirement has been computed. Using these figures the daily RDI for iron for various groups of the Indian population are given in Table 20.23.

Table 20.22: Iron requirements (μg/kg) per day of different physiological groups

Group	*Body wt kg*	*Basal*	*Growth*	*Menstrual blood*	*Total daily requirement*
Infant (0-2 yrs)	3.3-12.3	14	65		69
Children* (2-12 yrs)	12.2-35.4	14	15		29
Adolescent male (12-18 yrs)	35.4-57.1	14	12		26
Adolescent girls	31.5-49.9	14	8	8	30
Adult male	60	14	-	-	14
Adult female	50	14	-	16	30
Pregnant female	50	14	46	-	60
Lactating female	50	14	16		30

* Dietary iron absorption: Adult men, children and adolescent boys: 3%; Adult women, lactating women and adolescent girls: 5%; Pregnant women: 8%.

Table 20.23: Daily iron requirement of Indians

Group	Body wt (kg)	Basal iron requirement µg/kg	Basal iron requirement Total daily mg/day	Dietary iron* requirement on a mixed cereal diet (mg/day)
Adult: Men	60	14	0.840	28.0
Women	50	30	1.500	30.0
Pregnant woman	50	60	3.000	37.5
Lactating woman	50	30	1.500	30.0
Infants:				
0-6 months	4.5	70	0.315	
Children:				
1-3 yrs	12.2		0.354	11.5
4-6 yrs	19.0	29	0.551	18.4
7-9 yrs	26.9		0.780	26.0
Adolescents:				
10-12 yrs:				
Boys	35.4	29	1.027	34.2
Girls	31.5	30	0.945	18.9
13-15 yrs:				
Boys	47.8	26	1.243	41.4
Girls	46.7	30	1.401	28.0
16-18 yrs:				
Boys	57.1	26	1.485	49.5
Girls	49.1	30	1.497	29.9

* Dietary iron absorption: Adult men, children and adolescent boys: 3%; Adult women, lactating women and adolescent girls: 5%; Pregnant women: 8%.

VITAMINS (Tables 20.24 to 20.26)

Table 20.24: Recommended intake of vitamin A (µg/day)

Group	Retinol	β-carotene
Adult man and woman	600	2400
Pregnant woman	600	2400
Lactating woman	950	3800
Infants: 0-6 months; 6-12 months	350	1400
Preschool children: 1-5 yrs	400	1600
School children: 7-12 yrs	600	2400
Adolescents: 13-18 yrs	600	2400

Vitamin A

The recommended level of vitamin A (retinol) for an adult is 600 µg. In terms of beta-carotene, it will be 2400 µg, the conversion and bioavailability factors used being 1 mg beta-carotene = 0.25 µg retinol. In diets containing both retinol and beta-carotene, the vitamin A content can be expressed as follows:

a. Retinal content in µg= µg retinol +0.25 × µg beta-carotene, if retinol and beta-carotene are expressed in µg.
b. Retinol content in µg = vitamin A International Units (IU) × 0.3 + beta-carotene in IU × 0.15, if vitamin A and beta-carotene are expressed in International Units.

Table 20.25: Recommended allowances of thiamin, riboflavin and nicotinic acid

Thiamin	0.5 mg/100 kcal
Riboflavin	0.6 mg/1000 kcal
Nicotinic acid (Niacin equivalents)*	6.6 mg/1000 kcal

$$*\text{Niacin equivalents} = \text{Niacin (mg)} \frac{+\text{ Tryptophan (mg)}}{60}$$

Table 20.26: Suggested daily intake of pyridoxine, folate, vitamin B_{12} and ascorbic acid

	Pyridoxine µg	Folate µg	Vitamin B_{12} µg	Ascorbic acid (mg)
Adult man and woman	2.0	100	1	40
Pregnant woman	2.5	400	1	40
Lactating woman	2.5	150	1.5	80
Infant:				
0.6 months	0.3			
6-12 months	0.4	25	0.2	25
Preschool children:				
1-3 yrs	0.9	40		
4-6 yrs		50		
School children:				
7-9 yrs	1.6	60	0.2 to 1.0	40
10-12 yrs		70		
Adolescents:				
13-15 yrs	2.0	100		
16-18 yrs		100		

Thiamine, Riboflavin and Nicotinic Acid

The daily allowances for these vitamins are related to energy intake. The basic allowances per 1000 kcal are: thiamine 0.5, riboflavin 0.6 mg and nicotinic acid 6.6 mg niacin equivalent.

Niacin allowance also takes into account the contribution of tryptophan, assuming that 60 mg dietary tryptophan yield 1 mg of niacin in the body.

$$\underset{\text{(mg)}}{\text{Niacin equivalents}} = \underset{\text{(mg)}}{\text{Niacin content}} + \frac{\text{Tryptophan content in mg}}{60}$$

Folic Acid

Allowance for folic acid is given in terms of the free folate (*L. casei* activity) present in foods. RDA of folate in pregnancy will be 300 µg in addition to the normal requirement of 100 mg. Since such high levels of folate cannot be obtained through diet alone, therapeutic supplementation becomes necessary in pregnancy.

Vitamin B_{12}

Recommended intake of vitamin B_{12} is 1 µg/day. Since this vitamin is entirely derived from animal food, there is justification for including some animal foods in the daily diet.

Vitamin C

The recommendations for adults is 40 mg/day. For infants, the RDA is 25 mg/day.

Vitamin D

Vitamin D is now considered more as a pro-hormone than a vitamin. It can be synthesized in the body in adequate amounts by simple exposure to sunlight even for 5 minutes per day. Indian diets do not supply even one-tenth of the present recommendation and yet rickets is a very rare disease. Accordingly no recommendation for vitamin D is made by the committee.

In prescribing medicinal doses of vitamin D under certain situations where there is minimal exposure to sunlight, a specific recommendation of a daily supplement of 400 µg is made.

Nutrient Requirement in Health and Disease

Nutrient requirements discussed for healthy individuals with normal activity, living and working under normal comfortable environment do not cover persons living and working under unusual conditions are high altitudes or under very cold conditions as prevailing in Antarctica. These requirements also do not cover sports persons and athletes who perform high levels of sustained activity and are constantly under training. The requirement of nutrients under such conditions is nearly 2-3 times the normal requirements.

Recent research shows that several micro nutrients with antioxidant properties have important functions for ensuring health besides their well-established nutritional (metabolic) functions in the body. Intake of elevated dosages of some of the vitamins like, carotenes, retinol, ascorbic acid and vitamin E, are reported to be useful in the prevention of certain degenerative diseases like cancer, heart diseases and cataract. Although the quantitative requirement of nutrients for these functions are not precisely established, they may be 2-3 times the RDA.

Application of RDA Database

The nutrient requirements and the recommended dietary intakes of nutrients have several practical applications, the important among them are:

a. To assess the adequacy of national food supplies and to plan for food production both in terms of quantity and quality, e.g., agriculture planning.

b. To provide dietary guidelines for healthy living individuals and groups and to formulate balanced diets.

c. RDA can also be used for judging the adequacy of intake of individuals or groups in a preliminary way. In the case of adult individuals RDA has to be adjusted for the actual body weight while assessing the adequacy of intake.

STUDY QUESTIONS

1. What are the general guiding principles of arriving at recommended dietary allowances for various classes of nutrients?
2. How do you make use of factorial approach to assess the energy requirements for different life styles and stages?
3. How do you set RDAs for proteins for different age groups and physiological conditions?
4. How do you assess the dietary fat requirements for different age groups, life styles and physiological conditions?
5. How human mineral and vitamin requirements are assessed and daily dietary intakes are recommended? Explain briefly.

Diet Therapy

CHAPTER 21

Institutional Delivery of Nutritional Care

Chapter Outlines

- Hospitalization and nutrition
- Objectives of modified diets
- Patient-expert group interpersonal relationship
- Concept of all encompassing or comprehensive care
- Enteral and parenteral nutrition
- Study questions

The attributes of good nutrition and the principles and practices for achieving them have been discussed for all age categories. The adoption of the normal diet according to the needs of individuals with some pathologic conditions is the objective of therapeutic nutrition. This introduction presents an overview of the factors that may have a bearing on the nutritional status of hospitalized persons and the role of the nutrition care team in meeting their nutritional needs, prevalence of malnutrition in hospitalized patients and the role of nutrition care team in assessing, preventing and treating it. These some points are of much concern and call for the attention they require.

HOSPITALIZATION AND NUTRITION

Hard times and disease can strike anyone. Any acute or chronic condition can require hospitalization. Food often is the only aspect of the daily routine that is familiar to hospitalized patients. However, if the usual food intake is not permitted because of the need for a therapeutic diet, food may become a source of apprehension. Regardless of the diagnosis or the type of diet prescribed, the satisfactory intake of food by the patient is essential for maintenance of tissue structures and body functions so that recovery from illness is quick. Inadequate intake of the proper nutrients, or impaired ability to digest, absorb, or metabolize foods, leads to nutritional deficiency. This lowers the body's resistance and may initiate or aggravate diseases of non-nutritional origin. Illnesses, such as infections, injuries and metabolic disturbances, lead to deficiencies even in otherwise well nourished persons because of failure to ingest sufficient food or because the disease process greatly increases nutritional needs. Thus a vicious cycle of disease, malnutrition and delayed convalescence ensues.

OBJECTIVES OF MODIFIED DIETS

Most patients do not require dietary modifications. Good nutritional care for them consists of supplying a normal diet that furnishes their nutritional, psychologic, and aesthetic needs and taking measures to enable them to consume it. On the other hand, modified diets are the principal therapeutic agents in some metabolic diseases such as non-insulin dependent (NIDDM) diabetese mellitus. In other cases, diet therapy supports the overall therapeutic program; for example, a sodium restricted diet may be prescribed in addition to diuretics for some patients with hypertension. Modified diets are also used as preventive measures. One example of this is the fat controlled diet prescribed for individuals with elevated blood lipids who are at increased risk for ischemic (coronary) heart disease. For some conditions in which diet therapy formerly played a major role, drug therapy is now a more effective means of controlling symptoms. Use of cimetidine in peptic ulcer or allopurinol in gout has largely superseded the need for bland and purine restricted diets in patients receiving these medications. Nevertheless, these diets are still used in some circumstances.

Expert Group Delivery of Nutritional Care

Meeting the patient's nutritional needs involves the coordination of several hospital departments. The core team is composed of the physician, nurse, and dietitian. With the advent of enteral and parenteral feeding formulae and greater awareness of drug diet interactions, the role of the clinical pharmacist is becoming increasingly recognized. At times, other health professionals, such as the social worker or physical therapist become directly involved. The focus, of course, is on the patient who must actively participate, as far as possible, in his or her health care. The physician prescribes the diet and should also give the patient some information concerning the reasons that a modified diet has been ordered. The dietitian is the specialist who translates the physician's written order into practical products or formulae. The dietitian assesses and evaluates the patient's nutritional status; formulates nutritional care plans; designs meal patterns, individualizes them according to the patient's food habits and modifies according to the therapeutic need; and recommend appropriate proprietary formulae for enteral feeding. The dietary staff is also responsible for the preparation and service of food to the patient, the evaluation of the patient's response to the diet, and the subsequent counselling of the patient and family if a home diet is required. The clinical pharmacists formulate solutions for parenteral feedings and advise on nutritional effects of drug therapy.

The nurse is the member of the health team who has the most constant and intimate association with the patient and the direct services she gives to the patient differ from those of the physician and the dietician. Some specific means by which nursing personnel assist in nutritional care include the following.

1. Maintaining lines of communication with the physician and dietitian regarding the patient's dietary needs:
   (i) Obtaining a diet prescription if there is none, and arranging for food service to the patient.
   (ii) Providing the dietitian and physician with information regarding the patient's response to the diet.
   (iii) Serving as liaison between the patient and the physician and dietitian.
2. Assisting the patient at mealtimes:
   (i) Providing a pleasant environment conducive to eating.
   (ii) Preparing the patient for the meal.
   (iii) Giving assistance to the patient as needed, including feeding.
   (iv) Helping the handicapped to adjust to self-feeding
   (v) Giving encouragement and support to the patient.
3. Interpreting the diet to the patient:
   (i) Explaining the reasons for a modified diet and what may be expected of the diet.
   (ii) Answering questions about the diet.
4. Observing, recording and reporting the patient's response to diet:
   (i) Eliciting information regarding food habits, likes and dislikes, and attitudes toward diet.
   (ii) Noting adequacy of food intake.
   (iii) Reporting patient's response to dietitian and physician.
5. Planning for home care:
   (i) Identifying needs for outside assistance.
   (ii) Arranging for counselling regarding home diet with members of family as well as patient.

Factors to be Considered in the Study and Practice of Diet Therapy

In order to function effectively in the provision of nutritional care, students of nursing and dietetics must have an understanding of (1) acute and chronic conditions which require a change in diet; (2) the rationale for dietary changes, characteristics of the diet, its beneficial and possible adverse effects, nutritional limitations of the various modified diets, and indications and contraindications for use; (3) ways in which drug therapy may influence food intake or utilization; and (4) the patient's tolerance for food.

A correctly planned diet is successful only if it is eaten. The dietitian and nurse must be able to apply the principles pertaining to the preparation and service of appealing, palatable, and nutritious food. They must have the necessary understanding of the psychologic and emotional factors influencing food acceptance.

Patient care includes planning for full rehabilitation. For some patients, a modified diet is required for weeks, months, or even a life time; for others, guidance may be desirable in the improvement of a normal diet. Such planning necessitates a consideration of social, religious, and cultural patterns, availability of foods, cost of food, suitable methods of food preparation, and so on.

The hospital or regional diet manual is used as the basis for planning modified diets.

Illness and Food Acceptance and Utilization

It is proven that physiologic, psychologic and emotional factors govern food acceptance. Likewise, a number of cultural food patterns are preferred by the respective patient groups. Illness may modify or enhance the influence of any of these factors.

The Stress Factor

The sick person has many fears: those relating to the outcome of the illness itself; economic concerns for self and family; emotional adjustments of having to depend on others during the illness; anxiety about loss of love and self esteem. The sick person may express fears in a number of ways: by being angry, self conscious, talkative or reticent, uneasy, depressed, indifferent, impatient, hostile, apologetic for failure, or resentful.

When hospitalization becomes necessary, the sick person experiences additional stress. Some patients adjust easily to a hospital routine, but for others it is difficult. The patient is subjected to seemingly endless questions, physical examinations, laboratory tests, administration of therapy by a number of specialists and auxiliary workers who, too often, do not explain what is happening, thus causing much needless anxiety. On the other hand, the patient often experiences long delays when he or she requires attention to personal needs. Especially if primary care nursing is not provided, patients may feel that there is no specific person who owns the primary concern and responsibility for his or her care. The loss of privacy is a special embarrassment and even shocking to an elderly individual who has never before been in a hospital. Likewise, the loss of independence to eat when and what one wishes, to get out of bed or not, to come and go as one wishes, and so on, can be frustrating. Each member of the health team should be concerned that the patient is treated with dignity and that his or her rights are observed.

Illness Modifies Food Acceptance

Hospitalization itself may influence food acceptance. When the patient most needs the comfort and companionship of family and friends, he or she is relegated to eating alone. Perhaps the meal hours are different from those to which the patient is accustomed; the foods appearing on the tray may be unlike those usually eaten with respect to choice, or flavouring, or portion size. A single food to which the patient has a strong aversion may be so upsetting that he or she is unable to eat anything served with it. Managing a tray and the utensils for eating may be awkward when one is in bed. Further, the patient may perceive expressed needs being minimized or brushed aside. Some patients, under stress, use diet as a means of gaining attention from hospital personnel and later from family members. They may insist upon meticulous attention to the minutest of details, in order to be noticed.

The disease process itself may have a profound effect on food acceptance. Some foods may produce marked anorexia, others may be distending, and still others may be irritants to the gastrointestinal tract. Food preferences may revert to those of earlier years. These may be bland foods of childhood, but they might be the special dishes associated with one's ethnic origin.

Modified Diets Impose Additional Problems

When a patient is confronted with the need for a therapeutic diet, he or she may respond with comments such as these: "I just can't afford such food when I go home", "Who is going to prepare my food at home?" "I can't buy these foods at work". Remarks such as these may indicate unwillingness to accept change; anger at those associated with the diet–nurse, dietitian, physician, or even mother or spouse who has nagged about the food habits at home; or fears–of having to eat disliked foods; of having to forego favourite foods; of loss of social status and self esteem; or the feeling that diet is, in some way, a punishment.

The nurse and dietitian must try to allay the patient's fears by empathetic understanding and by providing help in budgeting, arrangements for food preparation, suggestions for making the diet more palatable, and other useful advice.

Nutritional Stress

Emotional stress, such as the taking of examinations, leads to increased losses of nitrogen and calcium. In fact, persons under such stress may achieve balance only with considerable difficulty. One may reasonably assume that the anxiety concerning illness may also accentuate such losses.

Immobilization is also a stressful situation in which nitrogen and calcium excretions are elevated. In long-term illness, immobilization may be responsible for serious demineralization of bones.

Any trauma to the body such as bone fracture, wound injury, or infection increases the losses of nitrogen and various electrolytes. The secretion of several hormones is often increased, thereby elevating the needs for vitamins required to carry on metabolic processes.

Effect of Drugs

Drug therapy may have profound effects on nutritional status by interfering with food intake, decreasing nutrient absorption, or altering metabolic responses. Frequent gastrointestinal manifestation of drug intolerance is anorexia, nausea and diarrhea. Because food and drug interactions are common, the pharmacist advises a patient regarding not only dosages, but also the time for taking the medication with reference to food intake.

PATIENT-EXPERT GROUP INTERPERSONAL RELATIONSHIP

Requirements of the Patient

Each patient has physical, psychologic, social and spiritual needs. The pathophysiologic aspects of illness are the immediate reasons for care by the health team, but other needs must not be overlooked. Each member of the health team has a unique contribution to make in providing for these needs. Some examples relating to nutritional care are as under:

1. Each person wants to be treated as an individual. He or she has specific needs and values that are unique for him or her, and care should be personalized rather than making the patient fit into a general mould.

   Thus those who care for the patient must learn to listen carefully–not only to the words themselves but also to their tone and tenor. By taking time to listen, one may be made aware of a legitimate complaint about something wrong with the meals a patient receives. Such details are relatively easy to correct, and the patient is thereby made quite comfortable and satisfied. The seemingly casual conversation with the patient may bring to light that the past diet has been inadequate for a long period of time because of lack of teeth, poor health, inadequate income, or the inability to prepare food.

2. Each person has a right to know what should be expected from the nutrition team and what is expected of the patient. If a modified diet is prescribed, the patient should be given some understanding of the reasons for it and what he or she may expect by way of needed change in food habits.

   Appropriate diets for obesity and diabetese are basic to treatment, but some patients may find the adjustment to the restrictions extremely difficult; to minimize the problems involved is to invite failure. A fat restricted diet may be helpful to the patient with gallstones, but it should never be held as a guarantee that surgery would not be required at a later time. Likewise, benefit may accrue to a patient with cardiovascular disease who is placed on a diet with modification of the amount and nature of the fat, but success is so variable that promises of marked improvement would be ill advised and rash.

3. Each patient should be helped to participate in his or her own care. A selective menu can be a useful tool to help in making good choices for a normal as well as modified diet. If dietary counselling has begun early, each meal helps the patient to learn what changes will be needed in the diet when the patient goes home. A patient who has a physical handicap should be helped to feed himself or herself as much as is possible, thereby increasing independence.

4. Each person expects that his or her behaviour during illness will be accepted as part of the illness.

5. Each person expects to be treated with kindness, thoughtfulness, and firmness. The work of the dietitians, nurses, or homemakers is often more successful if they can place themselves in the patient's role, although they must guard against over identification. They should interview the patient in a relaxed environment and non judgemental manner as they listen to him, and skillfully get the information elicited by interjecting questions now and then.

Nutritional Care Plans

The dietitian is responsible for the nutritional care plan for each patient. Many hospitals' dietary departments have developed forms for this purpose. Information from the medical record, such as the diagnosis, pertinent laboratory values and medications, height, and weight are entered as well as information obtained directly from the patient regarding the dietary history, food preferences, food allergies, and so on.

The care plan includes (1) an estimate of the adequacy of the patient's usual dietary intake; (2) any nutritional problems; (3) plans for resolving these; (4) objectives for patient education, stated in terms of patient outcomes; (5) progress notes; and (6) evaluation of nutritional care.

Making the Patient Partake Food

Environment for meals: Time and effort directed toward creating an atmosphere conducive to the enjoyment of food are well spent. Such an environment implies that the surrounding areas are orderly and clean; that ventilation i good; and that distracting activities such as treatment of patients and doctors' rounds are not occurring at meal time except for emergencies may arise.

Patients who are ambulatory, enjoy eating with others. In some hospitals a dining room is provided for patients, and in others food service may be easily arranged at small tables set up in the patients' lounge.

Readiness of the Patient

The patient should be ready for the meal whether in bed or ambulatory. This may entail mouth care, the washing of the hands, and the positioning of the patient so that eating can take place in comfort. If tests or treatment unavoidably delay a meal, arrangements must be made to hold trays so that the food can be fresh and appetizing when the patient is ready to eat.

When the meal preparations are complete, the tray should be placed so that it becomes easy for the patient to feed herself or himself or, if necessary, convenient for someone else to do the feeding. If the patient needs help, the napkin should be opened and placed, the bread spread, the meat cut, the eggs shelled, and the straw offered. The patient should be encouraged to eat and be allowed sufficient time. If the meal is interrupted by the physician, the tray should be removed and the food kept at proper temperatures in the kitchen. It should be served again as soon as the physician leaves.

The tray should be removed and the patient helped to brush her or his teeth when the meal is finished. The kinds and amounts of food refused, the time, the type of diet, and the patient's appetite should be recorded on the patient's chart after each meal. At times, the doctor may request an accurate report of the types and amounts of uneaten food.

Some patients require assistance at meals because they are too weak to feed themselves, while others need the encouragement to eat.

Feeding the Disabled Patient

If the patient is unable to feed herself or himself, the person doing the feeding should sit near the side of the bed. Small amounts of food should be placed toward the back of the mouth with a slight pressure on the tongue with the spoon or fork. If the patient is suffering from one sided paralysis, the food and drinking straw must be placed in the non-paralyzed side of the mouth. The patient must be allowed to help herself or himself as much as possible. If the patient begins to choke, help her or him sit up straight. Do not give food or water while the patient is choking. The patient's mouth should be wiped as needed.

Foods should be served at the proper temperature. Hot foods should be served on hot plates, protected with a cover, and cold foods should be served on chilled dishes.

A final check of the tray should establish that it fully meets the requirements of the diet order and that the patient's preferences have been implemented.

CONCEPT OF ALL ENCOMPASSING OR COMPREHENSIVE CARE

The provision of all necessary health services so that the patient can maintain or be restored to independent living is implied in the term comprehensive care. The components of comprehensive health care include screening, assessment, intervention, and follow-up. Careful evaluation and re-evaluation of the client's physical, psychologic, economic, and social needs are required so that referral is made to the appropriate personnel in essential services. The services may be provided on an in-patient basis, including hospital care for the acutely ill, a minimum care facility within a hospital, or convalescent care in a nursing home.

An important part of patient care involves adequate planning for the patient's discharge. Here the social worker shares information with the occupational therapist, nurse, physician and dietitian.

It is estimated that the majority of people with age 85 years and over have at least one chronic disease such as arthritis, osteoporosis, diabetes mellitus, cardiovascular disease, or mental disorder. These conditions affect their attitudes, physical activities, appetites and, thus, nutritional status. PCM is a major problem for this population.

Anaemia can develop if the patient has too little animal protein in the diet. It can contribute to confusion and depression, but may go unnoticed because one of its major symptoms, fatigue, may be simply thought to be a characteristic of old age. It is helpful to make sure there is sufficient animal protein food and vitamin C (an iron enhancer) in the patient's diet.

Decubitus ulcers (bedsores) can develop in bedridden patients. They develop in areas where there is unrelieved pressure on the skin so the blood cannot bring nutrients and oxygen and remove wastes. Healing requires treatment of the ulcer, relief of the pressure, and high energy diet with sufficient protein.

Constipation can be caused by inadequate fiber, fluid or exercise, by medication, reduced peristalsis, or former abuse of laxatives. It can be relieved by increased fluid, fiber and exercise (if possible).

Diarrhea can be caused by lack of muscle tone in the colon. It will reduce the absorption of nutrients and can contribute to dehydration. A high-kcal/high protein diet combined with supplemental vitamins and minerals may be helpful.

The sense of smell declines with age and diminishes the appetite. A reduced sense of taste can be caused by medications, disease, mineral deficiencies, or xerostomia (dry mouth). The addition of spices, herbs, salt and sugar (if allowed) can be helpful. The inadequate amount of saliva in these patients contributes to increased tooth decay.

Dysphagia (difficulty in swallowing) can result from a stroke or develop in patients with Alzheimer's disease. They may be able to take food as liquid through a bottle with a nipple or possibly as a slightly thickened liquid.

ENTERAL AND PARENTERAL NUTRITION

Enteral Nutrition

The term enteral nutrition means the forms of feeding that bring nutrients directly into the digestive tract. Oral feeding is the usual method and should be used whenever possible. When patients cannot or will not take food by mouth, but their gastrointestinal tract is working, they will be given tube feedings. Sometimes this may be necessary because of unconsciousness, surgery, stroke, severe malnutrition, or extensive burns.

Mechanical difficulties that make chewing and swallowing impossible or an intestinal disease that cannot make the patient digest or absorb food sufficiently also necessitate tube feeding.

Usually, for periods that don't exceed three or four weeks, tube feeding is administered through a nasogastric tube inserted through the nose and into the stomach or small intestine. When the tube cannot be placed in the nose or when tube feeding will be required for more than four weeks, an opening called an ostomy is surgically created into the esophagus (an esophagostomy), the stomach (gastrostomy), or the intestine (jejunostomy).

The tubes used for these formulas are available, with varying types and amounts of nutrients. Those patients able to digest and absorb nutrients can be given intact formulas containing proteins, carbohydrates, and fats that require digestion. Patients that have limited ability to digest or absorb nutrients may be given elemental or hydrolyzed formulas that contain the products of digestion of proteins, carbohydrates and fats. Modular formulas can be used as supplements to other formulas, or for developing customized formulas for certain patients.

Tube feedings usually are administered by the continuous infusion method with or without a pump. This means the feeding is continuous during a 16 to 24 hours period. Initially, it is usually diluted by half and given at a rate of from 30 to 50 ml per hour. This rate may be increased by about 25 ml every 8 to 24 hours until the desired amount is attained. The strength of the formula also is gradually increased until it reaches full strength.

When patients are ready to return to oral feedings, the transfer must be done gradually.

Problems Associated with Tube Feeding

The osmolality of a liquid substance means the number of particles per kg of solution. Solutions with more particles (high osmolality) exert more pressure than solutions with fewer particles. Solutions with high osmolality attract water from nearby fluids that contain lower osmolality. When a formula with high osmolality reaches the intestine, the body may draw fluid from the blood to dilute the formula. This can cause weakness and diarrhoea in the patient.

Aspiration can occur (some of the formula enters the lung), causing the patient to develop pneumonia. The tube may become clogged, or the patient may pull the tube out.

Obviously, patients requiring tube feeding need a great deal of patience and understanding. They have been deprived of a basic pleasure of life—eating. They may also be fearful, uncomfortable, and apprehensive about the tube.

Parenteral Nutrition

Parenteral nutrition is the provision of nutrients intravenously. It is used if the gastrointestinal tract is not functional or if normal feeding is not adequate for the patient's needs. It can be used alone or as part of a dietary plan that includes oral or tube feeding as well. When parenteral nutrition is used to provide total nutrition, it is called TPN for total parenteral nutrition.

Nutrient solutions are prescribed by the physician and nutrition specialist and are prepared by a pharmacist. They can be administered via a central vein or, for a period of two weeks or less, a peripheral (near the surface) vein. Typically, dextrose/amino acid solution and a separate fat emulsion are given. These two solutions are not combined until just before their entry into the vein because they don't form a stable solution together.

If patients require TPN for extended periods, it is provided via a central vein. When this is done, a catheter is surgically inserted, under sterile conditions, by a physician. It is inserted into the jugular or subclavian vein and then into the superior vena cava. The vena cava is used because the blood flow is high there. This facilitates the quick dilution of the highly concentrated TPN solution. This reduces the possibility of phlebitis (inflammation of a vein) or thrombosis (blood clot).

When parenteral nutrition is no longer necessary, the patient must be transferred gradually to an oral diet. Sometimes, patients can be given tube feeding before oral feeding as they are weaned from TPN.

Possible Complications Associated with Parenteral Nutrition

Infection can occur at the site of the catheter and enter the bloodstream, causing an infection of the blood called sepsis. Bacterial or fungal infections can develop in the solution if it is unrefrigerated for over 12 hours. Abnormal electrolyte levels may develop, as can phlebitis or blood clots. Careful monitoring of the patient is essential.

STUDY QUESTIONS

1. How does the behaviour and attitude of the attending person affect a patient's appetite? Explain.
2. How does long bed ridden illness affect the patient's nutrition? Explain.
3. Why should the patient be encouraged to feed herself or himself? Explain.
4. Discuss the importance of proper preparation of the patient as well as the room inhabitating him, before a meal.
5. Write a meaningful note on patient-expert group interpersonal relationship.
6. Explain the purpose of modified diets.
7. Explain the enteral and parenteral nutrition. Discuss their advantages and limitations.

CHAPTER 22

Underpinnings of Diet Therapy

Chapter Outlines

- An introduction to diet therapy
- Considerations for the appropriateness of the prescription diet
- Caloric and other requirements
- Study questions

AN INTRODUCTION TO DIET THERAPY

Despite the fact that the practitioners of modern medicine understand the scientific basis of dietary therapy, it is ironical that patients are generally not given adequate advice as to what to eat and what not to eat during the period of illness. It appears, there is so much dependence on drugs that the simpler, and yet very beneficial, approach of diet therapy is being ignored by the modern healers. It is high time that we reminded them of the advice of Sir William Osler, that if all the drugs were thrown into the sea, it will leave all the fish dead in the sea. This may be a strong statement against the use of modern drugs, but the fact remains that drugs alone don't cure disease. A proper diet is essential for the prevention and treatment of several diseases.

Diet therapy is based on rational and scientific approach. However, it is sad that most of the advice about food is influenced by a number of taboos and traditions, resulting in harmful effects on the patients. Some foods should not be taken after sunrise and others must be avoided after sunset. Scientific explanations lack for such recommendations. Often a serious condition is precipitated by withholding food for a long time by treating patients to starvation or semi-starvation diets. It is quite common that if a patient has diarrhoea or fever, only some local fluid diets of very low calorie values are permitted. In fact, near epidemics of marasmus and kwashiorkor have been precipitated by practising such measures for children with mild to moderate protein-calorie malnutrition and associated gastrointestinal or pulmonary infection.

Food provides us essential nutrients for growth, development, and functions of the different organs. A balanced diet has been recommended in reference to our physiological needs. This diet is to be modified to fulfil the special needs of sick persons, e.g., a child in stages of marasmus or kwashiorkor due to protein calorie malnutrition needs high calorie and high protein food, specially made so as to be digested, absorbed and assimilated. An elderly, obese, diabetic person is recommended low calorie and restricted carbohydrate diet for obvious reasons. Nutrient requirements and metabolic functions of sick persons are altered and, therefore, dietary therapy is planned in reference to the pathophysiology of the disease. The main objectives of this therapeutic measure are: (a) to provide for all nutrient requirements of the patients, which may be more or less than their recommended daily allowance, (b) to correct the metabolic alterations due to the functional abnormalities of different organs as a consequence of the disease process, and (c) to stimulate the recovery of the diseased organs. The nutrients can be provided by any of the following methods:

(a) Normal methods of oral feedings;

(b) Intragastric feeding with the help of Ryle's or Levine's stomach tubes (enteral nutrition);

(c) Intravenous feeding also known as hyperalimentation (parenteral nutrition).

CONSIDERATIONS FOR THE APPROPRIATENESS OF THE PRESCRIPTION DIET

Economic Considerations

The economic status of the patient is an important practical consideration in formulating a diet prescription. During an acute illness or convalescence, a few expensive items may be permissible, but for more prolonged or chronic illnesses, foods must be within means of the patient.

Cultural Considerations

Whether the patient is vegetarian or not must be known. If vegetarian, then the 'degree' of vegetarianism should be assessed; for instance, vegans don't eat even eggs or dairy products 'ovo vegetarians' eat eggs and fish but not animal flesh; and 'home vegetarians' are vegetarians at home, for family reasons, but relish meat or chicken at a restaurant or party.

Physiological Considerations

Many people cannot tolerate all foods; especially milk, pulses, spices, egg, meat, fish and prawn. Milk produces diarrhoea in some and constipation in others; those with colonic disorders are likely to get flatulence with pulses. Such foods should be restricted or excluded as and when necessary.

Depending on the disease, certain foods may have to be excluded. In peptic ulcer and gastritis, spices and chillies are not permitted. For a patient confined to bed, fried foods and pulses are best avoided as they produce flatulence.

Allergy: Hypersensitivity to food causes urticaria, abdominal cramps, or bleeding. The common allergens are fish and eggs, and need to be excluded.

CALORIC AND OTHER REQUIREMENTS

A person confined to bed tends to consume less calories than a person undergoing physical exertion as bed rest decreases appetite. For an average adult confined to bed, about 1500 kcal may be adequate. Fever increases the caloric needs considerably.

A diet high in calories is indicated for undernourished or convalescent patients. They are advised to take more cereals, butter and oils at the main meals, and snacks of milk, sandwiches or biscuits at mid morning, mid evening and at bed time.

A low calorie diet is indicated for all obese patients. A diet consisting of vegetables, fruits, egg, meat, fish, chicken, and skimmed milk, with a low intake of cereals provides bulk satiety, adequate proteins, and relatively few calories. Avoiding fat reduces weight.

Energy and Protein

Total intake of proteins is usually adequate in a standard non-vegetarian diet. For vegetarians, the important sources of proteins are milk, cereals and pulses. In diseases of the colon, whole milk usually produces diarrhoea while pulses produce flatulence. The protein requirements of vegetarians with colonic diseases can only be met by providing commercial protein foods, or by supplying skimmed milk powder which is usually more easily digested than fresh milk.

Cirrhosis, Nephrotic Syndrome, Pregnancy and Lactation

A high protein diet is prescribed to patients with low serum albumin, as in liver cirrhosis without liver failure and in nephrotic syndrome. It is also advisable to increase the protein intake during pregnancy and lactation. For a non-vegetarian, this can be done by increasing the quantity of meat, chicken, fish or egg. For the vegetarian, extra skimmed milk, cottage cheese and all pulses are advised. All pulses and groundnut are relatively inexpensive and palatable protein-rich foods.

Fat

Fats are a rich source of calories. Fats are not as indispensable as proteins, though prolonged deficiency of essential fatty acids leads to skin changes. A high calorie diet should contain fatty foods like butter, ghee and oil, and fats should be liberally used in cooking. A low calorie diet contains little fat.

Carbohydrate

Carbohydrate provides bulk, and together with fat, forms the chief source of calories. If a high calorie diet is to be prescribed, carbohydrates in the form of chapattis (of wheat or other cereals), bread and biscuits provide comparatively inexpensive nourishing foods. For a low calorie diet, they are used sparingly.

Vitamin Requirement

The best sources of vitamins are whole grain cereals, fruits, liver and yeast. Vitamin A is derived from egg, milk and butter, while carrots and green vegetables provide pro-vitamin A, into the form of carotene. Vitamin B-complex is derived from unrefined cereals and flesh foods. The best sources of vitamin C are fresh fruits, vegetables, and germinating cereals. Vitamin D can be easily converted from skin sterol by exposure of skin to the sun for about half an hour.

Mineral Requirement

Calcium is available from milk. The usual diet is normal in phosphorous. Iron is available from cereals, liver, kidney and egg. Sodium is easily provided by common salt added to food. A low-sodium diet may have to be prescribed during fluid retention, as in ascites, cardiac failure, or the nephrotic syndrome. The potassium intake can be increased with vegetables and fruits. A low potassium intake is advisable for patients with kidney failure.

Fluid Requirement

Inadequate fluid intake can lead to constipation. Fluid intake should be liberal enough to ensure the passage of 1.0 to 1.5 litre of urine per day.

Fluids need to be restricted when excretion is impaired, as in acute nephritis and kidney failure. The water requirement per day is then calculated as : 1000 ml a day to replace the insensible loss in respiration and perspiration, plus the volume of urine passed during the previous 24 hours.

Combination of Foods

The food combinations in a diet may improve or impair the quality of its constituents. A combination of cereals with milk provides amino acids which improve the quality of proteins. At the same time, the phytic acid in cereals decreases the amount of calcium or iron absorbed.

Thus, a general guidance suffices in formulating a diet. A diet prescription should be a blend of nutritional knowledge and common sense.

Diet prescription should express cooked foods in terms of serving measures. The food values given below are rounded off for simplicity.

Breakfast

Some of the following items are usually taken at breakfast:

- Toast, chapattis, paratha.
- Butter and jam.
- Cereals.
- Boiled eggs or omelette.
- Fruit.
- Tea, coffee or milk.

Bread or Chapattis

The amount of bread, paratha or chapattis prescribed varies according to the calories required and the economic status of the patient. Chapattis prepared from any cereal or millet supply 100 kcal for every 30 g flour used.

One medium slice of bread, or two thin wheat chapattis, or one chapatti of millet like bajra or jowar, supply about 80 kcal and 3 g protein.

Bajra and Jam

The quantity advised varies according to the calories required. One teaspoon of butter provides 30 kcal. A level teaspoon of jam provides 30 kcal.

Cereals

Cereals may be taken cooked in the form of dalia porridge, cornflakes, puffed rice and semolina. They are served with milk and sweetening agents such as sugar or honey, which increases the calorie intake. The usual helping of breakfast cereals provides about 100 kcal with 3.5 g protein. Milk and sugar provide additional calories.

Eggs

Eggs are served half boiled or poached; if more calories are required, fried eggs or eggs scrambled in fat are prescribed. An average hen's egg provides 50 kcal and about 4 g of protein.

Fruit

Fruit like orange, apple or banana may be available according to season. One average helping of fruits provides 50 kcal.

Tea or Coffee

One cup of tea or coffee with two tablespoons of milk and one teaspoon of sugar provides 50 kcal. Sugar, honey or jaggery is advised according to taste.

Lunch and Dinner

The prescription for lunch or dinner is selected from the following items, according to the dietary habit:

- Soup.
- Bread or chapattis.
- Rice.
- Curry.
- Pulses.
- Vegetable salad.

- Cooked vegetables, including potatoes.
- Milk or curd.
- Meat, fish or chicken.
- Fruit.
- Dessert.

Soup

A small quantity of thin soup may increase the appetite; a large helping just before meals decreases the appetite for other foods. However, the same and may become desirable in a low calorie diet. Thin soups are rich in minerals and vitamins. Thick soup prepared with the addition of cream, potatoes, peas or nuts has a high calorie value.

One cup of thin chicken vegetable soup provides 35 kcal.

Rice

The quantity of rice prescribed varies according to the dietary habit. Some eat it by the plateful as a main dish. A bowl (150 ml) of cooked rice provides 100 kcal.

Curry

Curry is made with spices and coconut with the addition of vegetable, meat, fish or egg. Curry is forbidden in digestive disorders because it is usually spiced.

Four tablespoons of curry provide 80-90 kcal.

Pulses

These are more difficult to digest than other foods. They form a rich source of protein and should form part of the meal for vegetarians; they are served as liquid (thin dal) or semisolid (thick dal). Dal water (ossaman), the supernatant water obtained after cooking dal, is taken by many as soup.

One cup of thin dal or half a cup of thick dal provides 100 kcal and 7 g protein.

Raw Vegetables

Raw vegetables are prescribed in large quantities if the aim is a low calorie intake. In a high calorie diet the quantity of salad is reduced. The usual salad vegetables–cucumber, radish, lettuce, tomato, carrots and shredded cabbage–are prescribed as available in season. Raw vegetables in large quantities are not well digested, and produce flatulence.

Cooked Vegetables

One or two cooked vegetables are prescribed with each meal. The usual helping of a vegetable is 100 g. Of the variety of vegetables available is 100 g. Of the variety of vegetables available—bitter gourd (karela), brinjal (egg plant), cabbage, cauliflower, carrots, French beans, ridge gourd (turya), lady's finger (okra), pumpkin, papri, spinach, tinda, yellow pumpkin—the ones in season are advised.

A single good helping of vegetable salad or cooked vegetables provide 100 kcal mainly as carbohydrate. Potatoes are served in many ways; mashed, baked, boiled, or fried as chips or wafers. The quantity may be increased or decreased, depending on the calories required.

One medium potato weighing 100 g provides 100 kcal with 20 g carbohydrate.

Milk, Butter Milk, Curd, Yoghurt

These are important for a vegetarian, mainly because of their protein content of high biological value. The calorie content of milk products is calculated from the original quantity of milk used for their preparation. If a low calorie diet is needed, skimmed milk is advised.

Small cup of whole cow's milk, or half a cup of whole buffalo's milk, provides 100 kcal with 7 g protein. A cup of skimmed buffalo's milk provides 90 kcal with 9 g protein.

Meat, Fish or Chicken

The edible portion of an average helping weighs about 100 g. Meat or chicken may be boiled, grilled, roasted, or minced and fried into cutlets.

One average helping of 100 g provides 100 kcal with 20 g protein.

Fruits

Fruits are prescribed according to season; they provide 50-100 kcal.

Dessert

Custard and pudding are made in various ways and flavours, usually from milk and sugar with eggs.

Ice cream provides 150-200 kcal.

Fat in Cooking

The daily amount of fat recommended for cooking depends on the caloric requirement.

One teaspoon of fat (10-12 g) such as butter, ghee or oil provides 90-120 kcal.

Snacks and Dry Fruits

Snacks include sandwiches, biscuits, cakes, samosa and kachori. They are prescribed with tea; as substitutes for a main meal when a regular cooked meal is not feasible; or between the principal meals, to increase the consumption of calories.

Fluids

A liberal intake of water—about 7-10 glasses daily—is advised unless otherwise indicated.

Fine Tuning to Give the Final Finish

After the menu making in household measures, its calorie equivalent and content of proteins, fats and carbohydrates are compared with the recommended intake. The calories are increased or decreased by varying the quantity of bread or chapattis, or fat used for cooking. If the protein intake is not adequate, the quantity of milk, skimmed milk powder, pulses (dal) wheat or fish is increased. The carbohydrate intake can be varied by adjusting the intake of cereals as bread or chapattis. As long as enough calories and proteins are provided, fats and carbohydrates are interchangeable.

STUDY QUESTIONS

1. Discuss the considerations that have to be undertaken while prescribing diets to the patients.
2. Explain why diet therapy becomes ineffective if we depart from rational and scientific approach.
3. What are the main objectives of diet therapy?

CHAPTER 23

Some Therapeutic Diets

Chapter Outlines

- Normal diet
- Therapeutic diet
- General diet
- Modified diet
- Study questions

NORMAL DIET

Diet-health relationship is cardinal. Because of essentiality of food for survival, human beings had the inherent belief since early times, that the amount and kind of food they eat, somehow influences their well-being. Whereas a balanced diet brings optimum nutrition, dietary imbalances cause malnutrition, which in turn permit and promote disease and dysfunction.

"Normal diet", the term refers to the diet which provides all the nutrients to the body that are necessary for growth, maintenance and optimum functioning of organ systems in right quantities and proportions in relation to each other.

THERAPEUTIC DIET

Therapeutic diets are mostly adaptations of the normal diet and are planned in such a way that they maintain and/or restore good nutrition in any given situation or ailment.

The normal diet may be subjected to the following modifications:

1. A change in consistency mostly in fluid and soft diets.
2. A change in the caloric content.
3. A variation in the amounts of one or more nutrients, for example high or low protein, low sodium diets.
4. A variation in the fiber content of diet.
5. Inclusion of foods bland in taste.
6. Addition or exclusion of specific foods as in allergic conditions.
7. Increase or decrease the time interval between feeding.

When the normal diet is used as the basis for planning therapeutic diets, it is easy to see what the effects of omissions or additions of specific foods may have on the nutritive value, for example, if an individual with lactose intolerance is also allergic to milk, it becomes immediately apparent that some other means must be sought to provide proteins, calcium and riboflavin.

The use of the normal diet as a basis for planning therapeutic diets is of immense psychological importance. When as much of the normal diet is retained as possible, the patient does not feel segregated from its family and friends.

Objectives of a Therapeutic Diet

The objectives of planning therapeutic diets are:

1. To give a diet in keeping with the ability of the body to metabolize certain food constituents, e.g., as in diabetes mellitus.
2. To give relief to a particular organ, for instance, fat content is reduced in diseases of the gallbladder.
3. To increase or disease body weight by the addition or restriction of calories.
4. To treat chronic malnutrition giving high protein diet.
5. To treat or to prevent oedema by restricting salt, as in cardiac and renal disease.

6. To make digestion easier by exclusion or removal of irritating substances or those which delay the emptying time of the stomach such as fiber, condiments and fried food as in certain diseases of gastrointestinal tract.

Principles of Therapeutic Diets

The principles that govern the planning of therapeutic diets are:

- The factors of height, age, gender, body weight and activity of patient.
- The nutrients amounts required for normal body needs and the foods that are the principal sources of these food constituents.
- The diet should be well balanced with respect to macro and micronutrients (carbohydrates, protein, fat, vitamins and minerals).
- Physiology and pathology of the body tissue or part affected and relationship to food metabolism and utilization.

Two types of diets are provided to the patients who come to the hospital.

Diets in the hospitals	
General diet	Modified consistency (soft or liquid diets)
• Full diet	Modified energy value (high or low calorie diet)
• Half diet	Modified nutrients (high protein/low sodium/low fat diet)
	Modified bulk (high or low fiber diet)
	Modified flavour (bland diet)
	Modified food content (elimination diet; diet in food allergy)
	Modified feeding interval (six and seven meals; peptic ulcer diet)

GENERAL DIET

1. **Full Diet:** This is a normal diet which provides all the nutrients in slightly higher amounts then recommended for a healthy sedentary worker. It can be used for an adult patient admitted to a hospital who does not need any dietary modification. This is also known as regular or general diet. This is well-balanced and nutritious diet.
2. **Half diet:** This diet provides the nutrients required for children upto the age of 10 years.

MODIFIED DIET

Following modified diets are provided in the hospital.

1. **Soft Diet:** This diet is soft in texture and consists of liquids and semi-solid foods. It is an intermediate step between the full and liquid diets. It is indicated in certain postoperative cases, in acute infections, in some gastrointestinal conditions and cardiac diseases etc. it is low in residue and is readily digested. Little or no spices and condiments are used in the preparation. Well-known examples of soft diets are khichri diet and milk and bread diets.
2. **Fluid Diet:** This diet is used when the patient is unable to tolerate solid food. The nutritional adequacy will depend upon the type of food given to the patients when they are actually ill, and have marked intolerance to food, nausea, vomiting, anorexia, distension, diarrhea etc. It consists of clear fluid only, i.e., light tea without milk, clear soups, carbonated beverages, glucose, electrolyte solution, cereal water, strained fruit juices. The diet is nutritionally inadequate and is used for short period of one or two days. The main aim is to maintain the fluid and electrolyte balance. This diet is not complete diet nutritionally.

   Full fluid diet on the other hand is a liquid diet which is nutritionally adequate if planned properly and can be as near to a normal diet as possible. Indicated for those patients who can't chew, swallow or tolerate solid foods.
3. **Bland Diet:** It is a diet which is non-irritating, chemically bland and inhibits gastric secretion. It can be used for patients with gastrointestinal irritation. This can be brought about with slight changes and reduction in fibre and fat content. It can also be used for various gastrointestinal diseases like diarrhea and ulcerative colitis.
4. **High Calorie Diet:** This is normal diet supplemented with high calorie foods in the form of concentrated carbohydrates or fats so that the bulk of the diet is not much increased. It is used in patients with fevers, convalescence after prolonged illness, leanness and hyperthyroidism etc.
5. **Low Calorie Diet:** It provides less calories than the total energy requirements for the day. It is used in obese patients with hypertension and obesity. Foods like concentrated sweets, fried foods, dry fruits and nuts, alcoholic drinks, cream and excess of fat in the diet should be avoided.

6. **Low Protein Diet:** It is used for patients with acute and chronic renal failures and also in hepatic encephalopathy patients.
7. **Low Fat Diet:** It is a normal diet modified to reduce fat content to approximately 30 g per day.
8. **Low Cholesterol Diet:** This diet is used for the treatment of patients with high cholesterol level and patients with coronary heart disease. The high cholesterol sources in the food like egg yolk, liver, red meat should be reduced in which the ratio of polyunsaturated, monounsaturated and saturated fatty acids should be 1:1:1. In general, ghee and oil should be used in 1:1 proportion.
9. **Low Sodium Diet:** This is normal diet with low sodium content and is used in conditions where there is hypernatremia as in oedema, nephritis, congestive heart failure etc. It can be salt free diet or moderate salt restricted diet and accordingly 1-5 g of salt may be allowed.
10. **Diabetic Diet:** The main purpose of the diet is to bring the blood sugar levels to as normal as possible and this is brought about by giving a balanced diet providing 60-65% of total calories from carbohydrates, 20-25% of total calories from fats and rest from proteins. More emphasis is on complex carbohydrates, high in fibre and avoiding refined carbohydrates source. In addition pure sugars should be avoided.

It is pertinent to mention the details of the menu planning of some diets provided to the patients in the following sections:

Full diet — **Sample diet**

Foodstuff	*Vegetarian* g.	*Non-vegetarian* g.
Cereal	400	400
Pulses	70	50
Green leafy vegetables	50	50
Other vegetables	100	100
Roots and tubers	100	100
Fruits	100	100
Milk	400	200
Flesh foods	–	100
Sugar	20	20
Oil (for cooking)	20	20

Energy and other nutrients provided by full diet

Calories	2450 kcal
Proteins	77 g.
Calcium	1.1 g
Iron	43 mg
Retinol	800 μg
Thiamin	9 mg
Riboflavin	1.4 mg

Cooked Measures: Non-vegetarians can include:

1. Eggs two or mutton or fish curry 1 katori.
2. Use 3 tbsp. of extra oil to cook and cut down 1cup of milk and dhal for one meal.

This is a normal diet, which is modified from the balanced diet recommended by ICMR. It provides all the nutrients in slightly higher amounts than recommended for a healthy male sedentary worker. It can be used for an adult patient (male or female) admitted in a hospital, which does not need any dietary modification.

This is also known as general or regular diet.

Principle: The following foods should be avoided while formulating the diet:

1. All bran, coarse cereals.
2. Too much of spices and condiments.
3. Fried foods.

Half Diet: This diet provides the nutrients required for children, upto the age of 10 years. It is a normal diet which is modified from the balanced diet recommended for children by ICMR. It can be used for children who do not need any specific diet. This is also known as children's diet.

Principle: The following foods should be avoided while formulating the diet:

1. All bran, coarse cereals.
2. Too much of spices and condiments.
3. Fried foods.

Sample diet

Foodstuff	*Vegetarian* g.	*Non-vegetarian* g.
Cereals	225	225
Pulses	60	40
Green leafy vegetables	25	25
Other vegetables	75	75
Roots and tubers	75	75
Fruits	100	100
Milk	400	200
Meat/fish/egg	–	50
Sugar	30	30
Oil (for cooking)	20	25

Distribution (in different meals)					
		South India	East India	West India	North India
Early morning breakfast	Tea	–	1 cup	–	1 cup
	Coffee	1 cup	–	1 cup	–
	Bread	–	6 slices	–	6 slices
	Butter	–	1 tbsp.	–	1 tbsp.
	Idli	4	–	4	–
	Chutney	2 tbsp.	–	2 tbsp.	–
	Milk	1 cup	1 cup	1 cup	1 cup
Lunch	Rice	4 K	2 K	–	4 K
	Chapatti	–	3	5	–
	Dal	–	1¾ K	¾ K	1½ K
	Sambar	1 K	–	–	–
	Green leafy vegetable with	¾ K	1 K	1 K	1 K
	tomato salad	1	1	1	1
	Tomato	1 K	½ K	1 K	½ K
	Curd	1	1	1	1
	Orange	4 K	2 K	–	4 K
Dinner	Rice	–	–	–	4 K
	Chapatti	–	1¾ K	¾ K	1½ K
	Dal	–	–	–	1
	Sambar	¾ K	1 K	1 K	1 K
	Rasam				
	vegetable with onions curd	½ K	–	½ K	–

This diet provides	
Calories	1800 kcal
Proteins	55 g
Calcium	972 mg
Iron	26 mg
Retinol	520 µg
Thiamin	1.3 mg
Riboflavin	1.1 mg

Distribution of the diet can be done as for full diet.

Soft Diet I–Khichri Diet: It is a soft diet which provides most of the nutrients required by a male adult. It is slightly deficient in iron, calories and riboflavin. It is a transitional diet between the liquid diet and full diet. The same diet for an adult female can be formulated by affecting appropriate reductions in keeping with reduced body weight.

Sample diet	
Foodstuff	*Amounts*
Rice	200
Green gram dal or lentil dal	70
Calabash cucumber	100
Potatoes and onions	100
Orange of sweet lime	200
Milk	400
Egg	2
Paneer or cheese	50
Sugar	30
Oil (for cooking)	20

This diet provides	
Calories	2000 kcal
Proteins	64 g
Calcium.	890 mg
Iron	19.5 mg
Retinol	785 µg
Thiamin	1.4 mg
Riboflavin	1.1 mg

Soft Diet II—Milk and Bread Diet: This is also soft diet which provides all nutrients except calories, iron and thiamin in the amounts required for an adult man. It is also a transitional diet between the liquid and full diet. It can be used for the patients who do not like khichri diet. (To formulate the same diet for adult female, make appropriate reductions in keeping with reduced body weight).

Sample diet

Foodstuff	*Amounts*
Milk	1000 ml
Bread	100
Potato	200
Banana	200
Egg	2
Paneer or cheese	50
Sugar	50
Butter	30

This diet provides	
Milk	1000 ml
Calories	2000 kcal
Protein	62 g
Calcium	1810 mg
Iron	8.4 mg
Retinol	1504 µg
Thiamin	101 mg
Riboflavin	1.7 mg

Liquid Diet: This diet is designed to give oral nourishment in the liquid form. It can be used for the patients who cannot tolerate or consume solid or semi-solid foods. Since this diet does not provide enough nutrients it should not be continued for more than necessary time.

Sample diet

Foodstuff	*Amounts*
Milk	1000 ml
Fruit juice	1000 ml
Egg	2
Sugar	50 g

This diet provides	
Calories	1400 Kcal
Protein	52 g
Calcium	1760 mg
Iron	11.1 mg
Retinol	1100 mg
Thiamin	1.4 mg
Riboflavin	1.8 mg

Bland Diet: A bland diet is a diet which is non-irritating chemically and mechanically and which inhibits gastric secretion. It can be used for gastric and duodenal ulcer patients after acute symptoms have subsided. With slight changes and reduction in fiber and fat content it can also be used for diarrhea and ulcerative colitis.

Principle: The following foods should be avoided while formulating the diet:

1. All bran, coarse cereals.
2. Skin and seeds of fruits.
3. Raw vegetables.
4. Vegetables like cabbage, beans, ladies fingers and bitter gourd etc.
5. Spices and condiments.
6. Fried foods.
7. Strong beverages.
8. Pickles, chutneys etc.
9. Tender coconut water.
10. Chocolates, puddings and similar preparations.
11. Meat extracts and soups.

Sample diet: Vegetarian	
Foodstuff	*g*
Rice	100
White bread	40
Pulses	40
Potatoes	75
Vegetables	100
Milk	1000 ml
Curd	300
Skimmed milk powder	15
Orange juice	150
Banana	50
Sugar	25
Butter	7
Ghee or oil	125

Note: Ovo-vegetarian can take a half-boiled egg instead of skimmed milk powder.

* This amount can be used for cooking purposes.

This diet provides	
Calories	2000 kcal
Protein	75 g
Fat	90 g
Carbohydrates	220 g

Distribution			
Cooked measures		*Cooked measures*	
7 A.M		1 P.M.	
Milk	1 glass	Soft boiled rice	2 bowls
Sugar	1 tsp	Sieved cauliflower and carrots	1½ bowls
Half boiled egg	1	Curd	1 bowl
Skimmed milk Powder to be Mixed with milk	3 tsp	Sieved green gram dal (dehusked)	¼ bowl
10 A.M.		4 P.M.	
Toast	2	Milk	1 glass
Butter	1 tsp	Sugar	1 tsp
Milk	1 glass	Biscuits	2
Sugar	1 tsp	Banana	half
7 P.M.		10 P.M.	
Soft boiled rice	2 bowls	Milk	1 glass
Sieved lentil dal	¼ bowl	Sugar	1 tsp
Mashed potato	½ bowl		
Curd	1 bowl		
Sieved orange juice	½ bowl		

High Calorie Diet: This is a normal diet supplemented with high calorie foods so that the bulk of the diet is not much increased. It can be used for fever, convalescence after prolonged illness, leanness and hyperthyroidism.

Principle: The following foods should be avoided if the patient is convalescing or having fever:

1. Fried foods.
2. Dry fruits and nuts.

Sample diet		
	Vegetarian	*Non-vegetarian*
Foodstuff	*Weight of raw ingredient (g)*	
Cereal	250	300
Pulse	100	50
Root and tubers	50	75
Other vegetables	50	50
Green leafy vegetables	100	100
Bread	60	60
Butter	10	20
Milk	750	300
Curd	100 ml	–
Sugar	50	50
Ghee or oil	30	30
Banana	150	250
Egg	–	1
Meat or fish	–	100

This diet provides	
Calories	2700 kcal
Protein	80 g
Fat	70 g

Low Calorie Diet: The diet provides less calories than the total energy requirements of the day; thus paving the way for depletion of body fat. It is used in cases of obesity, cardiac disturbances and hypertension in over-weight individuals.

Principle: The following foods should be avoided while formulating the diet:

1. Sweets, chocolates, jaggery, jam, honey, preserves, puddings, cakes etc.
2. Roots and tubers.
3. Fried foods.
4. Dried fruits and nuts.
5. Alcoholic drinks and soft drink unless they contain artificial sweetening agents instead of sugar.
6. Cream and free fats.
7. Fruits like banana, custard-apple dates etc.

Sample diet		
	Vegetarian	*Non-vegetarian*
Foodstuff	*Weight of raw ingredient (g)*	
Wheat flour	60	60
Rice	30	60
Other vegetables	200	200
Green leafy vegetables	200	200
Pulse	70	50
Citrus fruit or tomato	200	200
Milk (cow's)	600 ml	250 ml
Skimmed milk powder	20	–
Ghee or oil	7	12
Egg	–	1
Meat or fish	–	50

This diet provides	
Calories	1200 kcal
Protein	60 g
Fat	30 g
Carbohydrates	170 g

Low Fat Diet: This is a normal diet modified to reduce the fat content to approximately 30 g per day. It may be used in treating diseases with intolerance to fat such as gallbladder, liver and pancreatic diseases or in conditions of steatorrhea.

Principle: The following foods should be avoided in such diets:

1. High fat foods like nuts, cheese etc.
2. Fried foods.
3. Free fat and cream etc.

Sample diet		
	Vegetarian	*Non-vegetarian*
Foodstuff	*Weight of raw ingredient (g)*	
Cereal	200	250
Pulse	100	75
Milk (cow's)	–	100
Skimmed milk powder	50	–
Curd	200	–
Other vegetables	100	100
Green leafy vegetables	100	100
Potato	50	50
Sugar	50	50
Banana	75	75
Orange	100	100
Ghee or oil	17	15
Egg	–	1
Meat or fish	–	100

This diet provides	
Calories	2100 kcal
Protein	75 g
Fat	30 g
Carbohydrates	385 g

Low Cholesterol and Reduced Saturated Fat Diet: This is a normal diet formulated with increased polysaturated fats. It is adequate in all nutrients. It can help in lowering plasma cholesterol. Calories and protein can be changed as per individual needs.

Principle: The following foods should be avoided while formulating the diet:

1. Butter, hydrogenated fat and lard.
2. Coconut and coconut oil.
3. Foods cooked with these fats.
4. Fatty meats, visible fat on meat sausages etc.
5. Whole milk and cream.
6. Cheese.
7. Organ meats like liver, kidney and brain etc.
8. Shrimp.
9. Eggs more than one or, at the most, two per week.

Sample diet	
Foodstuff	*Amounts (g)*
Cereal	300
Pulse	50
Green leafy vegetables	50
Other vegetables	100
Roots and tubers	100
Fruit	100
Skimmed milk	400
Sugar	30
Ghee or oil	30

This diet provides	
Calories	2400 Kcal
Protein	70 g
Fat	55 g
Carbohydrates	400 g

Low Sodium Diet: This is a normal diet with a low sodium content. These food preparations for this diet are cooked without extra salt and high sodium foods are avoided. This is designed for use in conditions where there is sodium retention like oedema, nephritis, cardiac diseases, toxemia of pregnancy and hypertension.

Principle: These foods should be avoided while formulating the diet.

1. Salt in cooking or on table.
2. Sea fish, salted meat and salted dry fish, liver etc.
3. Salted butter and cheese.
4. All foods to which salt or baking soda has been added in cooking.
5. Pickles and chutneys.

Sample diet

Foodstuff	*Vegetarian*	*Non-vegetarian*
	Weight of raw ingredient (g)	
Rice	250	300
Dal	100	75
Other vegetable	200	200
Fruit	200	200
Milk (cow's)	600 ml	200 ml
Potato	100	125
Oil	30	30
Egg	–	1
Meat or fish	–	50
Sugar	30	50

This diet provides

Calories	200 kcal
Protein	70 g
Sodium	0.5 g

Diabetic Diet: This diet is as close to the normal diet as possible so as to meet the nutritional needs and the treatment of the individual patient. This diet is slightly low, but adequate in other food principles.

Sample diet

Foodstuff	*Vegetarian*	*Non-vegetarian*
	Weight of raw ingredient (g)	
Cereals	200	250
Pulse	60	20
Green leafy vegetables	200	200
Other vegetables	200	200
Fruit	200	200
Milk (dairy)	400 ml	200 ml
Oil	30	30
Fish	–	100

This diet provides

Calories	1600 kcal
Protein	65 g
Fat	40 g
Carbohydrates	245 g

Distribution

		Cooked measures	
		Vegetarian	*Non-vegetarian*
Breakfast	Coffee or tea	1 cup	1 cup
	Toast	2	2
	Butter	1 tsp	1 tsp
Lunch	Rice	2 K	2 K
	Sambar	1 K	1 K
	Green leafy veg.	1 K	½ K
	Curd	½ K	1 K
	Tomato	1	1
	Pickle	1 piece	1 piece
Evening	Tea	1 cup	1 cup
Dinner	Chapatti	3	4
	Dal	1 K	½ K
	Curd	½ K	1 K
	Other vegetable	1 K	1 K
	Fish/Chicken	–	1 K
	Roasted papad	1	1
	Tomato, cucumber	1	1
Before to bed	Milk	1 cup	1 cup

Principle: The following foods should be avoided in all diabetic diets:

1. Roots and tubers.
2. Sweets, pudding and chocolates.
3. Fried foods.
4. Dried foods.
5. Sugar.
6. Fruits like bananas, sapota, custard, apple etc.

Note: 5 tsp. of oil can be used in cooking.

Diet prescription in no less vital than drug prescription for a patient's recovery and convalescence. Likewise keeping a therapeutic diet schedule even for a brief period is no easy task and ask for a lot of patience and self-discipline on the part of the sick person, during illness nutritional requirements increase but appetite and inclination to eat decreases. Thus the patient's food should not only be catering to the requirements of his illness and physical condition but should also be relishable and enjoyable. It should be served in a soothing and congential environment.

STUDY QUESTIONS

1. What is the difference between a normal and therapeutic diet? What modifications a normal diet must undergo in order to acquire a specific therapeutic potential?
2. What are the objectives of therapeutic diets and what principles govern their planning?
3. Discuss different general and modified diets.

CHAPTER 24

Diet in Weight Management and PEM

Chapter Outlines

- Overweight and obesity
- Dietary management
- Surgical treatment of obesity
- Medicinal intervention in obesity
- Underweight
- Protein energy malnutrition
- Nutritional management of PEM
- Study questions

OVERWEIGHT AND OBESITY

Normal weight can be translated to read average, desired or standard. Normal weight is that which is appropriate for the maintenance of good health for a particular individual at a particular time or stage of life. Overweight is defined as weight 10 to 20 percent above average. Obesity is defined as excessive body fat, with weight 20 percent above average. Underweight is when the pendulum swings to the lower side or when the weight is 10 to 15 percent below average.

Body weight is composed of fluids, organs, fat, muscles, and bones so large variation exists among people. In addition to height, age, physical condition, heredity, sex, and general frame size (small, medium or large) are all critical factors in determining desired weight.

Some people can weigh more than normal and still be in good physical condition. Professional football players, because of the amount of muscle they develop, are examples of this. However, when they retire and reduce their physical activity and workouts, the same muscle can change to fat. If their weighs remain the same, they then will be considered over fat because the proportion of fat would become too high.

To measure body fat, a calliper is used. Because the fat under the skin on the stomach and the upper arm is representative of the percentage of overall body fat, it is usually measured when knowledge of the percentage of body fat is required. If it is more than/and 1/2 inches, one is considered overweight. If it is under ½ inch, one is considered underweight.

A moderate amount of fat is a necessary component of the body. It provides stored energy, protects organs from injury, and acts as insulation. The final determination of desirable weight depends on common sense with which one can strive for normal weight when one is overweight.

Overweight is a serious health hazard as it puts extra strain on the heart, lungs, mouth, bones and joints, and increases the susceptibility to diabetes mellitus and hypertension. It creates surgical risks, shortens the life causes psychological problems, and is associated with heart disease and some forms of cancers.

Causes

The most common cause of overweight is energy imbalance. People eat more than they need. Excess weight can accumulate during and after middle age because people reduce their activity and metabolism slows down with age. Consequently, weight accumulates unless energy intake is reduced. Hypothyroidism is a possible, but rare, cause of obesity. In this condition, the basal metabolic rate is lowered, thereby reducing the number of kcal needed for energy. Unless corrected, this can result in excess weight.

Although neither has been proven, there are two popular theories about weight loss: the fat cell theory and the set point theory.

According to the fat cell theory, obesity redevelops when the size decreases during a reducing diet. The individual is driven to eat or crave for more and eat more in order for the shrunken fat cells to regain their former size. Therefore, it is difficult to lose weight and keep it off.

According to the set point theory, everyone has a set point or natural weight at which the body is so comfortable that it does not allow for deviation. This is said to be the reason why some people cannot lose weight below a set point or why, if they do, they quickly regain to that set point.

DIETARY MANAGEMENT

Obviously, if the most common cause of overweight is overeating, the solution is to reduce one's food intake. This is seldom easy. To accomplish it, a weight reduction (low-energy) diet must be undertaken. For the diet to be effective, one must have a genuine desire to lose weight.

The simplest and, therefore, perhaps the best weight reduction diet is the normal diet based on the Food Guide Pyramid, but with the energy content controlled. If necessary, its consistency can also be adapted to meet individual needs by using a food processor or a blender.

The exchange lists provide another excellent method frequently used to healthfully control the kcal content of the diet. These lists were originally developed for the use of diabetic patients. They are organized to provide specific numbers of kcal and nutrients according to six lists.

A reduction of 3500 kcal will result in a weight loss of 500 g. Physicians frequently recommend that no more than 1000 g of weight be lost in one week. To accomplish this, one must reduce one's weekly kcal intake by 7,000 or daily intake by 1,000 kcal per day or the dieter will not receive the necessary nutrients. The diet should consist of 10-15 percent protein 55-65 percent carbohydrate and 20 percent fat, in other words, normal proportions of nutrients, but in reduced amounts. The number of meals and snacks each day should be determined by the dieter's needs and desires, but the total number of energy must not be exceeded.

There is no magic way of losing weight and maintaining the reduced weight, but there is a key to it. That key is revised eating habits. Infact, unless eating habits are truly revised, it is likely that the lost weight will be regained once the weight reduction has been accomplished because at that point the dieter may be euphoric about the weight loss and forget its cost. The cost of slimness is eating less than one might prefer.

A dietary scheme for the obese

Exchange	*No. of exchange*	*Protein*	*K calories*
Milk	2	16	340
Legumes and pulses	2	14	200
Veg. A	2	2	40
Veg. B	2	4	80
Fruits	2	–	80
Cereals	5	10	350
Fat	3	–	135
Sugar	10	–	40
Total		46	1265

Menu Plan

Breakfast	:	Milk 1 glass
		Milk with sugar
		Raw sandwich without butter
Lunch	:	Chapatti 2
		Thick dal 1 bowl
		Veg of bottleguard 1 bowl
		Curd 1 cup
		Fruit salad
Afternoon	:	Fruit
Dinner	:	Roti 2
		Dal 1 bowl
		Palak curry 1 bowl
		Curd 1 cup
		Vegetable salad

Food Selection

The dieter must learn to "eat lean". It is useful to learn the energy values of favourite foods, and to consider them before indulging. Energy counting is not necessary, however, if one learns the basic value of foods that are allowed on low kcal diets because of their low kcal values, it is beneficial.

Foods Allowed on a Low Kcal Diet

Skim milk, butter milk, low fat yogurt, cottage cheese and other skim milk cheeses, eggs, lamb, chicken, turkey, fish, all prepared using low fat cooking and clear soups.

Whole grain or enriched bread as allowed by doctor vegetables should be low in carbohydrate fresh fruits and those canned without sugar, coffee or tea, without milk and sugar salt, pepper, herbs, garlic and onions.

Foods to Avoid on a Low Calorie Diet

Cream soup	Nuts
Cream sauces	Jellies/jams
Cream in any form	Fatty meats
Gravies	Salad dressing
Rich desserts	Cakes
Sweet drinks/sodas	Cookies
Alcoholic beverages	Pastries
Candy	Oily fish
Fried foods	Whole milk

Substitution of foods with very low kcal contents should be made for those with high kcal contents whenever possible. The following are examples:

- Skim milk.
- Yogurt for sour cream.
- Lemon juice and herbs for heavy salad dressings.
- Fruit for rich appetizers or desserts.

Low Energy Foods that May be Used Freely on a Weight Loss Diet

Black coffee	Broccoli
Plain tea or tea with lemon	Cauliflower
Cantaloupe	Celery
Strawberries	Cucumbers
Lettuce	
Cabbage	Bean sprouts
Aspargus	Mushrooms
Tomatoes	Spinach

Cooking Methods

Right cooking methods should be considered. Baking, roasting, poaching or boiling are the preferred methods because they don't require the addition of fat, as frying does. Skimming of fat from the tops of soups, meat dishes, and vegetables reduces their fat content as does trimming fat from meats before cooking. The addition of extra butter or margarine to foods should be avoided.

Patience and encouragement are needed throughout the ordeal of the dieting. Temptation is everywhere, and the dieter should be forewarned.

Just one piece of chocolate cake should set the diet back for half a day (400 to 500 kcal) and lower resistance to future temptation. Breaking the diet one day will make it seem easy to break it a second day, and so on. Fresh vegetables and drinks of water may be used to harmlessly prevent or assuage the hunger pangs that are bound to appear. A short walk or a few minutes of exercise may help to turn the dieter's thoughts from food.

Exercise

Exercise, particularly aerobic exercise, is an excellent adjunct to any weight loss program. Aerobic exercise uses energy from the body's fat reserves as it increases the amount of oxygen the body takes in. Examples are dancing, jogging, bicycling, skiing, rowing, and power walking. Such exercise helps tone the muscles, burns kcal, increases the BMR so food is burned faster and is fun for the participant. Any exercise program must begin slowly and increase over time so no physical damage occurs.

Exercise alone can only rarely replace the actual diet, however. The dieter should be made aware of the number of calories burned by specific exercise so as to avoid overeating after the workout.

Do's for Those on Weight Reduction Diet

Record food for two weeks before diet. Figure calories and circle those items that could easily have been avoided.

1. Plan your weight loss diet to include some favourite foods.
2. Weigh regularly (for example, once a week) but not daily.
3. Don't wait too long between meals. Allow low calorie snacks.
4. Watch size of portions and eat slowly.
5. Use small plates.
6. Use low calorie garnishes.
7. Eat whole, fresh foods. Avoid processed foods.
8. Anticipate high eating days (e.g., banquets and holidays). "Undereat" before and after.
9. If something goes wrong, don't punish yourself by eating.
10. If there is no weight loss for one week, begin a new food diary and evaluate your diet sincerely.

11. As you near your goal, keep a diary and indicate adjustments for your new regimen of no further loss, but no gain either.
12. Write a lifetime diet plan to use after the weight loss. Allow for special occasions and treats.
13. If a binge does occur, don't punish yourself by continuing the binge. Stop it ! Go for a walk. Call a friend.
14. Adapt family meals to suit your needs. Avoid the heavy kcal items. Limit yourself to a spoonful of something too rich for a weight loss diet. Substitute something you like if–low in calorie content.

Crash Diets

A crash diet usually does result in an initial rapid weight loss. However, the weight loss is thought to be caused by a loss of body water rather than body fat. Sudden weight loss of this type is followed by a plateau period, that is, a period in which weight doesn't decrease. Disillusionment is apt to occur during this period and may cause the dieter to go on "eating binge". This can result in regaining the weight that was lost and sometimes more. This in turn causes the dieter to try another weight loss diet, creating a yo-yo effect.

Some popular reducing diets severely limit the foods allowed, providing a real danger of nutrient deficiencies over time, and their restricted nature makes them boring. Some provide too much cholesterol and fat, contributing to atherosclerosis. Some contain an excess of protein, which puts too great a demand on the kidneys. The powered varieties of weight loss diets available are not only expensive and inconvenient (if one is not at home to prepare them), they can be life threatening if they fail to supply sufficient potassium for the heart.

These diets ultimately fail because they defeat the dual purpose of the dieter, which is to lose weight and prevent its returning. To accomplish both, eating habits must be changed and crash diets do not do this.

SURGICAL TREATMENT OF OBESITY

When obesity becomes morbid (damaging health), and the individual lacks the self control to reduce weight by dieting, surgery could be indicated. Two of the surgical procedures used for this include the jejunoileal bypass and the gastric bypass. In the former, the jejunum (the middle section of the small intestine) is surgically attached to a small section of the ileum (the last part of the small intestine). This results in fewer nutrients being absorbed and consequent loss of weight.

Some obese people think that such procedure would be their salvation, believing that following them, they could eat as much as they wanted and still lose weight. It may not be salvation. Common complications of this type of surgery include diarrhea and consequent electrolyte and fluid imbalances, liver problems, kidney stones, and bone disease–the last probably caused by reduced absorption of minerals and vitamins.

Gastric bypass is a procedure in which the stomach is stapled so that it is reduced in size. This reduced stomach capacity reduces the amounts of food that can be eaten. Post surgery complications (nausea and vomiting) are fewer than with jejunoileal bypass surgery, but there is comparatively less weight lost.

MEDICINAL INTERVENTION IN OBESITY

Amphetamines (pep pills) have been prescribed for the treatment of obesity because they depress the appetite. However, it has been learned that their effectiveness is reduced within a relatively short time. The dosage must be regularly increased; they cause nervousness and insomnia; and they can become habit forming. Consequently, they are rarely prescribed now. Over-the-counter diet pills are available. They are intended to reduce appetite but are not thought to be effective. In addition to caffeine and artificial sweeteners, they contain phenylpropanolamine that can damage blood vessels and should be avoided.

Some people believe that diuretics (medications that cause frequent urination) and laxatives promote weight loss. They do, but only of water. They do not cause a reduction of body fat, which is what the dieter is seeking. An excess of either could be dangerous because of possible upsets in fluid and electrolyte balance. In addition, laxatives can become habit forming. They should not be used on any frequent or regular basis without the supervision of a physician.

UNDERWEIGHT

Underweight can cause complications of pregnancy and various nutritional deficiencies. It may lower one's resistance to infection, and if carried to the extreme, can cause death.

Causes

Underweight can be caused by inadequate consumption of nutritious food because of depression, disease, anorexia nervosa, bulimia, or poverty. It also can be caused by excessive activity, the tissue wasting of certain diseases, poor absorption of nutrients, infection, or hyperthyroidism (a condition in which the basal metabolism rate is increased) and consequently the number of kcal needed for energy is increased; unless corrected, it usually results in weight loss).

Dietary Management

Underweight is treated by a high calorie diet alone, or by a one combined with psychological counselling if the condition is of psychological origin as, for example, in depression or anorexia nervosa. In many cases, a high calorie diet will be met with resistance. It can be as difficult for an underweight person to gain weight as it is for an overweight person to lose it.

The diet should be based on the Food Guide Pyramid so it can be easily adapted from the regular, family menus, or to a soft textured diet. The total number of kcal prescribed per day will vary from person to person, depending on the person's activity, age, size, sex and physical condition.

If the individual is to gain some 500 g a week, 3500 kcal in addition to the individual's basic normal weekly kcal requirement are prescribed. This means an extra 500 kcal must be taken in each day.

Time will be needed to gradually increase the daily kcal value. In this diet, there is an increased intake of foods rich in carbohydrates, some fats and proteins. Vitamins and minerals are supplied in adequate amounts. If there are deficiencies of some vitamins and minerals, supplements are prescribed.

Nearly all nutritious foods are allowed in the high-calorie diet, but easily digested foods (carbohydrates) are recommended. Because an excess of fat can be distasteful and spoil the appetite, fatty foods must be used with discretion. Fried foods are not recommended. Bulky foods should be used sparingly. Bulk takes up stomach space that could be better used for more concentrated, higher calorie foods.

Those requiring this diet frequently have poor appetites so meals should be made especially appetizing. Favourite foods should be served, and portions of all foods should be small to avoid discouraging the patients. Many of the extra calorie needed may be consumed as snacks between meals, unless these snacks reduce the patient's appetite for meals and consequently reduce the total kcal intake. In some cases, the patient may consume more calorie each day if the number of meals is reduced, thereby increasing the appetite for each meal served. When the causes of underweight are psychological, therapy is required before the diet is begun, and the diet counsellor and therapist may well need to consult one another before and during treatment. Foods to be avoided in a high calorie diet are foods the patient dislikes, as well as, and bulky, low kcal foods.

Diet for the underweight

Exchange	*No. of exchange*	*Protein*	*K calories*
Milk	3	24	510
Legumes and pulses	3	21	300
Meat	1	7	70
Veg A	2	2	40
Veg B	2	4	80
Fruits	3	–	120
Cereals	10	20	700
Fat	4	–	180
Sugar	10	–	200
Total		78	2200

Menu Plan

Early morning	:	Biscuit
Breakfast	:	Grilled paneer sandwich Boiled egg
Mid-morning	:	Banana shake
Lunch	:	Chapatti 3 Rice 1 bowl Fried dal 1 bowl Dum aloo 1 bowl Curd 1 cup Orange 1
Afternoon	:	Fried finger chips or pakore
Late evening	:	Fruit salad
Dinner	:	Roti 2 Rice 1 bowl Rajma 1 bowl Palak curry 1 bowl Curd 1 cup Vegetable salad

Even for the most determined patients, a successful weight gain program will be charged with anxiety. There will be days of disappointment. It will take a long time to reach the ultimate goal. The health care professional will need to supply psychological support and nutritional advice. There may be times when sympathy over disappointing results will be the most important thing the health care professional could offer the dieter. It is essential that the health care professional see the problems, sympathises with the patient, and then effectively lead her or him back to the diet. The key word for the health care professional is support.

In a nutshell, excessive weight endangers health and should be lost by the use of a restricted calorie diet based on the Food Guide Pyramid. Such a diet helps the dieter revise eating habits and avoid regaining the lost weight. Excess weight is usually caused by energy imbalance. Exercise is beneficial to weight loss regimens but rarely can replace the restricted kcal diet. Fad diets are expensive, boring and conducive to nutritional deficiencies. They ultimately fail because they do not revise eating habits. Underweight is also dangerous to health, psychological counselling as well as a high calorie diet may be required for proper treatment.

PROTEIN ENERGY MALNUTRITION

Protein energy malnutrition (PEM) comprises an array of conditions which occur due to different degree of dietary deficiency of energy and protein accompanied by dietary deficit of other nutrients as well. Whereas a severe energy deficiency leading to one end of the extreme manifests as marasmus, a deficiency of protein of severe magnitude causes kwashiorkor, a condition on the other end. However, these two conditions making the two ends of the spectrum are seen rare with intermediary situation of varying energy and protein deficiency occur more commonly and are usually connotated by PEM children between the age span of 6 to 24 months are most vulnerable to PEM and the most common reason for this is inappropriate weaning.

The foremost symptoms of PEM are loss of weight due to wasting of muscle. As malnutrition also increases vulnerability to infection, there can be many more accompanying symptoms neither malnutrition nor infection enhancing each other in a vicious circle.

NUTRITIONAL MANAGEMENT OF PEM

To compensate for the muscle wasting and accompanying weight loss, both energy and protein requirements become high. Although energy requirement fall between 120-160 kcal/kg body wt, at the time of 'catch up' growth they may touch as high a value as 200 kcal/kg body wt. As for the protein requirements, they are set in keeping with the weight loss, being set between 3-4 g/kg body wt in severe form and between 2-3 g/kg body wt in moderate to mild malnutrition. Whereas in the initial acute stage, actual weight becomes the basis foe setting energy and protein requirement, but with the recovery process setting in, the basis for energy and protein requirements shift to ideal body weight. Additionally, the quality of the protein given must be good as confirmed by its high biological value (BV) and Net Protein Utilization (NPU). To keep protein from getting utilized for energy production, enough carbohydrates are included besides giving 25-30% of energy value in the form of fat depending on the child state. As a matter of fact, increment in protein and energy intake should not be abrupt so as to ensure the building up of tolerance for their utilization. Another point worthy of consideration is that along with protein and energy, other nutrients (mineral and vitamins) that become deficient during PEM are also given in sufficient quantities, sometimes even in amounts more than RDA values as per the demands of the situation. Likewise, to take care of intestinal absorption aspect, the promoters like vitamin C to ensure adequate iron absorption and fat to pave the way for the vitamin A absorption are also given alongside. Since a large number of PEM cases suffer from diarrhoea, an adequate fluid intake is also ensured. Paralleling this, a lowering down of dietary fiber intake is also brought about.

Dietary Pattern and Food Selection

1. Meals more in number and modest in quantity is the norm for dietary pattern. This strategy suits the best in meeting the high nutritional requirements of children suffering from PEM.
2. Choice of food, if made wisely from the family pot, can become convenient and long lasting. The food recipes prepared should be bland in taste and easily digestible and assailable.
3. The recipes should ensure high nutrient density in order to cater to the high requirement of energy and protein. Since children have small stomach capacities, they need to be given more nutrition in smaller volume of food. Moreover, the feeding period for the PEM children, who are often listless and anorexic cannot but be small.
4. In the event of lactose intolerance, milk and milk products are withheld and protein from other food

sources is given, judiciously selecting then if they happen to be only plant based.

5. To prevent and manage diarrhoea, fried as well as carbohydrate rich foods are sparingly given. Moreover, in the children suffering from diarrhoea, both body fluid level and nutrition are maintained by giving oral rehydration solution (ORS) along with breast and milk feeding.

STUDY QUESTIONS

1. Discuss overweight, obesity and underweight. What are some causes of overweight? Discuss why some people eat more than need. Discuss how this can be prevented or changed.
2. Explain why revised eating habits are essential to an effective weight loss program.
3. Describe three cooking methods that are preferred for people on low kcal diets and explain why they are preferred.
4. Name ten foods that should be avoided during a weight loss program. Tell why?
5. Describe the use of exercise during a weight loss program. Could it be used in lieu of the diet? Why?
6. Explain why a high calorie diet could be unpleasant for a patient.
7. Discuss the causes and dangers of underweight.
8. Discuss dietary management in Protein Energy Malnutrition.

CHAPTER 25

Gastrointestinal Tract Disorders and Nutrition

Chapter Outlines

- Disorders of the primary organs of GI tract
- Dyspepsia
- Diarrhoea
- Constipation
- Hiatus hernia
- Peptic ulcer
- Diverticulosis/diverticulitis
- Inflammatory bowel diseases
- Celiac disease
- Cholecystitis and cholelithiasis
- Pancreatitis
- Study questions

DISORDERS OF THE PRIMARY ORGANS OF GI TRACT

Whereas, primary organs of gastrointestinal tract include mouth, esophagus, stomach and small and large intestine, liver, gallbladder, and pancreas are accessory organs that are also involved in the processes, occurring in the GI tract. Many disorders of the gastrointestinal system cause distress to numerous individuals. Some problems are physiologically caused; others can be psychological in origin. At times; it is difficult to determine the cause of a "GI" problem. Consequently, controversy exists in some cases about appropriate treatment.

DYSPEPSIA

Dyspepsia or indigestion is a condition of discomfort in the digestive tract that can be physical or psychological in origin. Symptoms include "heartburn", bloating, pain, and sometimes, regurgitation. If the cause is physical, it can be due to hasty eating, over-rich foods, or it may be a symptom of another problem, such as appendicitis, kidney, gallbladder, or colon diseases and possibly, cancer. If the problem is organic, treatment of the underlying cause will be the normal procedure. On the other hand, psychological stress can also affect stomach secretions and trigger dyspepsia. Treatment in this case includes counselling to help the patient come out of the stress situation. One can save oneself from simple dyspepsia by allowing convenient time to relax and enjoy meals as well as by learning to improve eating habits

Diarrhoea and constipation are the most common disorders of gastrointestinal tract.

DIARRHOEA

Passage of stools with increased frequency, fluidity, or volume is known as diarrhoea. Severity of the disease can be understood from the fact that the number of stools range from several in a day to one every few minutes. Origin of diarrhoea is mostly infective, causative agents being bacteria, viruses or protozoa. Other agents could be medicinal side effects, toxic chemicals, shock and other psychological conditions and even dietary over or obsessive consumptions. Mostly the infection occurs through the oral faecal route. Acute diarrhoea persists for 1 to 2 days (24 to 48 hours) with a sudden onset. Chronic diarrhoea is the one that persists for weeks together. Rapid depletion of water and electrolytes in acute diarrhoea can make a person gravely ill or even proves fatal in infants and children and the aged due to dehydration. Undernourishment intensifies the symptoms and the two even occur in a vicious circle aggravating the nutritional deficiencies. Fluid and electrolyte loss beyond a limit due to this disease causes weakness, listlessness, vomiting and aversion to food or anorexia.

Dietary Management

Invariably, death occurs in diarrhoea due to dehydration, the prime aim of dietary management is replenishing lost fluid and electrolyte. UNICEF/WHO recommended oral rehydration formula with the following composition is used to give oral rehydration therapy. Glucose–20.0 g; Sodium chloride–3.5 g; Sodium bicarbonate–2.5 g; Potassium chloride–1.5 g; made into one litre with boiled water. The therapy can be given at home also by giving small and frequent doses of oral rehydration solution. Loss of fluids and electrolytes can also be made up by liberal intake of fluids in the diet.

Nutrient requirements during diarrhoea are based upon following points:

Energy: There is 25 percent increase in energy requirement in order to make up for the losses.

Protein: In case of chronic diarrhoea prolonging for a lòng time, there is depletion in tissue protein. To make up for that and to normalize blood plasma protein levels, a 25 percent increment in protein intake is advisable.

Fat: Since 'fat' is a nutrient which requires an elaborate process for digestion, it is important to include moderate amount of fat based on the daily requirement levels, so as to meet the enhanced energy requirements. Inclusion of middle chain triglycerides (MCT) in the diet is advised but may not be possible to follow under household settings.

Vitamins and Minerals: There is always need to be liberal in the intake of micronutrients. To affect this, vitamin and mineral supplements can also be used along with dietary sources.

In essence, a good nutritious soft diet abundant in energy, protein and micronutrients with liberal amount of fluids should be given.

Dietary Pattern and Food Selection

1. Small frequent and soft bland meals make one better cope with the disease.
2. Whereas complex carbohydrates should go to make a large proportion of daily diet, fiber content of the diet should be as low as possible.
3. Among milk and milk products, curd and butter milk should be preferred as milk is ill tolerated in this disease condition.
4. Desserts, fried fatty foods, strongly flavored foods are better avoided.
5. Fruit and fruit juices, vegetable and pulse soups, as a source of potassium, should find place in the diet.
6. There should be liberal inclusion of foods like low fiber fruits, low fiber refined cereal flours, dehusked pulses and lean meat.
7. To keep dehydration away, a discrete use of oral rehydration solutions (WHO based and improvised ones) is necessary.

CONSTIPATION

It is difficult in the elimination of excretory material resulting from gastrointestinal digestion and absorption of foods. Alternatively, constipation could be defined as hardening of stool that results in its infrequent or difficult evacuation of faeces. Persistent constipation can cause headache, anorexia and halitosis or foul breath. It also causes scratches or damages in the anal passage leading to bloody faeces. Causes of constipation can be faulty eating habits in resorting to refined, low fibre foods with inadequacy in fluid intake. Sometimes irregularity or inadequacy in sleep, remaining in sitting posture for long hours and irregular elimination habits also cause this malady.

Nutritional Management

Although nutritional requirements do not change but inclusion of fibre and liberal intake of fluids are definitely helpful. Thus by including raw green vegetable salads, fruits and whole cereals, beans and pulses, clear soups and ones with cream, one can remain free from constipation. In addition, a liberal intake of fluids including 8-10 glasses of water per day will not let people suffer from this disease.

HIATUS HERNIA

Hiatus hernia is a condition in which a part of the stomach protrudes through the diaphragm (a muscular sheet separating the abdominal cavity from the chest cavity) into the thoracic cavity. This prevents the food from moving normally along the digestive tract, although it does mix

Diet for constipation			
Exchange	*No. of exchange*	*Protein*	*K calories*
Milk (slim)	2	16	340
Legumes and pulses	3	21	300
Meat	½	3.5	35
Veg A	4	4	80
Veg B	2	4	80
Fruits	3	–	120
Cereals	10	20.0	700
Fat	5	–	225
Sugar	6	–	120
Total		66.5	2000

Menu Plan

Breakfast	:	Digestive biscuit 4
		Boiled egg
		Guava 1
Lunch	:	Veg soup
		Chapatti 2 (whole meal flour)
		Rice 1 bowl
		Dal 1 bowl
		Aloo methi 1 bowl
		Curd 1 cup
		Vegetable salad
Afternoon	:	Lassi
		Sprout Bhel
Dinner	:	Cabbage soup
		Roti 2
		Rice 1 bowl
		Palak curry 1 bowl
		Dal 1 bowl
		Curd 1 cup
		Vegetable salad with fruit

somewhat with the gastric juices. Sometimes the food will move back into the esophagus, creating a burning sensation ("heartburn"), and sometimes food will be regurgitated into the mouth. This condition can be very uncomfortable.

The problem can sometimes be alleviated by serving small, frequent meals (from a well balanced diet) so the amount of food in the stomach is never large. If the patient is obese, weight loss may be recommended to reduce pressure on abdomen. It may also be helpful if patients avoid lying down soon after eating. When they do lie down, they may be more comfortable sleeping with their heads and upper torso somewhat elevated. If discomfort cannot be controlled, surgery may be necessary.

PEPTIC ULCER

An ulcer is an erosion of the mucous membrane. Peptic ulcers may occur in the stomach (gastric ulcer) or the duodenum (duodenal ulcer). The specific cause of ulcers is not clear, but some physicians believe that a number of factors including genetic predisposition, abnormally high secretion of hydrochloric acid by the stomach, anxiety, excessive use of aspirin or ibuprofen (NSAID), cigarette smoking, and possibly a bacteria may contribute to their development.

The active principle of chillies, capsaicin, causes shedding of surface cells and increases acid secretion when in used in the stomach. Clinicians generally agree that peptic distress is reduced by avoiding chillies.

Helicobacter pylori is a bacterium commonly found in the stomach. It is now suspected to be an agent in the causation of chronic gastritis, non ulcer dyspepsia, duodenitis, duodenal ulcer, and even gastric ulcer and cancer.

Cigarette smoking damages the mucosa and may even increase acid secretion. Smoking interferes with attempts to reduce gastric acid and pepsin secretion with drugs. It also causes pyloric incompetence and reflux of duodenal juice into the stomach. These may explain the inflammation and ulcers in heavy smokers. Tobacco chewing also causes shedding of the stomach lining, and may have a role in the production of peptic ulcers.

Mental tension, or not being able to 'let off steam', is usually associated with peptic ulcer. Brooding, frustrations and inner resentment regarding matters connected with the family or place of work may not only predispose an individual to ulcer, but also contribute to the perpetuation of symptoms and subsequent recurrences.

Ulcers are generally treated with drugs such as cimetidine, which inhibit acid secretion in the stomach and thus help to heal the ulcer. Antacids can also be prescribed to neutralize any excess acid. Rest and counselling to help the patient learn to deal with pressure and stress are also useful in the treatment of ulcers.

In the past, diet therapy typically began with the sippy diet, which originally included hourly servings of milk and cream only, and was later liberalized to include some soft foods. It is rarely used today because while whole milk does initially neutralize the gastric acid, certain type of protein that it contains stimulates the stomach to secrete additional acid. When it is used, whole or skim milk are now advised because of the danger of atherosclerosis from the cream. Generally, the diet therapy for peptic ulcers has been vastly liberalized and the effectiveness of soft or bland diets has become controversial.

However, it is still used as a first hand option in peptic ulcers. A bland diet includes food that are simply prepared, have little fibre, are mild flavoured, and are not known to increase the production of stomach acid. Such a diet should not irritate the gastrointestinal tract chemically or mechanically.

Sufficient protein should be provided, but not in excess because of its ability to stimulate gastric acid secretion. It is recommended that patients receive no less than 0.8 gram of protein per kilogram of body weight. However, if there has been blood loss, this may be increased to 1 or 1.5 grams per kilogram of body weight. Vitamin and mineral supplements, especially iron, if there has been haemorrhage, may be prescribed.

Although fat inhibits gastric secretions, because of the danger of atherosclerosis, the amount of fat in the diet should not be excessive. Carbohydrates have little effect on gastric acid secretion.

While coarse foods were previously prohibited to the ulcer patients because it was thought that the roughage irritated the ulcer, this is no longer the case now. Generally, caffeine and alcohol are to be avoided. Light foods may be eaten as per toleration levels.

Coffee, tea, or anything containing caffeine, stimulates gastric secretion. Alcohol and aspirin irritate the mucous membrane of the stomach, and cigarette smoking decreases the secretion of the pancreas that buffers gastric acid in the duodenum.

Currently, a well balanced diet of three meals a day consisting of foods that do not irritate the gastric mucosa of the patient is generally recommended.

Diet in peptic ulcer

Exchange	*No. of exchange*	*Protein*	*K calories*
Milk	2	16	340
Legumes and pulses	3	21	300
Meat	½	3.5	35
Veg A	2	2	40
Veg B	2	4	80
Fruits	2	–	80
Cereals	10	20	700
Fat	5	–	225
Sugar	4	–	80
Total		66.5	1880

Menu Plan

Breakfast : Milk 1 glass
Dal pitha
Fruit

Lunch : Chapatti 2
Rice 1 bowl
Moong dal 1 bowl
Cabbage curry 1 bowl
Curd 1 cup

Afternoon : Boiled egg
Biscuit

Dinner : Roti 2
Rice 1 bowl
Arhar dal 1 bowl
Potato curry 1 bowl
Curd 1 cup

DIVERTICULOSIS/DIVERTICULITIS

Diverticulosis is an intestinal disorder characterized by little pockets in the sides of intestines. When food collects in these pockets instead of moving on through the intestines, bacteria may breed, an inflammation and pain can result, causing diverticulitis. If a diverticulum ruptures, surgery may be needed. This condition is thought to be caused by diet lacking in sufficient fibre. A high fibre diet is commonly recommended for patients with diverticulosis.

Diet therapy for diverticulitis may begin with a clear liquid diet, followed by a low residue or even minimum residue diet, and very gradually (over several weeks) progress to a high fibre diet as it increases stool volume, reduces the pressure in the colon, and shortens the time the food is in the intestine, giving bacteria less time to grow.

Residue Regulated Diets

Fibre is indigestible carbohydrates found in plants. Residue is the solid part of faeces. Residue is made up of all the undigested and unabsorbed parts of food (including fibre), connective tissue in meat, dead cells, and intestinal bacteria and their products. Most of this residue is composed of fibre.

Dietary fibre refers to the non-digestible carbohydrates present in a food when it is eaten. Examples are corn kernels, strawberry seeds, and celery seeds, and celery strings. Crude fibre is the amount of fibre remaining in a plant food after it has been treated with various acids and alkalies in the laboratory. In this process, much of dietary fibre is destroyed. Therefore, crude fibre is just an approximation accurate measurement of the dietary fibre in food.

Diets can be adjusted to increase or decrease fiber and residue. The specific names of these diets vary among health care facilities. The specific foods allowed and, thus, the amount of fibre and residue allowed will depend on the physician's experience and the patient's condition.

High Fiber Diet

High fiber diets are believed to help prevent diverticulosis, constipation, hemorroids and colon cancer. They also are helpful in the treatment of diabetes mellitus and atherosclerosis.

It is currently estimated that the normal diet in the United States contains about 20 grams of dietary fibre each day. A high-fiber diet is often 20 to 30 grams and can be as much as 50 grams a day. The recommended foods for this diet include coarse and whole grain breads and cereals, bran, all fruits, vegetables (especially) raw and legumes. Milk, meats, and fats don't contain fiber. This diet is nutritionally adequate. High fiber diets must be introduced gradually to prevent the formation of gas and the discomfort that accompanies it.

Low Residue Diet

The low residue diet is intended to reduce the normal work of the intestines by restricting the amount of dietary fiber and reducing food residue. Low fiber or residue restricted diets may be used in cases of severe diarrhoea, diverticulitis, ulcerative colitis, intestinal blockage, and in preparation for and immediately after intestinal surgery.

In some facilities, these diets consist of food that provide no more than three grams of fibre a day and that do not increase faecal residue. Some foods that do not actually leave in the colon are considered "high residue" foods because they increase stool volume or provide a laxative effect. Milk and prune juice are examples of them. Milk increases stool volume and prune juice acts as a laxative.

The Minimum Residue Diet

The minimum residue diet is extremely restrictive and can contain no more than one gram of fiber per day. Generally,

Foods to allow/avoid on low residue foods	
Foods to be allowed in low residue diet Milk, butter milk (limited to two cups daily)	Foods to be avoided Fresh or dried fruits and if physicians allows cottage cheese and some mild cheese as vegetables
Flavourings in small amounts butter and margarine eggs, except fried Tender chicken, fish, sweetbreads, ground beef, and ground lamb (meats must be baked, boiled, or broiled) Soup broth	Whole grain breads and cereals nuts, seeds, legumes, coconut and marmalade
Cooked, mild flavoured vegetables without coarse fibers; strained fruit juices (except for prune); apple sauce; canned fruits including white cherries, peaches and pears; pureed apricots, ripe banana refined breads and cereals, white crackers, macaroni, spaghetti and noodles custard, sherbet, vanilla ice cream, junket and cereal puddings when considered as part of the 2-cup milk allowance	Tough meats rich pastries milk, unless physician allows
If physician allows; plain gelatine; angel cake sponge cake; and plain cookies coffee, tea, cocoa, carbonated beverages salt, sugar, small amount of spices as permitted by the physician	Meats and fish with tough tough connective tissue

fruits or vegetables are not allowed except for limited amounts of fruit and vegetable juices. Whole grain breads and cereals are not allowed, and milk may be prohibited. Because of the severe limitations of foods allowed, this diet may be inadequate in vitamins and minerals. If this diet may be used for a period of time, the physician may prescribe the vitamin and mineral supplements.

Minimum Residue Foods

Foods allowed in a minimum residue diet	*Foods to be avoided*
1 cup or less milk, if allowed	Fruits and vegetables
Cottage cheese, if tolerated and in small amounts	Fried foods
Margarine	Coarse, whole grain
Eggs, except fried	Breads and cereals
Tender chicken and fish; ground	Quick breads,
lamb	Fibrous meats
Soup broth	Milk unless permitted
Vegetable juice	Physician nuts, seeds, legumes
Fruit juice	
Refined breads and cereals,	
white crackers	
Macaroni, spaghetti and noodles	
Sherbet, gelatine, plain cake and	
plain cookies	
Tea, coffee (if physician permits)	
Small amounts of salt and sugar	

INFLAMMATORY BOWEL DISEASES

Inflammatory bowel diseases are chronic conditions causing inflammation in the gastrointestinal tract. The inflammation causes malabsorption that often leads to malnutrition. The acute phases of these diseases occur at irregular intervals and are relatively free of symptoms. Neither cause nor cure these conditions are known.

Two examples are ulcerative colitis and Crohn's disease. Ulcerative colitis causes inflammation and ulceration of the colon, the rectum or, sometimes, the entire large intestine. Crohn's disease can occur in any part of the gastrointestinal tract. The ulcers can penetrate the entire intestinal wall, and the chronic inflammation can thicken the intestinal wall causing obstruction.

Both conditions cause bloody diarrhea, cramps, nausea, anorexia, malnutrition, and weight loss. Electrolytes, fluids, vitamins, and other minerals are lost in the diarrhea, and the bleeding can cause loss of iron and protein.

Treatment may involve anti-inflammatory drugs nutritional therapy. Usually a low residue diet is required to avoid irritating the inflamed area and to avoid the danger of obstruction. When tolerated, the diet should include about 60-70 g of protein, additional cal vitamins and minerals.

In severe cases, total parenteral feeding (directly into the superior vena cava;) may be necessary for a period. As a patient begins to regain health, the diet may be increasingly liberalized to suit the patient's taste while maintaining good nutrition.

CELIAC DISEASE

Celiac disease, also called non-tropical sprue or celiac sprue, is a disorder characterized by malabsorption. It is thought to be due to hereditary reasons.

Symptoms include diarrhoea, weight loss and general malnutrition. Stools usually foul smell, light colored and bulky. The cause is unknown, but it has been found that the elimination of gluten (a protein found in grains) from the diet gives relief. Untreated, it leads to decreased absorption of all nutrients, hence the malnutrition and weight loss.

A gluten controlled diet used in treatment of celiac disease. All products containing wheat, buck wheat, barley, rye and oats are disallowed. Rice and corn may be used. A reduction in the fiber content is also frequently recommended. If the patient is under weight, the diet should also be high in kcal, carbohydrates and protein. Fat may be restricted until bowel function is normalized. Vitamin and mineral supplements may be prescribed.

The avoidance of food products containing wheat is not a simple thing to do. Breads, cereals, crackers, pasta products, desserts, gravies, white sauces and beer contain wheat or other cereal grains with gluten. The patient will have to learn to read food labels carefully and to avoid restaurant foods such as breaded meats or fish, meat loaf, creamed vegetables and cream soups.

The dual function of the gallbladder is the concentration and storage of bile. After bile is formed in the liver, the gallbladder concentrates it to several times its original strength, and stores it until needed. Fat in the duodenum triggers the gallbladder to contract and release bile into the common duct for the digestion of fat in the small intestine. If this flow is hindered, there may be pain.

Source of gluten

Food groups	*Foods that contain gluten*	*Foods that may contain gluten*	*Foods that do not contain gluten*
Beverage	Cereal beverages (e.g.), Postum, malt, Ovaltine, Beer and ale	Commercial chocolates milk; cocoa mixes; other beverage mixes: dietary supplements	Coffee; tea; decaffeinated coffee; carbonated beverages; cocoa; chocolate drinks made with pure powder; wine; distilled liquor
Meat and meat substitutes	Commercially breaded meats	Meat loaf and patties, cold cuts and prepared meats, stuffing, cheese foods and spreads; commercial Soufflés, omelets and Fondue; soy proteins Meat subsitutes	Pure meat, fish, fowl, egg, cottage cheese and peanut butter
Fat and oil	Commercial gravies, white and cream sauces	Commercial salad dressing and mayonnaise, non-dairy creamer	Butter, margarine, vegetable oil
Milk	Milk beverages that contain malt	Commercial chocolate milk	Whole, low fat and skim milk; butter milk
Grains and grain products	Bread, crackers, cereal and pasta that contains wheat, oats, rye, malt, malt flavouring, gram flour, durham flour, pastry flour, bran or wheat germ; barley; millet; pretzels; communion wafers	Commercial seasoned rice and potato mixes	Specially prepared breads made with wheat starch, rice, potato, or soyabean flour or cornmeal; pure corn or rice cereals; hominy grits; white, brown and wild rice; popcorn; low protein pasta made from wheat starch
Vegetables	Commercially breaded vegetables or vegetables with a cream or cheese sauce	Commercial seasoned vegetables mixes; canned baked beans	All fresh vegetables; plain commercially frozen or canned vegetables
Fruit		Commercial pie fillings	All plain or sweetened fruits; fruit thickened with tapioca or cornstach
Soup	Most commercial soup; soup mixes; soup that contains barley, wheat pasta; soup thickened with wheat flour or other gluten-containing grains	Broth	Soup thickened with corn starch, wheat starch, or potato, rice or soyabean flour; pure broth
Desserts	Commercial cakes, cookies and pastries; commercial dessert mixes	Commercial ice cream sherbet, puddings	Gelatin; custard; fruit ice; specially prepared cakes, cookies and pastries made with gluten free flour or starch; pudding and fruit filling thickened with tapioca, cornstarch, or arrow root flour
Sweets		Commercial candies, especially chocolates	
Miscellaneous		Ketchup; prepared mustard; soy sauce; commercially prepared meat, sauces and pickles; white vinegar; flavouring, syrups (syrups for pan cakes or ice cream)	Monosodium glutamate; salt; pepper; pure spices and herbs; yeast; pure baking chocolate or cocoa powder

The precise etiology of gallbladder disease is unknown, but hereditary factors may be involved. Women develop gallbladder disease more often than men do. Obesity, total parenteral nutrition (TPN - feeding entirely via a vein), the use of esterogen, and various disease of the small intestine are frequently associated.

CHOLECYSTITIS AND CHOLELITHIASIS

Cholecystitis (inflammation of the gallbladder) and cholelithiasis (gall stones) may inhibit the flow of bile and cause pain. Cholecystitis can cause changes in the gallbladder tissue which in turn can affect the cholesterol (a constituent of bile), causing it to harden and form stones. It is also thought that chronic overindulgence in fats may contribute to gallstones because the fat stimulates the liver to produce more cholesterol for the bile, which is necessary for the digestion of fat. In addition to pain, which can be severe, there may be indigestion and vomiting, particularly after the indigestion of fatty foods.

Treatment may include medication to dissolve the stones and diet therapy. If medication neither does nor succeed, surgery to remove the gallbladder (cholesystectomy) may be indicated.

Diet therapy includes abstinence during the acute phase. This is followed by a clear liquid diet, and gradually, a regular but fat restricted diet. Amounts of fats allowed run from 20 to 60 grams, with the amount being increased gradually. In chronic cases, fat may be restricted on a pemanent basis. For the obese patients, weight loss is recommended in addition to a fat restricted diet.

PANCREATITIS

In addition to the hormone insulin, the pancreas produces other hormones and enzymes that are important in the digestion of protein, fats and carbohydrates. When food reaches the duodenum, the pancreas sends its enzymes to the small intestine to aid in digestion.

Pancreatitis is an inflammation of the pancreas. It may be caused by infections, surgery, alcoholism, biliary tract (includes bile ducts and gallbladder) disease, or certain drugs. It may be acute or chronic.

Abdominal pain, nausea and steatorrhea (fat in the stool) are symptoms. Malabsorption (particularly) of fat soluble vitamins and weight loss occur, and in cases where the islets of Langerhans are destroyed, diabetes mellitus may result.

Diet therapy is intended to reduce pancreatic secretion and bile. Just as fat stimulates the gallbladder to secrete bile. Just as fat stimulates the gallbladder to secrete bile, protein and hydrochloric acid stimulate the pancreas to secrete its juices and enzymes. During acute pancreatitis, the patient is nourished strictly parenterally. Later, when the patient can tolerate oral feedings, a liquid diet consisting mainly of carbohydrates is given because, of these three nutrients, carbohydrates have the least stimulatory effect on pancreatic secretions.

As recovery progresses, small frequent feedings of carbohydrates and protein with little fat or fiber are given. The fat is restricted because of the deficiencies of pancreatic lipase. The patient is gradually returned to a regular diet as tolerated. Vitamin supplements may be given. Alcohol is forbidden in all cases.

In a nutshell, disturbances of the gastrointestinal tract require a wide variety of therapeutic diets. Peptic ulcers are treated with drugs, and diet therapy generally involves only the avoidance of alcohol and caffeine. Diverticulosis may be treated with a high fiber diet, while diverticulosis is treated with a gradual progression from clear liquid to the high fiber diet. Ulcerative colitis may require a low residue diet combined with high protein and high kcal. Cirrhosis requires a substantial, balanced diet, with occasional restrictions of fat, protein, salt or fluids. Diet therapy for hepatitis may range from parenteral to a full, well balanced diet, although protein may be restricted, depending upon the patient's condition. Cholecystitis and cholelithiasis require a fat restricted diet, and in cases of overweight, a kcal restricted diet as well. Pancreatitis diet therapy ranges from parenteral to a regular diet, if tolerated.

STUDY QUESTIONS

1. Discuss dyspepsia. Include its probable causes and the suggested therapy for it.
2. Describe hiatus hernia. Name its symptoms and possible treatment.
3. Define ulcers. Where are they found in the gastrointestinal system and how are they treated? What substances should not be allowed an ulcer patient? Why?
4. Explain the difference between diverticulosis and diverticulitis. How are these conditions treated?
5. Discuss the high fiber diet. For what conditions might it be used? Compare it to the low and minimum residue diets.
6. Discuss ulcerative colitis. What causes it and how is it treated?
7. Explain the salient features of nutritional management in diarrhoea and constipation.

CHAPTER 26

Dietary Management of Liver Disorders

Chapter Outlines

- Hepatitis
- Cirrhosis
- Fatty liver
- Metabolic disorders of the liver
- Study questions

The liver is of major importance to, and plays many roles in, metabolism. Except for a few of the fatty acids, all nutrients that are absorbed in the intestines are transported to the liver. The liver dismantles some of these nutrients, stores others, and uses some to synthesize other substances.

The liver synthesizes plasma proteins, enzymes and urea. It changes the simple sugars to glycogen, provides glucose to body cells, and synthesizes glucose from amino acids if needed. It converts fats to lipoproteins and synthesizes cholesterol. It stores iron, copper, zinc, and magnesium as well as the fat soluble vitamins and B vitamins. The liver synthesizes bile and stores it in the gallbladder. It detoxifies many substances such as barbiturates and morphine.

Liver disease may be acute or chronic. Early treatment can lead to complete recovery.

HEPATITIS

Hepatitis is an inflammation of the liver. It is caused by viruses or toxic agents such as drugs and alcohol. Necrosis (tissue death due to loss of blood supply) occurs, and the liver's normal metabolic activities are restricted. It may be acute or chronic.

In mild cases, the cells can be replaced. In severe cases, the damage can be so extensive that the necrosis leads to liver failure and death. There can be bile stasis (stoppage or slowing) and decreased blood albumin levels. Patients experience nausea, headache, fever, fatigue, tender and enlarged liver, anorexia and jaundice (yellow caste of the skin and eyes). Weight loss can be pronounced.

Thus infective hepatitis is a disease which produces inflammatory and degenerative changes in the liver. Most prevalent has been viral type occurring as A, B or C. Type A is transmitted through oral fecal route, type B through parenteral route with improperly sterilized needles, saliva, blood and semen causing the transmission. Type C mostly occurs due to post transfusion hepatitis. Viral hepatitis A is most common and usually mild and rarely progresses to the chronic stage. However, type B is often more serious and often progresses to the severe chronic hepatitis. Type C can be put somewhere in between A and B in terms of severity and progression. Different types of the viral hepatitis produce similar non-specific symptoms such as anorexia, exhaustion on exertion, fatigue, vomiting, diarrhoea, fever, weight loss and abdominal discomfort. These symptoms are followed in time course by jaundice which consists of a yellow pigmentation of the skin and body tissues due to the accumulation of bile pigments in the blood. This happens as hepatitis progressives with hepatic cell injury and necrosis denting their capacity to incorporate bilirubin and other bile pigments into bile. In fact, synthesis and secretion of bile itself is impaired due to the damaged liver cells. Whereas symptoms take 1 to 3 weeks to subside, it takes several months for a person to recover completely. Main points of treatment include complete rest especially retraining from physical exertion and intake of nutritious diet which though provides for all nutrient requirements yet spares the liver from excessive metabolic work including that of lipid metabolism and distribution. Infact, mainstay of treatment is usually bed rest, plenty of fluids and diet therapy. During early treatment, a full liquid diet may be prescribed.

Objectives of the Dietary Management

To prevent further hepatic damage and help in regenerating hepatic tissue. Thus a nutritious diet is a must for promoting recovery and preventing a relapse. Since anorexia is a frequent problem, the patient is encouraged to eat through counselling as well as good preparation and consideration for individual preferences within the dietary prescription. The role of attractively served food is no less in promoting intake.

Nutritional Management

A diet low in fat but abundant in energy and protein plays a key role in the regeneration of liver cells.

Energy: During the acute phase of the disease normal energy requirement need to be fulfilled. In the event of weight loss, energy may even be increased by 10 to 20%. As the patient improves and accepts food, the diet should provide 35 to 40 kcal per kilogram of body weight. Most of these should be provided by carbohydrates; there should be moderate amounts of fat.

Protein: The intake should be normal during the acute phase and in the event of weight loss, linked by 10 percent. If the necrosis has not been severe, upto 50 to 60 grams of protein for cell regeneration. If the necrosis has been severe and the protein cannot be properly metabolized, it must be limited to prevent the accumulation of ammonia in the blood. Patients may prefer frequent, small meals rather than three large ones.

However, due to hepatic damage, a too high protein diet is not given.

Carbohydrate: A liberal intake of carbohydrate in the range of 300 to 400 g for an adult is to be ensured. Carbohydrate as abundant energy source can exercise protein sparing action along with hepatic glycogen storage which acts to protect the liver from further damage.

Fat: The other extreme of dietary prescription has to be exercised during the acute phase, i.e., withholding fat during the acute phase. However, small amounts need to be added as the symptoms begin subsiding. Beginning with 10 g/day the amount can be gradually increased to the normal levels. Even emulsified fats are given sometimes to obviate the role of emulsification.

Minerals and Vitamins: To ensure regeneration, their intake needs to be liberal. Supplements of vitamins B complex and C are often given. Vitamin K is also recommended in chronic cases.

Fluid: Fluid intake should be liberal to compensate for symptoms of gastrointestinal (GI) tract.

Dietary Pattern

1. Bland foods need to be taken so as to cause least strain on liver during the acts of digestion and absorption.
2. Diet should be low fat, high carbohydrate.
3. Small and frequent meals are well tolerated.
4. Foods with strong flavour, desserts and dishes based on cream, fried and high fat foods and alcohol are better avoided.
5. Low fat milk and milk products, cereals, pulses, lean meats, fruits, starchy vegetables, sugarcane juice and table sugar can be the foods of choice.
6. Consistency can be as per convenience and tolerance; liquid, soft or semi-solid.

Diet in hepatitis

Exchange	*No. of exchange*	*Carbohydrate*	*Protein*	*K calories*
Milk	3	–	24	510
Legumes and pulses	3	51	21	300
Meat	½	–	3.5	35
Veg. A	2	7	2	40
Veg. B	2	14	4	80
Fruits	4	40	–	160
Cereals	10	150	20	700
Fat	2	–	–	90
Sugar	10	50	–	200
Total		312	74.5	2115

Menu Plan

Tea	:	1 cup
Breakfast	:	Fruit milk shake 1 glass
		Biscuit 2
		Boiled egg 1
Lunch	:	Roti 3
		Thick dal (moong) 1 bowl
		Methi curry 1 bowl
		Rice 1 bowl
		Curd 1 cup
		Papad roasted

Afternoon	:	Apple
		Tea 1 cup
Dinner	:	Roti 3
		Thick dal (arhar) 1 bowl
		Vegetable salad
		Rice 1 bowl
		Curd 1 cup
		Vegetable of brinjal and potato 1 bowl
Bed time	:	Macroni salad

CIRRHOSIS

Cirrhosis is a general term referring to all types of liver disease characterized by cell loss. Alcohol abuse is the most common cause of cirrhosis, but it can also be caused by congenital defects, infections, or other toxic chemicals.

Although the liver does regenerate, the replacement during cirrhosis does not match the loss. In addition to the cell loss during cirrhosis, there is fatty infiltration and fibrosis (development of tough, stringy tissues). These developments prevent the liver from functioning normally. Blood flow through the liver is upset and a form of hypertension, anaemia, and haemorrhage in the esophagus can occur. The normal metabolic processes will also be disturbed to such a degree that in severe cases, death may result.

The dietary treatment of cirrhosis provides at least 35 to 50 kcal or more, and 1 to 1.5 grams of protein per kilogram of weight each day, depending on the patient's condition. If hepatic coma appears imminent, the lower amount is advocated. Supplements of vitamins and minerals are usually needed. In advanced cirrhosis, 50 to 60 percent of the kcal should be from carbohydrates.

In some forms of cirrhosis, patients cannot tolerate fat well, so it is restricted. In another form, protein may not be well tolerated so it is restricted to 30 to 35 grams per day. Sometimes cirrhosis causes ascites (accumulation of fluid in the abdomen). In such a case, sodium and fluids may be restricted. If there is bleeding in the esophagus, fiber can be restricted to prevent irritation of the tissue. Smaller feedings will be better accepted than larger ones. No alcohol is allowed.

FATTY LIVER

When fat content of liver becomes more than 5 percent from the usual 3 percent, it is called fatty liver.

Fatty liver usually occurs in malnourished or semistarved individuals. In children, fatty liver has been described: (i) with skin and mucous membrane changes (as in kwashiorkar) in the poor communities of Asia and Africa. Infact, fatty liver is one of the most striking features of kwashiorkor; (ii) without skin and mouth changes in Jamaica; and (iii) with iron deposits in South Africa.

Fatty liver is usually noted in adult chronic alcoholics, or after massive small intestinal resection for Crohn's disease or gangrene, or intestinal bypass surgery for gross obesity. Fatty liver may also be associated with diabetes mellitus, obesity, or ulcerative colitis. Long term intravenous feeing causes fatty liver due to choline deficiency; this is reversed by lecithin supplement. It also occurs in pregnancy, and can be diagnosed by ultrasonography.

Methionine and choline contain a methyl group, and are known as 'lipotropic factors' and they not only prevent deposition of fat, but also aid in removal from the liver.

The requirement of protein increases directly with the calorie intake. Clinical manifestations of kwashiorkor, therefore occur, when, along with a low protein intake, the total ingestion of carbohydrates (calories) is increased.

Alcohol increases the total calorie intake (1 g supplies 7 kcal). With excessive alcohol consumption, the protein intake that may be adequate for average needs, becomes relatively deficient. Moreover, fatty changes due to direct liver cell injury with alcohol occur despite adequate protein intake. The source of increased liver fat is not definitely known.

(i) It may be due to overload of dietary fat;
(ii) Mobilization of free fatty acids from the body fat depots to the liver by excessive alcohol consumption;
(iii) Enhancement of fatty acid synthesis by alcohol;
(iv) Decreased fatty acid oxidation; or
(v) Reduced lipid removal from the liver.

Deficiency of body proteins reduces synthesis of lipoproteins which transport fat from the liver to distal sites. With deficiency of lipoproteins, fat is not transported and accumulates in the liver.

The liver becomes enlarged, smooth and soft with the liver cells becoming laden with fat. Adjoining fatty liver cells coalesce to produce fatty cysts. Occasionally, all the liver cells appear to be replaced by fat. Four weeks of adequate dietetic treatment may show remarkable recovery.

Fatty liver following chronic alcoholism may be associated with fibrosis or cirrhotic changes. Withholding alcohol and supplying adequate nutrition removes fatty changes, but the fibrosis or cirrhosis does not regress.

The condition may be totally asymptomatic; it may be detected on a routine examination for other indications. Malnourished patients may come with complaints of ascites or oedema of the leg, which may appear gradually or suddenly after diarrhoea.

On examination, the patient is found pale and poorly nourished. The abdomen is distended if ascites is present, but the abdominal veins are not visible. The liver is palpable two to three centimetres below the costal margin, and is soft. The spleen is not usually enlarged. The skin shows a fine scaling. There is moderate hypochromic anemia. The serum albumin may be less than 2 g per 100 ml. Transaminases show some change. Liver function tests may show mild to moderate deterioration because of associated cirrhosis.

Nutritional management is done by giving a high protein diet. A marked improvement in fatty change within 3-4 weeks is seen. In alcoholic fatty liver associated with cirrhosis, the fat disappears with refrain and adequate nutrition, but the ultimate prognosis is that of cirrhosis.

A 2000-2500 kcal diet is prescribed. Protein (about 70 to 100 g daily) is served mainly as milk, eggs, meat or fish. Other protein rich foods are skimmed milk, pulses, including Bengal gram and groundnuts. Preparations of wheat, such as chapattis, bread and biscuits provide 10% protein.

The lipotropic factors methionine and choline, and fat restriction, are necessary with an adequate protein diet. About 60 g fat is advised. Iron, folic acid, vitamin B_{12} or multivitamins are injected when needed. For ascites, thiazide or frusemide diuretics are useful. As a matter of fact, patients with liver disease require a great deal of encouragement because their anorexia and consequent feelings of general malaise can be severe. Their recovery takes patience, rest and time.

METABOLIC DISORDERS OF THE LIVER

Certain congenital and hereditary metabolic disorders of hepatitis tissue need continuous dietary alterations so as to minimize in deleterious effects. A brief overview of the same is given hereunder:

Hereditary Tyrosinaemia

This results from defective, tyrosine aminotransferase enzyme. If not corrected, it leads to cirrhosis. Dietary restriction of tyrosine and phenylalanine by selecting appropriate foods is beneficial in some cases.

Galactosaemia

It results from Galactose-1-Phosphatase uridyl transferase deficiency, and leads to prolonged cholestasis and secondary biliary cirrhosis. Dietary exclusion of galactose can totally arrest the disease.

Hereditary Fructose Intolerance

It results from Fructose - 1 phosphate aldolase deficiency. If not recognised early and without dietary management, it leads to cirrhosis. Early recognition and restriction of fructose can reverse the hepatic changes.

Glycogen-Storage Disorder Type-I

It results from glucose phosphatase deficiency. Clinical manifestation is marked hypoglycaemia. In liver, only histological changes are observed. Dietary manipulations in infants include nocturnal intragastric feeding with high glucose elemental formulae via nasogastric tube. In older patients, uncooked corn starch food serves as a constant source of glucose.

Phenylketonuria (PKU)

Phenylketonuria is a group of inherited disorders of phenylalanine metabolism caused by impaired phenylalanine hydroxylase activity. This enzyme is mainly expressed in liver. If not treated before three weeks of age, the metabolic imbalances result in irreversible mental retardation. Hence screening is necessary to detect the infants suffering from the disorder. The aim of the therapy is to maintain phenylalanine levels close to normal, i.e., 40-50 moles/L in order to prevent mental retardation and at the same time ensuring adequate protein intake for somatic growth. This objective can be met by using combination of proprietary, chemically defined medical and natural foods. It is not possible to supply low phenylalanine content diet as natural proteins contain 2.5 to 9% of phenylalanine by weight. Hence commercial therapeutic preparations are the only alternative. Some clinicians even discontinuance of this therapy after the age of 12-14 years as they argue that phenylalanine utilization metabolism begins thereafter. However, others have found diminished intelligence in patients who do away with the therapy.

STUDY QUESTIONS

1. Explain the role of nutrition in the management of infective hepatitis and cirrhosis.
2. Chart out the relationship of alcoholism and fatty liver and discuss the dietary management of the latter.
3. Discuss briefly the metabolic disorders of liver and their dietary management.
4. Explain the role of liver as a central tissue of metabolism.

CHAPTER 27

Dietary Management of Diabetes Mellitus, Atherosclerosis and Hypertension

Chapter Outlines

- Diabetes mellitus: Symptoms and diagnosis
- Laboratory tests for diabetes mellitus
- Dietary management
- Atherosclerosis: Risk factors and diet plan
- Hypertension: Occurrence and nutritional management
- Study questions

DIABETES MELLITUS: SYMPTOMS AND DIAGNOSIS

The disease was initially named diabetes in ancient times which meant to follow through, due to the large volume of urine formed in the patients. The word 'mellitus' (meaning honeyed) was added to it to make diabetes mellitus due to the presence of sugar in the urine. Two major types of diabetes mellitus; Type 1 or insulin dependent diabetes mellitus (IDDM), earlier known as juvenile onset diabetes mellitus, due to its occurrence mostly before 20 years of age; and Type 2 or non-insulin dependent diabetes mellitus, earlier known as adult onset diabetes mellitus due to its occurrence mostly after 40 years of age are prevalent. A third type, gestational diabetes occurs in some women during pregnancy especially in the last trimester. Likewise, secondary diabetes mellitus occurs infrequently due to the disease of pancreas or due to the intake of corticosteroids or antihypertensive medicines. Of late there have also been reports of the occurrence of diabetes mellitus due to malnutrition. Whereas the prevalence of IDDM is only 10 to 20% that of NIDDM is 80-90%. Among IDDM and NIDDM, the former is treated through dietary modification and insulin therapy and the latter through dietary modification alone or in combination with oral hypoglycemic drugs.

Classic Triads of Symptoms in Diabetes Mellitus

The triad of symptoms includes increased craving for food or polyphagia, increased urination or polyuria and the symptoms of excessive thirst or polydipsia which occurs to compensate for increased water loss due to frequent urination.

Acute and Chronic Complications of Diabetes Mellitus

First acute complication include hypoglycemia or lower than normal level of sugar in blood. This occurs due to an imbalance between diet and insulin in IDDM patients and between diet and hypoglycemic drugs in those with NIDDM. This can also become life threatening in extreme situations. Second acute complication is termed as ketoacidosis, which is acidosis because of high concentration of ketone bodies in blood as a consequence of poor dietary and medicinal management of the disease.

This can prove equally disastrous, even to the extent of being fatal. Chronic complications occurring due to diabetes mellitus include diseases of the eye, kidney, heart and nervous system. Besides, ill managed diabetes mellitus can cause a kind of ulceration in the feet of diabetics which eventually culminate as gangrene necessitating amputation of foot or a part thereof. This condition is termed as diabetic foot.

LABORATORY TESTS FOR DIABETES MELLITUS

Blood Tests

Fasting Blood Sugar: The subject's 12 hours fasting sample is obtained for the purpose of blood sugar estimation. Normal fasting blood sugar level lies between 80 to 120 mg/100 ml and a level above 140 mg/100 ml is indicative of diabetes mellitus.

Glucose Tolerance Test: A measured amount of glucose (generally 100 g) is given orally or intravenously to the subject after obtaining a fasting blood sample. Thereafter, further blood samples are drawn at specific intervals (1/2, 1, 2, 3 hours). A non-diabetic person's blood sugar level doesn't exceed beyond 180-200 mg/100 ml l at any of these intervals. Higher levels point towards the diagnosis of diabetes mellitus as positive.

Glycated Hemoglobulin: Glucose can chemically add to the hemoglobulin in an irreversible reaction to make glycated hemoglobulin. Whereas in persons having normal blood sugar level, the percentage of glycosylated hemoglobin is 4 to 8 percent, it is higher in diabetics in keeping with the degree of hyperglycemia. Glycated hemoglobulin level of 10 percent or more is indicative of a poor glycemic control or moderate diabetes mellitus and that beyond 15 percent of very poor glycemic control or severe form of the disease.

Urine Tests

Urine Sugar: In most of the human beings, kidneys start spilling glucose into the urine at a blood sugar concentration of 180-200 mg/100 ml. This level of blood sugar is known as renal threshold for glucose. Thus a qualitative presence of sugar in urine could be indicative of diabetes mellitus. However, the test is not fully reliable as renal threshold varies from individual to individual and even change in the given person with falling kidney function.

Urine Acetone: As a consequence of an enforced fat metabolism in a diabetic individual, there is an excessive production of ketone bodies which spill into urine as acetone in severe diabetes mellitus.

Thus an acetone positive urine is indicative of one suffering from a severe form of diabetes mellitus and the condition of presence of acetone in urine is known as ketonuria.

Major objectives of the therapy in this disease essentially remain as under:

1. To maintain the patient's blood glucose level within normal limits as it is the hyperglycemia which majorly becomes the cause of further, and often dreaded, complications.
2. To provide optimal nutrition to the patient for a protective limiting.
3. To cheque the development of hypoglycemia in patients on insulin or oral hypoglycemic agents.
4. To make the diabetics lead as much a normal life as possible.

DIETARY MANAGEMENT

Management of diet plays a pivotal role in controlling the disease. Though nutritional requirements of diabetics and healthy persons do not vary much, yet due consideration needs to be given to affect subtle variations in menu planning and meal scheduling.

Distribution of calories derived from carbohydrate, protein and fat, the three macronutrients in the diet should be more or less as under:

Carbohydrate 60-65%, protein 15-20%, fat 15-25%.

Calculation of energy requirements per kg/bodyweight should be as per the following scheme:

Nutritional status	*Types of activity*		
	Sedentary	*Moderate*	*Heavy*
Underweight	35	40	45
Normal	30	35	40
Obese	25	30	35

Carbohydrate: Complex carbohydrate containing foodstuffs remain the only choice for including into diet. Foodstuffs comprising sugarcane juice, table sugar, dextrose and jam furnish simple sugars which instantly increase blood sugar levels and thus need to be avoided.

Protein: They can be both from animal and plant sources. However, in the event of proteins coming exclusively from plant sources, the principles of mutual supplementation (cereal-pulse combination) need to be applied.

Fat: Since diabetes mellitus makes people vulnerable to coronary heart disease, fat component should not exceed the prescribed limit.

The three types of fatty acids comprising the dietary fat should be in equal proportion as:

SFA: MUFA: PUFA.

Vitamin and Minerals: Their requirements remain similar to those of non-diabetics.

Diet for diabetes mellitus

Exchange	*No. of exchange*	*Carbohydrate*	*Protein*	*Fat*	*K calories*
Milk	2	24	16	20	340
Legumes and pulses	2	34	14	–	300
Meat	1	–	7	5	70
Veg. A	4	14	4	–	80
Veg. B	1	7	2	–	40
Fruits	1	10	–	–	40
Cereals	3	45	6	–	210
Fat	2	–	–	10	90
Total		134	49	35	1070

Menu Plan

Breakfast	:	Papaya milk shake 1 glass
		Toasted bread 2
		Boiled egg 1
Lunch	:	Small roti 2
		Thick dal 1 bowl
		Drumstick curry 1 bowl
		Vegetable salad
Afternoon	:	Sprout chat
Dinner	:	Small roti 2
		Egg curry 1 bowl
		Vegetable salad
Bed time	:	Milk without fat and sugar 1 glass

Fiber: The diabetes need to take more of fiber, even as much as 50 g per day with soluble fiber making the bulk of it as its presence in the diet makes the person exercise a better glycemic control.

Other 'do must' instructions for the diabetics are as follows:

1. To observe the prescribed dietary regimen regularly.
2. Neither to miss a meal nor to indulge in overeating as both can prove patently harmful.
3. To consume the permitted fruits (non-sweet) and vegetables as they provide dietary fiber and neutraceuticals. Fruits like gooseberry, pomegranate, apple, guava and papaya should become the articles choice. Watermelon and muskmelon with large water content are also most beneficial to a diabetic person.
4. To avoid fried foods and exercise preference for steamed boiled and baked foods.
5. To use some proven hypoglycemic substances such as bittergourd (Karela), fenugreek (methi) seeds.
6. To follow some exercise schedule daily. Regular exercise is another factor which proves very helpful in the management of diabetes mellitus. However, type, extent and duration of the exercise has to be carefully decided in consultation with physician/physiotherapist. In general, morning/evening walks in keeping with one's stamina can be undertaken regularly to keep weight under check as well as to enhance carbohydrates utilization. Exercise also tends to become helpful against cardiovascular risk factors such as hypertension and hypercholesterolemia.
7. To follow the distribution of calories among various meals (breakfast, lunch, tea, dinner, bed-time) as per the prescription of physician/dietician. This becomes necessary depending on the fact whether the patient's disease is managed by diet alone, or diet and oral hypoglycemic drugs, or diet and insulin. As far as insulin therapy is concerned, various types of insulins (short, intermediate and long acting) are used in keeping with the state of disease in an individual. Normally when on dietary, or dietary and oral hypoglycemic drugs, the three meal pattern with equal distribution of calories is followed.
8. To use side effect free artificial or non-caloric sweetner like aspartame for sweetening tea, coffee and other beverages.

Use of Food Exchange System

To ensure a non-variable daily caloric intake by diabetics in general and IDDM patients in particular, food exchange system is made use of. This system provides for groups of foods that furnish similar amount of foods calories, carbohydrates, protein or fats in a group. Such enlisting of groups provides variety in the diet keeping the total nutrient intake constant. Each exchange list has a number of food items which can be interchanged within the group. In this way, a number of exchange lists such as cereals, legumes, milk, fat, flesh foods, vegetables and fruits exchange have been developed.

ATHEROSCLEROSIS: RISK FACTORS AND DIET PLAN

No single but the following multiple factors cause atherosclerosis:

1. Hypercholesterolemia or high blood cholesterol level.
2. Hypertension or high blood pressure.
3. Cigarette smoking and alcoholism.
4. Obesity.
5. Lack of regular exercise.
6. Diabetes mellitus.
7. Family history of heart disease.
8. Stress.
9. Personality behaviour pattern.

The first five factors can well be modified to reduce the risk of developing atherosclerosis and ensuing heart attack. Whereas the role of high blood cholesterol and hypertension is obvious in atherosclerosis development, the role of smoking is due to the presence of nicotine in cigarette smoke which after entering bloodstream not only constricts small blood vessels but also stimulates the adrenal gland to over secrete epinephrine and norepinephrine that cause increase in heart rate and blood pressure. Obese people develop extra capillaries (44 million per 100 g of adipose tissue) to nourish adipose tissue which cause heart to work harder to pump blood this extra distance. Regular exercise betters cardiac efficacy and output. Other factors that contribute to heart disease are high blood levels of fibrinogen which promotes blood clot formation and renin which increases blood pressure. High blood uric acid level is another factor.

Major risk factor for developing atherosclerosis is high blood cholesterol level. It goes to build fatty plaques in the arterial walls narrowing the arterial passage way for blood and promoting blood clotting which eventually can cut off blood flow altogether. If a blockage occurs in one of the coronary arteries, the blood vessels that supply blood to the heart muscle, it results in heart attack and the disease is termed as coronary artery or coronary heart disease (CAD or CHD). In fact, CAD refers to conditions, such as atherosclerosis, that cause narrowing of coronary arteries so that blood flow to the heart is reduced. This results in CHD. Generally, symptoms begins when there is around ¾th narrowing of a coronary artery and range from a mild chest pain to a full scale heart attack depending upon the extent of blockage. The principle causes of narrowing are atherosclerosis, coronary artery spasm, or a clot in a coronary artery.

To understand atherosclerosis, we need to begin with arteriosclerosis which refers to a group of diseases with thickening of the walls of arteries and loss of their elasticity as the main characteristics. One form of arteriosclerosis is atherosclerosis, a process in which smooth muscle cells proliferate and fatty substances or the neutral fat (cholesterol and triglycerides) deposit in the walls of medium sized and large arteries. The first event in atherosclerosis of course, whose causes are not well understood, is damage occurring to the endothelial lining of the artery. Two more events follow this endothelial damage, again within the arterial wall; first proliferation of smooth muscle fibers and building up of lipid both within the endothelial cells as well in the interstitial spaces. This accumulated cholesterol, triglycerides and cells form a lesion called atherosclerotic lesion or plaque. With its growth, the plaque occludes the arterial lumen and blocks the blood flow in the affected artery and consequently, tissues supplied by the artery suffer damage which could be a heart attack (myocardial infarction). More or less, similar dietary considerations hold good for atherosclerosis as become applicable in diabetes mellitus.

The major dietary modifications for subjects with atherosclerosis involve fat (lipid) in general and cholesterol in particular in terms of quantity. In addition to weight control, sodium reduction also applies, especially for subjects suffering from hypertension. For cholesterol lowering, there are step I and step II diets that are practised on hypocholesterolemic subjects whether they suffer or not from atherosclerosis.

Step I diet is prescribed first to the afflicted subjects. Most of the times, from 10 to 20 percent reduction in total and LDL cholesterol levels has been the expected outcome after 3 months of practising step I diet. If no change is observed in total. LDL cholesterol level of the subject is referred to a registered dietician for instruction and practising step 2 cholesterol lowering diet. If the results do not improve even after 6 months of intensive dietary therapy and counselling, drug therapy, including therapy with statins is started.

HYPERTENSION: OCCURRENCE AND NUTRITIONAL MANAGEMENT

Hypertension or high blood pressure in simple terms is an increased blood pressure above the normal value of 120/80 in a healthy adult. A high blood pressure predisposes a person to coronary artery disease (CAD). Primary (essential) hypertension is persistently high blood pressure that cannot be attributed to any particular organic cause.

Diet in atherosclerosis				
Exchange	*No. of exchange*	*Protein*	*Fat*	*K calories*
Milk (slim)	2	16	–	340
Legumes and pulses	3	21	–	300
Meat	1	7	5	70
Veg A	2	2	–	40
Veg B	2	4	–	80
Fruits	2	–	–	80
Cereals	3	6	–	210
Fat	1	–	5	45
Sugar	3	–	–	60
Total		56	10	1225

Menu Plan

Breakfast : Milk 1 glass
Apple
Bread with boiled egg

Lunch : Chapatti 1
Thick dal 1 bowl
Palak curry 1 bowl
Curd 1 cup

Afternoon : Dhokla

Dinner : Veg soup without butter 1 cup
Roti 1
Dal 1 bowl
Bottlegourd vegetable
Curd 1 cup

Bed time : Fruit salad

About 90% of all hypertension cases fall into this category only remaining 10% belong to secondary hypertension having an identifiable underlying cause such as kidney disease or adrenal hyper secretion. Aldosteronism, the hypertension of aldosterone due to a tumor of adrenal cortex, may also cause hypertension. Likewise, pheochromocytoma, the tumor of adrenal medulla, produces and releases into blood stream, large quantities of epinephrine and norepinephrine, both of which raise blood pressure. Hypertension, as is well-known, is a disease that needs to be taken with seriousness and concern because of the damage it can cause to the heart, brain and kidneys.

Objectives of the Nutritional Management

1. To keep nutritional status of the person normal as also maintain bring the body weight towards normal.
2. To keep blood plasma lipids especially total and lipoprotein cholesterol as well as triglycerides within normal level or to attain normal level in the event of these being elevated.
3. To keep the blood pressure within normal limits.

In view of the effect of different dietary components on the level of blood lipids and blood pressure, the following guidelines could be used to take stock of the nutritional requirements:

a. Energy intake should commensurate with energy expenditure, and even in the case of the person being overweight, less than the expenditure to affect weight reduction.

b. As a matter of fact, excess energy ingested in one or the other macronutrient form eventually gets converted into fat and stored causing overweight and obesity. Moreover, overweight directly promotes other risk factors for atherosclerosis or CHD such as diabetes mellitus and hypertension. Thus maintaining ideal body weight or even a shade lower than that goes a long way in preventing or managing hypertension, diabetes mellitus and CHD. Since animal foods are rich in saturated fat and cholesterol it is absolutely essential that diet in the middle adulthood becomes based on plant foods as a major some of calories. Cereal pulse based diets with an abundance of fruits and vegetables as well as low fat dairy products can well provide the requisite nutrients without adding much energy to the diet.

c. Whereas a normal intake of proteins is sufficient for adequate nutrition proteins of vegetarian origin with fat free milk, lean meats and egg white should become protein sources.

d. Not more than 20 percent of the total energy requirement should come from fat, with an equal ratio of saturated fatty acids (SFA), monosaturated fatty acids (MUFA) and polyunsaturated fatty acids (PUFA) making up for them a-linolenic acid (ALNA) present in plant foods and long chain n-3 fatty acids (eicosapentanoic and docosahexanoic acids) present in fish prove beneficial anti-thrombotic effects. Besides, they also reduce blood triglycerides levels and are thus protective in nature. In general, a total of 20-25 g of visible fat should make for the fat intake with two or more visible fat making for it. Since animal foods such as whole milk, butter, ghee, red meat and eggs are abundant in saturated fatty acids which promote cholesterol synthesis, it is prudent to restrict these foodstuffs in the diet. Similarly cholesterol containing foods like organ meats and egg yolk should be restricted as total daily cholesterol intake from diet should not exceed 200 mg. Further calorie distribution need not be different from that for the diabetic diet with complex carbohydrate making up the carbohydrate making up the carbohydrate making up the carbohydrate component of 60-65% of total caloric intake.

e. In addition, mineral intake should become adequate with an emphasis laid on minerals like potassium and calcium. To control hypertension, it is important to restrict sodium to 100-200 mg/day for a moderate hypertensive and 500-1000 mg/day for a severe one.

f. Besides, adequate vitamin intake along with antioxidants like β-carotene, tocopherols and l-ascorbate levels in the diet are also important.

g. Further, about 50 g of dietary fiber, abundantly of soluble nature derived from fruits, gums and pectins should also be included in the daily diet. Another factor that we neglect often is the intake of clean potable water. A minimum of 2.0 to 2.5 litre water must become part of the daily diet.

Furthermore, dietary management also calls for a consistent dietary pattern with judicious distribution of nutrients and meal spacing. Some other points worthy of consideration have been given below:

1. Overeating is not desirable and meals small in quantity and more in frequency.
2. Fat requirement is met more from plant based foods so as to ensure more of MUFA and PUFA and less of SFA. The overall limit of fat intake must be observed.
3. Requirement for carbohydrate should be fulfilled from foodstuffs supplying complex carbohydrates. Table sugar or foods rich in it should not provide more than 10% of total calories.
4. Pressure cooked, boiled and baked foods should get precedence over fried and fatty foods.
5. Utmost discretion exercised to avoid processed foods, sodium rich foods and table salt in the diet.
6. Whole fruits and vegetables are liberally included in the diet for getting antioxidant and other photochemical.

Following is the list of foodstuffs that could be taken liberally sparingly and rarely respectively:

In a nutshell, dietary management can certainly reduce the risk of CHD and hypertension through a balanced diet which has been normalized for energy, quality and content of fat (SFA:MUFA:PUFA) cholesterol, vitamins and minerals, fiber, salt and antioxidants. Inclusion of natural and whole in terms of cereals, millets, legumes and pulses with fat free milk and products thereof with an attendant abundance of fruits and vegetables, work wonders.

STUDY QUESTIONS

1. What precautions might one take to prevent hypertension and atherosclerosis?
2. What occurs in severe myocardial infarction or heart attack? Explain.
3. Discuss the dietary management in diabetes mellitus.
4. Write a note on hypertension and its nutritional management.
5. Explain the various types of diabetes mellitus describe laboratory diagnosis of the disease.
6. Discuss the dietary management of diabetes mellitus.
7. Discuss the occurrence of atherosclerosis.
8. Explain hypertension and its dietary management.

CHAPTER 28

Diet in Renal Disorders

Chapter Outlines

- Renal functioning
- Types of renal disorders
- Nutritional treatment of renal disorders
- Study questions

RENAL FUNCTIONING

Uropoiesis, the urine formation, takes place in kidney tubules or nephrons by a process involving ultra filtration of blood to yield glomerular filtrate. This filtrate gets transformed into urine after going through tubular reabsorption and active secretion.

The kidneys are intricate and efficient processing systems that excrete wastes, maintain volume and composition of body fluids, and secrete certain hormones. To accomplish these tasks, they filter the blood, cleansing it of waste products, and recycle other usable substances so that the necessary constituents of body fluids are constantly available.

Each kidney contains approximately one million working parts called nephrons. Each nephron contains a filtering unit called a glomerulus in which there is a cluster of specialized capillaries (tiny blood vessels connecting veins and arteries). Approximately 180 litres of fluid or filtrate (substance) to be filtered are processed each day. As the filtrate passes through the nephrons, the kidneys are able to concentrate or dilute it to meet the body's needs. This enables the kidneys to help maintain both the composition and the volume of body fluids and, consequently, fluid balance, acid base balance, and electrolyte balance. The waste materials are sent via two tubes called ureters from the kidneys to the bladder from which they are excreted in urine. These include end products of protein metabolism (urea, uric acid, creatinine, ammonia and sulphates), excess water, dead renal cells, and toxic substances. The recycled materials are resorbed (taken back) by the blood. They include amino acids, glucose, minerals, vitamins and water.

The kidneys synthesize and secrete certain hormones as needed. For example, it is the kidneys that make the final conversion of vitamin D into its active form 1 ? 25 - dihydroxy D3, so it can play its role in the absorption of calcium. The kidneys indirectly stimulate the bone marrow to produce red blood cells.

As the kidneys excrete waste products of the body in general, and the end-products of protein metabolism in particular, urea is one of the major end-products of protein metabolism (breakdown). The normal daily excretion of urea is about 30 g (500 mol), which is more than that of any other solid excreted in the urine. On a mixed diet, about half the urinary urea is derived from ingested food and the rest from breakdown of tissue proteins. The maximum capacity of the kidney to concentrate urea is 4%. In order to excrete 30 g of urea at the maximum concentration (4%), the minimum urine voided should be 750 ml.

At the onset of acute kidney disease, the urine output is markedly diminished. Urea and the other end-products of protein metabolism are retained. The formation of these waste products can be considerably diminished by restricting the intake of dietary proteins and diminishing the breakdown of tissue proteins by supplying 'protein sparers' like carbohydrates and fats.

The intake of proteins cannot be restricted indiscriminately. Urea clearance is diminished on a low protein vegetarian diet, and the function of the kidney improves on a high protein diet. Adequate proteins should therefore be supplied as soon as the kidney recover and normal urinary flow is resumed.

TYPES OF RENAL DISORDERS

Kidney disorders can be initially caused by infection, degenerative changes, cardiovascular disorders, cysts (growths), renal calculi (stones), or trauma (surgery burns, poisons). When they are severe, renal failure may develop. It may be acute or chronic. Acute renal failure occurs suddenly and may last a few days or a few weeks. It is caused by another medical problem such as a serious burn, a crushing injury, or cardiac arrest. It can be expected in some of these situations so preventive steps may be taken.

Chronic renal failure develops slowly with the number of functioning nephrons constantly diminishing. When renal tissue has been destroyed to the point that the kidneys are no longer able to filter the blood, excrete wastes, or recycle nutrients as needed, uremia occurs. Uremia is a condition in which protein wastes that should normally have been excreted are instead circulating in blood. Symptoms include nausea, headache, coma, and convulsions. Severe renal failure will result in death unless dialysis (machine filtration to remove toxic substances) is begun or a kidney transplant is performed.

Nephritis is a general term referring to the inflammatory disease of the kidneys. Nephritis can be caused by infection, degenerative processes, or vascular disease.

Glomerulonephritis is a nephritis affecting the capillaries in the glomerular. It may occur acutely in conjunction with another infection and is self-limiting, or it may expand and lead to serious renal deterioration.

Nephrosclerosis is the hardening of renal arteries. It is caused by arteriosclerosis and hypertension. Although it usually occurs in older people, it sometimes develops in young diabetics.

Polycystic kidney disease is a relatively rare, hereditary disease. Cysts form and press on the kidneys. The kidneys enlarge and lose function. Although people with this condition have normal kidney function for many years, renal failure may develop near the age of 50 years.

Renal calculi or nephrolithiasis is a condition in which stones develop in the kidneys, the ureters, or the bladder. The size varies from that of a grain of sand to much larger. Some remain at their point of origin and others move. While the condition is sometimes asymptomatic, symptoms include hematuria (blood in urine), infection, obstruction and, if the stones move, intense pain. The stones are classified according to their composition - calcium, uric acid, cystine (amino acid), and oxalic acid. They are associated with metabolic disturbances and immobilization of the patient.

Most commonly kidney diseases may manifest as in one of the following forms:

1. Acute glomerulonephritis, characterized by red blood cells and casts in the urine, scanty urine, swelling of the body, and high blood pressure. The most common cause of this is acute nephritis (Ellis type I), which is possibly an allergic reaction in the kidneys to streptococcal infection, with complete recovery in the vast majority.
2. Nephrotic syndrome (type II nephritis), characterized by gradual onset of body swelling with massive protein loss in the urine. Complete recovery is infrequent. There is usually no retention of nitrogenous waste products in the early stages. The total quantity of urine excreted may be normal.

   Nephrotic syndrome is defined by excretion of more than 3.5 g protein per day in the urine; serum albumin concentration below 30 g per litre; total serum protein below 60 g per litre; raised serum cholesterol values; and presence of oedema without any other apparent cause. There is increase in synthesis of low density lipoprotein B and its normal catabolism.

   Causes include Kimmelstiel-Wilson syndrome, disseminated lupus, and bilateral renal vein thrombosis especially secondary to amyloid disease, amyloidosis, malaria and syphilis.
3. Chronic renal failure is characterized by decrease in urine output or increased urine of low specific gravity, high blood pressure, heart failure, mental confusion and dehydration.

NUTRITIONAL TREATMENT OF RENAL DISORDERS

Dietary Treatment of Renal Disease

The dietary treatment of renal disease can be extremely complicated. It is intended to reduce the amount of excretory work demanded of the kidneys while assisting them in maintaining fluid, acid base, and electrolyte balance. Patients require sufficient protein to prevent malnutrition and muscle wasting. Too much, however, can contribute to uremia. Typically, the patient with chronic renal failure will have protein and sodium, and possibly potassium and phosphorous, restricted.

It is essential that renal patients receive sufficient kcal–35 to 40 kcal per kilogram of body weight–unless they are overweight. Energy requirements should be fulfilled by carbohydrate and fat. The fat must be polyunsaturated to prevent or check hyperlipidemia. If the energy requirement is not met by carbohydrate and fat, ingested protein or body tissue will be metabolized for energy. Either would increase the work for kidneys because protein increases the amount of nitrogen wastes the kidney must handle. The diet may limit protein to 20 grams. The specific amount of protein allowed is calculated according to the patient's glomerular filtration rate (GFR) and weight. Rarely, protein may be increased in an effort to increase blood protein, and the requirement can go as high as 125 grams.

Sodium may be limited if the patient tends to retain it. Retained sodium and water could contribute to oedema, hypertension and congestive heart failure. Fluids are typically restricted for renal patients.

Calcium supplements may be prescribed. In addition, vitamin D may be added and phosphorous limited, to prevent osteomalacia (softening of the bones due to excessive loss of calcium). Phosphorous appears to be retained in patients with kidney disorders, and a disproportionately high ratio of phosphorous to calcium tends to increase calcium loss from bones.

Potassium may be restricted in some patients because hyperkalemia (high blood potassium) tends to occur in renal failure. Excess potassium can cause cardiac arrest. Because of this danger, renal patients should not use salt substitutes or low sodium milk because the sodium in these products is replaced with potassium. Potassium restriction can be especially difficult for a renal patient who probably must limit sodium intake. Potassium is particularly high in fruits–one of the few foods a patient on a sodium restricted diet may eat without concern.

Renal patients often have an increased need for vitamins B, C and D and supplements are often given. Vitamin A should not be given because the blood level of vitamin A tends to be elevated in uremia. If a patient is receiving antibiotics, vitamin K supplements may be given. Otherwise, supplements of vitamin E and K are not necessary. Iron is commonly prescribed because anaemia frequently develops in renal patients. To ensure enough energy, it is sometimes necessary to increase the amount of simple carbohydrates and fats.

Diet in acute and chronic glomerulonephritis

Exchange	*No. of exchange*	*Protein*	*Sodium*	*K calories*
Milk	2	16	40	340
Legumes and pulses	2	14	30	200
Meat	½	3.5	–	35
Veg A*	2	2	20	40
Veg B*	2	4	20	80
Fruits*	2	–	20	80
Cereals	10	20	250	700
Fat	5	–	–	225
Sugar	4	–	–	80
Total		59.5	370	1780

* Vegetables and fruits containing sodium less than 10 mg % should be used.

Menu Plan

Breakfast	:	Milk 1 glass
		Bread 2 bread
		Omlett
		Fruit (banana)
Lunch	:	Chapatti 2
		Rice 1 bowl
		Dal 1 bowl
		Veg of bottleguard 1 bowl
		Curd with sugar 1 cup
Afternoon	:	Upma
		Fruit (Orange)
Dinner	:	Roti 2
		Rice 1 bowl
		Dal 1 bowl
		Vegetable 1 bowl
		Curd 1 cup

Diet in nephrotic syndrome				
Exchange	*No. of exchange*	*Protein*	*Sodium*	*K calories*
Milk	2	16	40	340
Legumes and pulses	4	28	60	400
Meat	1	7	–	70
Veg A*	2	2	20	40
Veg B *	2	4	20	80
Fruits*	2	–	20	80
Cereals	10	20	250	700
Fat	5	–	–	225
Sugar	5	–	–	100
Total		77	400	2035

* Vegetables and fruits containing sodium less than 10 mg % should be used.

Menu Plan

Breakfast : Rice kheer
Fruit
Boiled egg
Lunch : Chapatti 3
Rice 1 bowl
Dal 1 bowl
Vegetable 1 bowl
Curd 1 cup
Afternoon : Dalia
Dinner : Roti 2
Rice 1 bowl
Dal 1 bowl
Vegetable 1 bowl
Curd 1 cup

Diet in chronic renal failure				
Exchange	*No. of exchange*	*Protein*	*Sodium*	*K calories*
Milk	2	16	40	340
Legumes and pulses	2	14	30	200
Meat	1/2	3.5	–	35
Veg A	3	3	30	60
Veg B	3	6	30	120
Fruits	3	–	30	120
Cereals	10	20	250	700
Fat	5	–	–	225
Sugar	4	–	–	80
Total		62.5	410	1880

Menu Plan

Breakfast : Methi paratha
Banana shake
Lunch : Chapatti 2
Rice 1 bowl
Dal 1 bowl
Vegetable curry 1 bowl
Curd 1 cup
Afternoon : Omlett sandwich
Fruit
Dinner : Roti 2
Rice 1 bowl
Dal 1 bowl
Palak curry 1 bowl
Curd 1 cup
Late night : Fruit

Diet During Dialysis

Dialysis patients may need additional protein, but the amount must be carefully controlled to prevent the accumulation of protein waste between treatments.

Potassium levels will vary and must be carefully monitored. Some patients will require supplements, whereas other patients will have potassium restricted. Fluids and sodium are usually restricted to prevent fluid retention. There is often a need for supplements of water soluble vitamins, vitamin D, calcium and iron.

Diet After Kidney Transplant

After kidney transplant, there may be a need for extra protein or for the restriction of protein. Carbohydrates and sodium may be restricted. The appropriate amounts of these nutrients will depend largely on the medications given at that time.

Additional calcium and phosphorous may be necessary if there has been substantial bone loss before the transplant. There may be an increase in appetite after transplants. To prevent excessive weight gain, fats and simple carbohydrates may be limited.

Dietary Treatment of Renal Calculi

Because the causes of renal calculi have not been confirmed, their treatment of them may vary. Generally however, large amounts of fluid–at least half of its water–are helpful in diluting the urine, as is a well balanced diet. Once the stones have been analyzed, specific dietary modifications may be indicated.

Alkaline ash and acid ash diets are sometimes used in an effort to change the pH of the urine and consequently, the incidence of stones. In these diets, foods are labelled by the ash they leave after oxidation. If the ash is acid, the food is labelled acid ash; if alkaline, it is labelled alkaline as. Foods that cause the urine to become acidic (a pH below 7) are called acid ash and those that cause the urine to become alkaline (a pH above 7), alkaline ash. Both diets become tedious and difficult to follow.

Calcium Stones

About two thirds of the kidney stones formed contain calcium. If the patient has a history of calcium stones, this mineral is restricted in the diet, but not usually to less than 600 mg per day. Obviously, foods rich in calcium will have to be limited.

Uric Acid Stones

When the stones contain uric acid, purine rich foods may be restricted. Purines are the end products of nucleoprotein metabolism and are found in all meats, fish and poultry. Organ meats, meat extracts and soups are especially rich sources of them.

Oxalic Acid Stones

Stones containing oxalic acid are thought to be partially caused by a diet especially rich in oxalic acid, which is found in broccoli, aspargus, chocolate, tea and spinach. Evidence also indicates that deficiencies of pyridoxine, thiamine, and magnesium may contribute to the formation of oxalic acid kidney stones.

Cystine Stones

Cystine is an amino acid. Cystine stones may form when the cystine concentration in the urine becomes excessive due to a hereditary metabolic disorder. The usual practice is to increase fluids and recommend an alkaline ash diet.

Purine rich foods

Avoid	*Limit*
Liver	Meats
Kidneys	Fish
Sweetbreads	Poultry
Brains	Meat soups
Heart	
Sardines	
Meat extracts	
Broth	

The High Protein Diet

The high protein diet is a regular diet with increased protein content. The protein is provided by normal protein rich foods and may be further increased by the addition of skim milk powder to soups, cream sauces, gravies and baked products. It is highly nutritious. It may be used for patients following surgery or during convalescence from burns.

The Low Protein Diet

When a low protein diet is prescribed, it is important that the protein be equally distributed among the three meals. This diet contains insufficient protein, minerals, vitamins, and in some cases, kcal.

Table Foods Included in a High Protein Diet

Milk in large amount (3 to 4 cups)

Cheese

Eggs

Lean meats, fish and poultry

Vegetables

Fruits

Cereals (whole grain or enriched) and breads as desired

Patients Deserving Consideration From a Health Care Professional

The patient with renal disease has a severe burden. Anger and depression are common among these patients. These feelings complicate management of the disease if they contribute to the patient's unwillingness to learn about his or her nutritional needs. These complications then add to the patient's problems.

The health care professional can be extremely helpful if he or she can develop a trusting relationship with the patient. Such a relationship can be established by listening to the patient's complaints, needs, and concerns and responding with sincere understanding and sympathy. This can ultimately help motivate the patient who wants to learn how to manage his or her nutritional requirements and help the nutrition counsellor assist the patient.

STUDY QUESTIONS

1. Discuss the three main tasks of the kidneys.
2. Define nephrons and explain what they do.
3. Discuss some causes of kidney disease.
4. What is nephritis, glomerulonephritis and nephro-sclerosis?
5. Why is diet therapy of renal disease so complex?

CHAPTER 29

Nutrition in Surgery, Burns, Infections and AIDS

Chapter Outlines

- Repercussions of physical stress or trauma
- Nutritional care of surgical patients
- Nutritional care of burns patients
- Nutritional therapy in infections and fevers
- Role of nutrition in infections
- Diet in typhoid
- Diet in tuberculosis
- Nutritional care of AIDS patients
- Study questions

REPERCUSSIONS OF PHYSICAL STRESS OR TRAUMA

Normally the human body operates in a state of homeostasis (balanced, stable condition) but when the body experiences the trauma (serious physical stress) of surgery, severe burns, or infections, this balance becomes upset and the body reacts in an attempt to restore itself back to homeostasis.

During its response to physical stress, the body sends the signals to the endocrine system, which activates a self-protective, hypermetabolic response. This causes an increase in the energy output. The intensity of the response depends on the severity of condition. The mediators of response, human are a pair of small golden colored glandular structures called 'Adrenals' that lie over the top of the kidneys. The glands mediate stress response through their hormonal secretions. Each gland comprises two portions, outer cortex and central medulla. Interestingly, the two portions secrete two different kinds of hormones differing in action, stimulus and chemistry. The cells of medulla are known to secrete hormones epinephrine and norepinephrine, collectively known as catecholamines. They bring about a number of biochemical changes that enable an individual to adapt as much as possible to a sudden short term stress. The hormonal secretions of the cortex, on the other hand, aid the body to adapt itself to a long-term stress. Also, in a sharp contrast to the rapid fire action of catecholamine, the cortical hormones act in a slow, steady and sustained manner. As a consequence of adrenal hormonal interplay, catabolism occurs, causing the rapid breakdown of energy reserves to provide glucose and other substances necessary for the anabolic phase of wound healing and tissue maintenance. Proteins, fats and minerals are lost in the catabolic phase just when there is an increased need for them to rebuild tissues. When the condition includes hemorrhage and vomiting, these losses are compounded. Sufficient nutrients, fluids, and calories are required as soon as possible to replace the losses, build and repair tissues and return the body to the native state of homeostasis. Obviously, nutrition has to play an important role in the upkeep of patients undergoing surgery or of those who suffer from burns or infections.

NUTRITIONAL CARE OF SURGICAL PATIENTS

Presurgery Nutritional Care

Surgery becomes a kind of stress for the patient regardless of whether it is routine or emergency. If routine, the patient's nutritional status should be evaluated before surgery, and if improvement is needed, it should be undertaken. A good nutritional status before surgery enhances recovery. A nutritional assessment of the patient before surgery will be helpful to the dietician in providing foods that will be accepted by the patient after surgery when appetite and inclination to eat are poor.

Improvement of nutritional status means providing extra protein, carbohydrates, vitamins and minerals. The extra protein is needed for wound healing, tissue building, and blood generation. Extra carbohydrates are be converted to glycogen and stored, to help provide energy after surgery, when needs are high, and when patients may not become able to eat normally. The B vitamins are needed for the increased metabolism, vitamin A and C for wound healing, vitamin D for the absorption of calcium and vitamin K for proper clotting of the blood. Iron is necessary for blood building, calcium and phosphorous for bones, and other minerals for maintenance of acid base, electrolyte, and fluid balance in the body.

In cases of overweight, improved nutritional status includes weight reduction before surgery whenever possible. Excess fat is a surgical hazard because the extra tissue increases the chances of infection and fatty tissue tends to retain the anaesthesia longer than other tissues. Food usually is not allowed to the patients after the evening meal on the day before surgery. This ensures that the stomach contains no food, which could be regurgitated and then aspirated (taken into the airway), during surgery. Likewise, a low residue diet may become the object of choice for a few days before surgery. This is intended to reduce intestinal residue and thus the need for defecation.

Post-Surgery Nutritional Care

Surgery patients are examples of persons with increased needs who may inadvertently be starved. Often a surgical patient must be starved for 8 hours to 24 hours before surgery. In the process of anaesthesia for surgery, the peristalsis of the gut slows down. All muscle movement, including the swallowing mechanisms, are anaesthetized. It is not safe for a patient to try to eat a normal meal immediately after surgery because the digestive tract needs time to begin functioning normally again. Ordinarily this means that what the diet provided is inadequate to meet the patient's elevated needs. Depending on the surgery, recovery may be slow and some studies have indicated that upto 50% of all surgical patients have some degree of protein-calorie malnutrition. Malnutrition may result from increased needs, difficulty in adequate eating, digesting, or absorbing nutrients, starvation, or the complications that can result from surgery. The most common and potentially most dangerous complication is infection.

The post surgery diet is intended to provide energy and other nutrients in amounts sufficient to fulfil the patient's increased metabolic needs and to promote healing and subsequent recovery. In general, for the 24-hours immediately following surgery, most patients are given intravenous solutions only. These solutions contain water, 5 to 10 percent dextrose, electrolytes, vitamins, and medications as needed. The maximum number of energy supplied by them is about 400 to 500 kcal per 24-hour period. The estimated daily kcal requirement for adults after surgery is 35 to 45 per kilogram of body weight. A 50 kg individual would require at least 2000 kcal per day. Obviously, until the patient can take enough food, there will be a considerable energy deficit each day. Body fat will be used to provide energy and to spare body protein, but the energy intake must be increased to meet energy demands as soon as possible.

Because protein losses following surgery can be significant and the fact that protein is especially needed then to rebuild tissue, control edema, avoids shock, resist infection, and transport fats, a high protein diet of 80 to 100 grams a day may be recommended. In addition, extra minerals and vitamins are needed. When peristalsis returns, ice chips may be given and, if they are tolerated, a clear liquid diet can follow.

Normally in postoperative cases, patients proceed from the clear liquid diet to the regular diet. Sometimes this is done directly, and sometimes by way of the full liquid, soft, or residue restricted diets. It depends on the patient and the type of surgery. The average patient will be able to take food within one to four days after surgery. If the patient cannot take food then, parenteral or tube feeding may be necessary. Sometimes following gastric surgery, dumping syndrome occurs within 15 to 30 minutes after eating. This is characterized by dizziness, weakness, cramps, vomiting and diarrhea. It is caused by food moving too quickly from the stomach into the small intestine.

To prevent dumping syndrome, the diet should remain high in protein and fat with carbohydrates remaining somewhat restricted. Foods should contain little fibre or concentrated sugars and only limited amounts of starch. Complex carbohydrates are gradually reintroduced. This is recommended because carbohydrates leave the stomach faster than do proteins and fats. Fluids should be limited to 100 ml at meals, or, even restricted completely. They can be taken 30 minutes after meals. The total daily food intake may be divided and served as several small meals rather than the usual three meals, in an attempt to avoid overloading the stomach. Some patients do not tolerate milk well after gastric surgery so its inclusion in the diet will depend on the patient's tolerance or lack of it. The food habits of the postoperative patients should be closely observed because they will affect recovery. When the patient's failing appetite is notified, and efforts made to offer nutritious foods than the patient eats. The patient should be encouraged to eat and to eat slowly to avoid swallowing air, which can cause abdominal distension and pain.

NUTRITIONAL CARE OF BURNS PATIENTS

In cases of serious burns, the loss of skin surface leads to enormous losses of fluids, electrolytes and proteins. Water moves from other tissues to the burn site in an effort to compensate for the loss, but this only compounds the problem. This fluid loss can reduce the blood volume and thus blood pressure and urine output. Fluids and electrolytes are replaced by intravenous therapy mainly to prevent shock. Glucose should not become part of these fluids for the first two or three days after the burn because it could cause hyperglycemia.

Burns cause tremendous losses. The greatest loss is fluids, and fluid replacement is usually the first, most immediate treatment. Fluid losses can quickly lead to electrolyte imbalances, shock and death. Treatment, therefore, usually begins with fluids, often the fluids called Lactated Ringer's solution, a mixture of sterile water and electrolytes but without any nutrients providing energy.

As soon as the immediate crisis is over, nutrition support is started.

The hypermetabolic state after a serious burn continues until the skin is largely healed. This means an enormous increase in energy is needed for the healing process. Energy needs can be more than 3500 kcal per day because of the increased metabolic rate and to spare protein for tissue building. Daily protein needs can be as high as 150 g or more. A high-protein, high-energy diet is used. There is an increased need for vitamin C for healing and B vitamins for the metabolism of the extra nutrients.

Also, it is essential that badly burned patients have sufficient fluids to help the kidneys hold the unusual load of wastes in solution and to replace those lost.

If the patient can eat, oral feedings are advisable. Liquid commercial formulas may be used at first, and solid food may be added during the second week following the burn. If the patient cannot eat, tube feedings will be necessary. In some cases, parenteral feeding is required.

The foods served should be those the patient likes, and services should be as attractive as possible. Burn patients need a great deal of encouragement. They may be in pain, worried about disfigurement, and know they face along, costly, and painful hospital stay, with the possibility of surgery.

NUTRITIONAL THERAPY IN INFECTIONS AND FEVERS

Infection is the successful invasion, establishment and growth of microorganisms in the tissues of the host. A healthy person has adequate immunity to infections. However, this ability is reduced by a poor nutritional status and malnourished person easily infectious becomes victim of an infection which weakens the immune response of a person as it also deteriorates the nutritional status of a person.

Defence Mechanisms of the Body

The body has two types of defence mechanisms: Specific and Non-specific as per the details given below:

The common health deteriorating adverse effects of infection are as follows:

Specific and non-specific defence mechanisms of human body

Specific	*Non specific*	
• Cell mediated immunity	• Skin	• Hormonal factors
T-lymphocytes	• Mucous membranes	• Iron binding protein
• Humoral immunity	• Collagen	• Nutrients like vitamin A, C
B-lymphocytes	• Body secretions	• Protein
• Plasma accessory cells	• Pyrexia (fever)	• Zinc
• Antibodies	• Intestinal micro flora	• WBC

1. There are increased losses of nitrogen, some electrolytes like potassium and phosphates and other elements such as magnesium and zinc.
2. If there is fever along with an infection, then the energy needs are increased since the metabolic rate also increases with high temperature.
3. There is decrease in food intake due to nausea and loss of appetite.
4. Loss of nutrients is increased due to increased perspiration, vomiting and diarrhoea.
5. There is a decrease in the absorption of nutrients especially in case of enteric infections such as typhoid fever.

ROLE OF NUTRITION IN INFECTIONS

People with poor nutritional status are not only prone to infection but they also take a longer time to recover from infection whenever they fall prey to it. In our country, infants and preschoolers form the most vulnerable group to malnutrition. Immunity, as is well-known, is a complex result of many components, some native and heritable, others acquired. Specific antibodies fight the infection. Since antibodies are made up of proteins; the protein status of an individual determines his/her capacity to resist the invading infection. Obviously, poor nutritional status results in lowered resistance to infections.

Fever and Its Effects on Metabolism

Pyrexia or fever is increase in body temperature above the normal (37° C) which may occur in response to an infection or due to unknown causes as pyrexia of unknown origin (PUO).

The agents that cause fever may be microorganisms, the bacteria, viruses or fungi or antigen-antibody reactions, cancer of a tissue or malaria or tissue graft rejection reactions. Further, a fever can be of short duration–as in acute infection which last for a few hours or a few days like colds, influenza etc or of long duration–as in malaria, tuberculosis and typhoid which last from several days to several weeks.

Fever typically accompanies an infection. Fevers and infections may be acute or chronic. Fever is a hypermetabolic state in which each degree of fever on the Celsius scale raises the BMR 12 percent. If extra kcal is not provided during fever, the body first uses its supply of glycogen, then its stored fat, and finally its own muscle tissue for energy.

Sepsis is that kind of infection that spreads throughout the body; is always caused by bacteria. Infection can affect a small area, such as the area directly opened by the surgery, or it can become severe. If the bacteria that cause the infection spread to other areas or enter the blood (septicemia), it may become very difficult to control the process as they cause great damage, and lead to many more days in the hospital before the patient recovers fully. Fever is usually a sign that in a section of patients is present somewhere. Minor infection may raise the resting metabolism by 15%-40%, but severe sepsis may cause basic needs to rise 40-50% and almost double nitrogen losses. Since the body's immune system is composed of proteins that will work well only as long as they do not need to be used for energy, nutrition is a vital partner to medical (usually antibiotic) treatment used in fighting sepsis.

Effects of Fever on Metabolic Processes in the Body

Fever affects all the metabolic processes of the body as given in brief below:

1. The metabolic rate increases by 13% for every degree Celsius rise in body temperature. This increases the energy needs of the body during fever.
2. Glycogen stores of the body are depleted along with the fat stores since they provide for the increase in the caloric needs.
3. Due to an increase in the breakdown of proteins, there is an increase in excretion of protein wastes by the kidneys.
4. There is an excess loss of body fluids due to high rate of perspiration.
5. There is increased excretion of the electrolytes, sodium and potassium.

Effects on Nutrient Requirements

1. Even in the absence of fever, protein catabolism increases.
2. Energy requirement is increased by 10 to 30% during and after acute infections. Vitamin requirements are also increased to support high metabolism.
3. Requirement of zinc and iron increases since both are involved in the immunity process. Zinc excretion in urine is increased and destruction of the red blood cells cause zinc and iron losses respectively.

Nutrient Alterations

1. **Energy:** The intake of energy should be increased to one and a half times in case of high fevers lasting for

long periods. Since fever tells upon the patient's appetite and digestion may also be affected, hence to make up for this the maximum number of calories that can be utilised without discomfort should be given.

2. **Carbohydrates:** They should be high and given as liberal as possible. It is a must to add glucose in all liquids and fruit juices given to the patient.
3. **Protein:** Just as the energy needs increase, so does the need for protein. A high protein diet supplying about 1.25 to 1.5 g proteins per kg body weight should be given. Protein supplements, given blended with beverages, could prove useful. Protein intake should be increased during fever to one or two grams per kilograms of body weight. Protein is needed to replace body tissue and to produce antibodies to fight the infection. Minerals are needed to help build and repair body tissue and to maintain acid base, electrolyte, and fluid balance. Extra energy is needed for the increased metabolic rate. Extra vitamins are also necessary for the increased metabolic rate and to help fight the infection causing the fever. Extra liquid is needed to replace that lost through perspiration and possibly vomiting and diarrhea that can accompany the infection.
4. **Fats:** These can be used liberally by prudently including foods which contain large amount of fats.
5. **Minerals:** Loss of electrolytes, sodium and potassium, should be made up. Sodium in the form of salt in soups, dals and curries and broths should be given liberally.

   Potassium, which is also needed in greater amounts, should be given through fruit juices and milk which are good sources of potassium.
6. **Vitamins:** All vitamins may be given as supplements to the patients.
7. **Fluids:** Since loss of body fluids through perspiration and excretion is high, plenty of water, fruit and vegetable juices and soups need be given.
   1. **Texture and Consistency of the Diet:** Soft texture and fluid to semi solid consistency are desirable to promote appetite and help the patient to consume a diet which is nutritionally adequate. The feedings should be small and as many as possible.
   2. Generally six to eight feedings become sufficient. Patients usually have very poor appetites with fever, but they will often accept ice water, fruit juice, and carbonated beverages.

Usually, the diet during fever and infection progresses from the liquid to the regular diet with frequent, small meals recommended. It should be high protein, high kcal, and high vitamin. In some cases, parenteral and enteral feedings are necessary.

DIET IN TYPHOID

Fever in typhoid is of a long duration. The rise in temperature is very high, thus causing significant damage to the nutritional status of the person. Antibiotic therapy helps a lot to curb the fever but howsoever short the period of antibiotic therapy may be, protein losses are very high, glycogen stores of the body are depleted to a very large extent and the water balance too may be affected severely. The antibiotic therapy also kills the beneficial symbiotic bacterial flora of the intestines.

In typhoid or enteric fever the intestines are the worst affected part of the body. They become inflamed and irritated and in several cases diarrhoea may be a frequent complication. If sufficient care is not taken, ulceration of the intestines may take place which may lead to bleeding, and the intestine may perforate in worst cases a resulting in the death of the patient.

Dietary Modifications

Dietary modification is similar to those given in case of fevers of short duration. However, caution must be exercised in preventing inclusion of irritating dietary fibres. All whole grain cereals and cereal products, leafy vegetables, raw vegetables and fruits should be eliminated from the diet. Tender meat, fish and poultry, potatoes, soft cooked vegetables and simple preparations restricting the use of excessive fat and spices is advised. A diet recommended in typhoid goes as under:

Diet in typhoid

Exchange	*No. of exchange*	*Protein*	*K calories*
Milk	2	16	340
Legumes and pulses	3	21	300
Meat	1	7	70
Veg A	2	2	40
Veg B	2	4	80
Fruits	4	–	160
Cereals	10	20	700
Fat	4	–	180
Sugar	6	–	120
Total		70	1990

Menu Plan

Breakfast	:	Milk 1 glass
		Biscuit 2
		Boiled egg 2
		Apple 1
Lunch	:	Chapatti 3
		Rice 1 bowl
		Dal 1 bowl
		Veg of bottleguard 1 bowl
		Curd 1 cup
Afternoon	:	Dal pitha
		Mosambi juice
Dinner	:	Roti 2
		Moong khichdi
		Palak curry 1 bowl
		Curd 1 cup

DIET IN TUBERCULOSIS

Pulmonary or lung tuberculosis is accompanied by cough, spitting of phlegm, fever, exhaustion, wasting of tissue etc. in many cases it leads to pneumonia which can be fatal, or to a slow wasting disease in the bone causing deformities. Tubercular meningitis becomes frequently fatal.

Dietary Modifications

The energy needs are markedly increased due to wasting of tissues. A diet providing 3000 to 3500 kcals, about 75-100 g protein and large amounts of calcium and iron (if there is bleeding) and vitamins A and C are advised for fast recovery and quicker tissue regeneration. B-complex vitamins, especially pyridoxine and folic acid, are prescribed in larger amounts. This is so because the drug, isoniazid, which is commonly used in the treatment of tuberculosis, is an anti-metabolite of pyridoxine and prevents folate dependent reactions.

NUTRITIONAL CARE OF AIDS PATIENTS

Acquired immunodeficiency syndrome (AIDS) is an infectious (contagious) and eventually, a fatal (resulting in death) disease. It is caused by the human immunodeficiency virus (HIV).

As it is well-known that among infectious agents, viruses (Latin virus, venom or poison) are unique as they have simple, a cellular organization and pattern of reproduction. A virus particle or virion is made up of one or more molecules of DNA or RNA enclosed in a coat of protein called capsid, and at times, other layers derived from host cell membranes. A virus is unable to reproduce on its own. Therefore, it needs host cell's machinery in order to reproduce or make multiple copies of itself.

Virus consists of genetic material (RNA or DNA) and the protein envelope shell that encapsulates the genetic material. All cells in the human body have DNA or Deoxyribonucleic acid as their genetic material. A virus whose genetic material is DNA would infect a host cell by injecting its viral DNA into the cell. Then, through a series of events, the viral DNA becomes part of the cellular DNA. The cells, when out to make copies of their own genetic material, inadvertently make copies of virus nucleic acids as well. In this way, the cells of host become a virus nucleic acid factory and eventually make a number of virus particles in the body. Not all viruses have DNA as their genetic material. Some of them also have RNA and such viruses are known to belong to the class of retroviruses. The human immunodeficiency virus (HIV) also belongs to this class. The RNA of this virus gets converted into DNA in the human host cells by the action of the enzyme of virus named reverse transcriptase. Like all viruses, HIV relies on its capacity to subvert cells of the host to make multiple viral copies. Thereafter, one of the main targets of marauding HIV arming is a white blood cell type called a CD4+ T lymphocyte. This damage and destruction of CD4+ T lymphocyte makes the human victim (host) immunodeficient, becoming crippled as far as the defence against infections is concerned.

Since the HIV infection has made large inroads into the developing world, where majority of the population is malnourished, the extent of devastation it is causing in deprived masses is unimaginable. Since long duration of malnutrition operates in a vicious circle of malnourishment and infection, an exposure to HIV makes the lives of teeming masses inhabiting these countries most difficult. Whatever its origin, malnutrition weakens the immune system and heightens vulnerability to infection. An infectious episode leads, in turn, to profound metabolic changes and a decline in nutritional status. This vicious circle of malnutrition and infection can only be broken by acting the favour of nutrition and against infection by identifying and making medicines to combat not only HIV but also to treat malaria, tuberculosis and hepatitis.

Malnutrition is a determining factor of vulnerability to HIV—which directly attacks the cells responsible for immune response—and the more or less rapid onset of AIDS. Adults infected with HIV who have one or more nutritional deficiencies have more pronounced clinical symptoms and a greater propensity to contract AIDS, pregnant women infected with HIV who also have vitamin A deficiency carry a higher risk of transferring the virus to the child during gestation or nursing. HIV/AIDS undermines nutritional status owing to metabolic change brought on by infection and indirectly reduces food supply because of lower working capacity and agricultural production. It is, therefore, imperative to address all forms of nutritional deficiency and to prevent opportunistic infections like pneumonia, tuberculosis and malaria. Access to a proper balanced diet would help people infected with HIV maintain satisfactory nutritional status and improve their quality of life. Since the HIV infection is fraught with dangerous consequences in the undernourished, illiterate sections of the society, women of child bearing age in particular and expectant mothers, if infected with AIDS, carry the double burden of disease on themselves certainly and for their progeny, potentially. Nutritionists have a responsibility to make a special contribution to elevating the suffering of these individuals because good nutrition, do not though cure can help in prolonging life.

As this virus affects the T cells which are white blood cells that protect the body from infections. When T cells cannot function normally, the body offers no resistance to opportunistic infections. Opportunistic infections are caused by microorganisms that are present but don't normally affect people with healthy immune systems. The disease spreads in the following manner:

- Through sexual contact.
- By transfusion of contaminated blood.
- By use of contaminated needles during injections of illegal drugs.
- From infected mothers to their infants before birth.

Symptoms include fever, swollen lymph nodes, anorexia, diarrhoea and weight loss. Patients can develop infections of the lungs, skin, gastrointestinal and central nervous systems. A type of cancer called Kaposi's sarcoma, pneumonia, or severe diarrhea can result in death.

The infections increase the metabolic rate, and thus, nutrient and energy needs, but decrease the appetite and frequently reduce the body's ability to absorb nutrients. Weight loss, hypoalbuminemia (reduced amount of protein in blood) and malnutrition result. The immune system is further damaged by insufficient amounts of proteins and energy. The hazards of giving non-sterile food are enormous and make food selection and preparation for the patient a challenging task.

Feeding Problems

Although a high kcal/high protein diet is advisable, the patient may not accept it. The ravages of the diseases plus the nausea caused by medications contribute to anorexia.

When possible, medications should be given after meals to reduce the possibilities of nausea. Sores in the mouth or oesophagus can make eating painful, and soft foods may be better accepted than others. For the same reasons, spicy or highly acidic foods or foods with extreme temperatures may be rejected. In some cases, it may be useful to discuss food intake and nutritional care with the patient.

Frequent small meals, and sometimes, liquid formulas may be helpful. Additional sugar and flavouring may increase the acceptability of liquid formula. Because of the nausea and diarrhoea, sufficient fluids are essential. If the patient has difficulty swallowing or simply cannot eat, tube feeding may be necessary. The patient should be helped to eat as much as possible. The diet should be as much sterile and germ free as body's immune system is permanently paralyzed and any infection can bloom and cause disease in the face of lack of resistance.

Some patients may want to try unconventional diets, thinking these diets will help or even cure them. Unless these diets are obviously harmful, they can be used. In some cases, the idea of improvement may help the patient's appetite.

Those patients who could be benefited no further from either medication or nutrition can still be helped by the health care professional who shows support, understanding and respect for them.

In a nutshell, surgery, burns, fevers and infections are traumas that cause the body to react hyermetabolically. This creates the need for additional nutrients at the same time that the injury causes a loss of nutrients. Care must be taken to provide extra fluids, proteins, kcal, vitamins, minerals and carbohydrates as needed in these situations. When surgery is elective, nutritional status should be improved before surgery, if necessary. When food cannot be taken orally, tube or parenteral nutrition should be used. Likewise, in AIDS, nutritional intervention is aimed at preventing the erosion of nutritional status so as to make the immunocompromised body battle this vicious disease.

STUDY QUESTIONS

1. In what ways might diet history of a presurgical patient be helpful?
2. Explain why a burn patient needs extra protein. What happens when the extra protein is not provided?
3. Why does a surgical patient need extra minerals?
4. Describe dumping syndrome and tell how it may be alleviated.
5. Define fever and explain its effects on metabolism.
6. Give a brief account of specific and non-specific defence mechanisms of human body.
7. Write briefly the nutritional alterations made in fever.

CHAPTER 30

Nutrition in Cancer

Chapter Outlines

- Cancer eludes etiology
- Cancer-food connection
- Symptoms and treatment options
- Nutritional care of the cancer patients
- Study questions

It is a disease characterized by abnormal cell growth, and can occur in any organ. In some way the genes lose control of cell growth and reproduction becomes unstructured and excessive. The developing mass caused by the abnormal growth is called a tumour or neoplasm (new growth). Cancer is also called neoplasia. Cancerous tumors are malignant (life threatening), affecting the structure, and consequently the function of organs. When cancer cells break away from their original site, move through the blood, and spread to a new site, they are said to metastasize. The mortality rate for cancer patients is high, but cancer does not always cause death. When it is found early in its development, prompt treatment can irradiate it. Oncology is the study of cancer.

CANCER ELUDES ETIOLOGY

The precise etiology of cancer is not known, but it is thought that heredity, viruses, environmental carcinogens (cancer causing substances), and possibly emotional stress contribute to its development. Cancer is not inherited, but some families appear to have a genetic predisposition (inherited tendency) toward it. When such seems to be the case, environmental carcinogens should be carefully avoided and medical check-ups made regularly. Environmental carcinogens include radiation (whether from X-rays, sun, or atomic wastes); certain chemicals ingested in food or water; some chemicals that touch the skin regularly; and certain substances that are breathed in, such as tobacco smoke and asbestos.

Carcinogens are not known to cause cancer from one or even a few exposures, but after prolonged exposure. For example, skin cancers doesn't develop after one sunburn.

CANCER-FOOD CONNECTION

While the relationships of food and cancer have not been proven, there appear to be associations between them—both good and bad. Certain substances in foods, for example, are thought to be carcinogenic. Nitriles in cured and smoked foods such as bacon and ham can be changed to nitrosamines (carcinogens) during cooking. Regular ingestion of these foods is associated with cancers of the stomach and esophagus. High-fat diets have been associated with cancers of the uterus, breast, prostrate and colon. The regular, excessive intake of kcal is associated with cancers of the gallbladder and endometrium (mucous membrane of the uterus). People who smoke and drink alcohol immoderately appear to be at greater risk of cancers of the mouth, pharynx, and esophagus than those who do not.

On the positive side, it is thought that diets high in fibre help to protect against colorectal cancer. Diets containing sufficient amounts of vitamin C rich foods may protect against cancers of the stomach and esophagus. Diets containing sufficient carotene and vitamin A rich foods may protect against cancers of the lung, bladder and larynx.

Cancer: Initiation and Progression

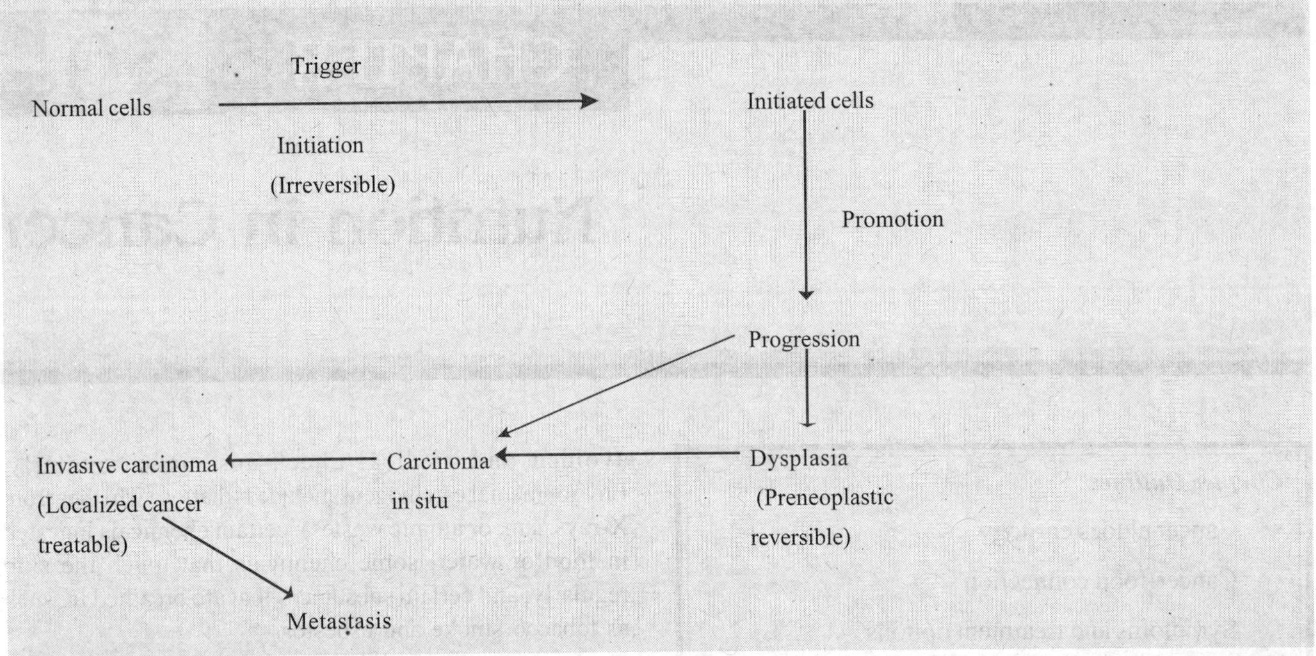

Possible causes of cancer		
Contributing factors	*Chemical factors*	*Biological factors*
Genetics	Industrial agents	Viral
Physical	Mycotoxins	Parasite infestations
Ionizing radiation	Diet-related chemicals	Chronic infections
Ultraviolet radiation (solar)	Tobacco, alcohol	
Asbestos		

Appropriate amounts of protein foods are essential for the maintenance of a healthy immune system. An immune system that has been damaged—possibly through malnutrition—may be a contributing factor in the development of cancer. Excessive protein intake, however, may be a factor in the development of cancer of the colon.

The obvious bottom line here is moderation. The regular, excessive use of carcinogenic foods may contribute to cancer. Vitamins that are thought to prevent cancer should be ingested in foods that naturally contain them. Excessive intake of vitamin supplements can be harmful.

SYMPTOMS AND TREATMENT OPTIONS

One of the first indications of cancer may be unexplained weight loss. This is because the tumor cells use for their own metabolism and development the nutrients the host has taken in. The host may suffer from weakness, and anorexia may occur, which compounds the weight loss. The weight loss includes the loss of muscle tissue and hypoalbuminemia (low albumen content of the blood), and anaemia may develop. The sense of taste and of smell may become abnormal in cancer patients. This may be because of nutrient deficiency. A zinc deficiency, often form aversions to those particular foods. These aversions result in limited acceptance of food and contribute further to the patient's malnutrition. It is preferable that chemotherapy be withheld for two or three hours before and after meals. The appetite and absorption usually improve after chemotherapy so the patient can improve nutritional status between chemotherapy treatments.

Obviously, diet plans for cancer patients require special attention. The patient's diet history should be taken, as usual, at the outset of hospitalization. Kcal and nutrient needs must be determined by the diet counsellor, and the patient's diet plan made in consultation with the patient. It is essential that favourite foods, prepared in familiar ways and served attractively, be included. Nutritious food beautifully served is useless if the patient refuses it. If chewing is a problem, a soft diet may be helpful. If diarrhea is a problem, allow residue diet may help. Patients should be evaluated continuously, but inconspicuously.

If the patient is scheduled to undergo radiation or chemotherapy, these factors must be included in the diet planning.

High protein and high-energy diets may be recommended. Energy demands are high because of the hypermetabolic state often caused by cancer. Calorie needs will vary from patient to patient, but 45 to 50 kcal per kg of body weight may be recommended.

Carbohydrates and fat will be needed to provide this energy and spare protein for tissue building and the immune system. Patients with good nutritional status will need from 80 to 100 grams of protein a day. Malnourished patients may need from 100 to 200 grams of protein a day. Vitamins and minerals are essential for metabolism, tissue maintenance, and appetite, and they may be supplied in supplemental form. Fluids are important to help the kidneys eliminate the metabolic wastes and the toxins from drugs.

The patient's food habits can require change if, before the illness, the patient has scrupulously avoided desserts and high kcal foods to maintain normal weight.

Sometimes patients may be willing to eat foods that are brought from home. Some may find cold foods more appealing than hot foods. Meats may taste bitter so milk, cheese, eggs, and fish may be more appealing. If foods taste less sweet to the cancer patient than to the well person, sugar may be added to juices and fruits. This may please the patient and add kcal to the diet.

Supplementation with high kcal, high protein, liquid foods between meals may be useful, but should not be used if their consumption reduces the patient's appetite at meals.

If the patient suffers from dry mouth, salad dressings, gravies, sauces and syrups appropriately served on foods can be helpful. Several small meals may be better tolerated than three large meals. It is preferable to serve the nutritionally richer meals early in the day because the patient is less tired and may have a better appetite at that time. If nausea or pain are a continuous problem, drugs to control them, particularly at meal times, may be helpful. While oral feedings are definitely preferred, enteral or parenteral feedings may become necessary if cachexia is extreme. Sometimes an oral diet may be used in conjunction with parental feeding. As the patient improves, kcal and nutritional content of the diet should be gradually increased for example, affects the sense of taste. Foods may taste less sweet and more bitter than they would to healthy people. Cancer patients become satiated earlier than normal, possibly because of decreased digestive secretins. Insulin production may be abnormal and hyperglycemia (high levels of blood sugar) can delay the stomach's emptying and dull the appetite. Some cancers cause hypercalcemia. If this is chronic, kidney stones and impaired kidney function can occur.

The effect(s) of cancer on the host is/are particularly determined by the location of a tumor. For example, an esophageal or intestinal tumor can cause blockage in the gastrointestinal tract, causing malabsorption as well. If the cancer is untreated, the continued anorexia and weight loss will create a state of malnutrition, which in turn can lead to cachexia (severe wasting) and ultimately death.

Medical treatments of cancer can include surgical removal, radiation, chemotherapy (drug), or a combination of these methods. These treatments, unfortunately, have side effects that can further undermine the nutritional status of the patient.

Surgery on the mouth, for example, might well affect the ability to chew or swallow. Gastric or intestinal resection (partial removal) can affect absorption and result in nutritional deficiencies. The removal of the pancreas will result in diabetes mellitus.

Radiation can change the senses of taste and smell, particularly if it is done for cancer of the head or neck. It also can cause a decrease in salivary secretions, which cause dry mouth (xerostomia) and difficulty in swallowing (dysphagia). This reduction in saliva also causes tooth decay and sometimes the loss of teeth. Radiation reduces the amount of absorptive tissue in the small intestine. In addition, it can cause bowel obstruction or diarrhea.

Chemotherapy reduces the ability of the small intestine to regenerate absorptive cells, and it can cause hemorrhagic colitis. Both radiation and chemotherapy depress appetite. They may cause nausea, vomiting and diarrhea leading to fluid and electrolyte imbalances. This can lead to fluid retention.

However, when the therapy is completed and the patient is able to return to a well balanced diet, these problems may disappear.

NUTRITIONAL CARE OF THE CANCER PATIENT

The nutrient and kcal needs of the cancer patient are actually greater than they were before the onset of the disease. The cancer causes an increase in the metabolic rate; tissue must be rebuilt; and the nutrients lost to the cancer must be replaced. Patients who can maintain their weight or minimize its loss increase their chances of responding to treatment, and thus, their survival. Patients on high-protein and high kcal diets tolerate the side effects of therapy and higher doses of drugs better than those who cannot eat feel better than those who cannot.

Despite their nutritional needs, however, anorexia is a major problem for cancer patients. It is particularly difficult to combat because cancer patients tend to develop strong food aversions that are thought to be caused by the effects of chemotherapy. Patients receiving chemotherapy near mealtime associate the foods at the meal with the nausea caused by the chemotherapy. The diet counsellor should be at hand to:

1. Explain why it is important that the patient eat.
2. Encourage him/her to eat foods he/she enjoys.
3. Recommend that he/she avoids eating at the time of day when nausea typically occurs.
4. Refrain from serving foods that give off odors and thus which contribute to nausea.

In essence, cancer is a disease characterized by abnormal cell growth. It can strike any body tissue. Energy needs increase because of the hyper metabolic state and the tumor's needs for energy nutrients at the same time anorexia occurs in the patient. Its cause is not known. It causes severe wasting, blockages, anaemia and various metabolic problems. Treatment of cancer includes surgery, radiation and chemotherapy. Improving the patient's nutritional state is difficult because of the illness and anorexia. Parenteral or enteral nutrition may be necessary.

STUDY QUESTIONS

1. Discuss cancer, telling what it is and how it affects body functions and nutritional status.
2. Explain why cancer patients lose weight.
3. Why is the anorexia of cancer patients especially difficult to combat? What causes it?
4. How does one attempt to improve the nutritional status of a cancer patient?

CHAPTER 31

Dietary Management in Ageing

Chapter Outlines

- Introduction
- Nutritional and social interventions to combat ageing
- Dietary management of the elderly
- Study questions

INTRODUCTION

Ageing is a biological process which makes an organism more susceptible to disease and debility because of a gradual erosion in its adaptability to the environment. Though the term ageing implies 'deterioration' and the lexical meaning of the word is 'the process of growing old'; yet to a naïve the word means an increase in the number of years in age. Hence ageing (physiological ageing) may precisely be defined as regression of physiological functioning accompanying advancement of age and chronological or calendar ageing (age in years) is not its best indicator. Ageing is a characteristic of all multicellular organisms. Ageing sums up all the changes that take place in a person leading to a decrease in his functional capacity as he ages ahead of adulthood.

Normal physiological ageing, therefore, begins after the completion of the growth and development period, and the changes occur slowly, yet surely, over time and are influenced by life events, such as illness, both acute and chronic, genetic heritage, stress, socio-economic status, accessibility of health care, nutrition and environment.

As a matter of fact, ageing is analogous to the phenomenon of projectile motion the pathway taken by a stone hurled at the soaring sky at an acute angle. The stone first ascends with a high speed slowing down progressively when it tends to reach the highest point on its flight and finally setting on a descending course to reach the ground ultimately. Just as the flight course trajectory of a projectile (stone thrust upwards at an acute angle) depends, among other things, upon its weight, force and angle at which it is launched, the pace and the intensity of ageing also varies from person to person owing to many reasons, a good number of which remain undiscovered as yet. The average life span of human species has increased due to advances made in technology, health care and the delivery of good nutrition. With fruits of development reaching out to the masses, average life span has increased from 50 to 70 years in developed countries and a similar trend has been observed in developing countries as well. The massive demographic shift from a population that is mostly young to the one that includes a large number of the old, presents humanity with one of its most dramatic challenges. In an effort to prove equal to this challenge, the science of ageing or 'gerontology' has been brought into sharp focus to conduct purposeful study and research on the different aspects of ageing. Three broad areas have been identified where systematic efforts can help elderly lead vigorous, fulfilling and independent lives. The first one concerns the study of ageing at the biochemical, molecular and physiological levels in the pursuit of finding the precise cause of ageing and to subsequently devise remedial measures to delay and slowdown this process. The area falls in the domain of biochemists, nutritionists, molecular biologists and physiologist. The other area deals with the diseases of old age and comes in the purview of clinicians and is also known by the name 'geriatrics'. Still another area, the third one, addresses itself to the social and psychological problems besetting the old and retired people and devises welfare, relief and rehabilitation strategies for them.

NUTRITIONAL AND SOCIAL INTERVENTIONS TO COMBAT AGEING

Current research suggests that nutrition plays a central role in health maintenance of older adults, for most of them suffer from inadequate or imbalanced nutrition. The poor health standing of the aged in the rural populations is the result of poverty, insanitation, malnutrition and infection, all parts of a vicious circle.

Here it is worthwhile to examine the value of nutritional interventions in coping with the ageing process, to regarding caloric intake in the elderly, it may be justified to mention that a decrease in body cell mass, including muscle mass, cause a decrease in energy requirement owing to a sure decline in basal metabolism. A decrease in energy requirement also results due to a reduced physical activity in the elderly. This calls for an appropriate reduction in the caloric intake.

A few guidelines given hereunder will go a long way in combating the nutritive vulnerability and promotion the health of the aged.

1. The right combination of foods including fruits, vegetables, grains, legumes, low fat and dairy products.
2. To fight infection and chronic diseases, take nutrients that strengthen immune system—vitamin E and vitamin B6 and traces of zinc. They are available from whole grains, legumes, green leafy vegetables, sea food, lean meats and vegetable oils.
3. To prevent bones from becoming porous and brittle, choose vitamin D and calcium rich foods. Since bone growth slows down in adolescence and reverses after mid 30's when demineralization takes place; to combat this change, low fat dairy products (skimmed mild yoghurt, cheese) and vitamin D fortified milk are to be taken.
4. Since an important route to one's health is through one's stomach, so it is necessary to take at least 20-30 gm of fiber in the daily diet so as to ensure an active, constipation free and regular digestive system. It becomes available in fruits, dark leafy vegetables, grains and legumes.
5. To help safeguard vision, abundant intakes of provitamin A (from B carotene), vitamin C and vitamin E (antioxidant nutrients) become desirable. Antioxidant nutrients become instrumental in combating damaging effects of oxidation in the body in general and on visual process in particular, prominent among which is development of cataract. Yellow and green vegetables and citrus fruits are rich in such ingredients.
6. To treat elderly women as especially vulnerable group and to evolve a system of care for the aged by reinforcing traditional family system with pragmatism encouragement and incentives like tax concession and allowances to those who care for their elderly. Alternatively, state sponsored collective arrangements, like old age homes, should also be set up.
7. To promote geriatrics as the medical specialty dealing with the health problems of the aged.
8. The society, on its part, should also make honest endeavors to prove equal to the vulnerabilities of the aged by encouraging family support and warmth to them by ensuring the adequate nutritive values of their diet in the context of a reduced caloric and fat intakes and higher protein, vitamin and mineral intakes.

We all should strive hard to give meaning and reality to the words of Dulcey-Ruiz, a Columbian psycho-geriatrician, who says 'let us seek to change the idea of ageing as being passive, useless, dependent and isolated into an ageing that is active, autonomous and socially participative.

Let us all also live up to the famous upanishad prayer Uivemah Saradah Shatam, Pasyemah Saradah Shatam, Shrunnyamah Saradah Shatam' for living long and strong upto one hundred years with all our senses performing adequately and make others do so.

DIETARY MANAGEMENT OF THE ELDERLY

It is true that as age advances, old people have problems of chewing food and digestion. Their diets need to be modified according to the type of activity (sedentary/ moderate/heavy) and general health condition. The Indian Council of Medical Research (ICMR), in the year 1989, suggested a reduction in the energy requirements of the elderly (aged 60 + years) compared to that of adults (below 59 years), based on the body weight, basal metabolic rate and physical activity. This worked out to be 18% (for males) and 11% (for females) less than that of adults. Accordingly, balanced diets for the elderly are worked out based on the recommended dietary intakes for Indians suggested by ICMR, 1981. Energy and other nutrients provided by these diets are given in the tables below.

Recommended foodstuff intakes for the elderly		
Foodstuffs	*Male (g/day)*	*Female (g/day)*
Cereals	325	270
Pulses	40	40
Green leafy vegetables	100	100
Other vegetables	50	50
Roots and tubers	50	50
Milk and milk products	200	200
Sugar and jaggery	20	20
Fats and oils	20	20
Fruits	100	100

Note: Any seasonal fruit (about 100 gm) can be included in the daily diet.

Recommended nutrient intake		
Nutrients	*Male (g/day)*	*Female (g/day)*
Calories	1973	1785
Protein (g)	55	45
Calcium (mg)	881	865
Iron (mg)	42	38
Vitamin A retinol (mg)	998	996
Thiamin (mg)	1.2	1.2
Riboflavin (mg)	1.1	1.0

Different menu patterns can be worked out for North, East, West and Southern regions depending on their food habits. A sample menu pattern worked out for a South Indian elderly male (sedentary worker) is provided below.

Sample menu		
Early Morning	Biscuits	Two
	Tea	1 cup
Breakfast	Idli	Two
	Chutney	1 tbsp
	Milk with sugar	1 cup
Mid morning	Fruit	1
	Banana	1
	Orange	1
Lunch	Rice	3 cups
	Sambhar	1 cups
	Vegetable curry	1 cups
	Curd	1 cups
	Salad	2 tbsp
Evening tea	Upma	1 cup
	Tea	1 cup
Dinner	Rice	3 cups
	Vegetable curry	1 cup
	Curd	½ cup
	Salad	2 tbsp
	Lime	½ cup

Note:

1. Cup = 150 ml of volume.
2. Non-vegetarians can include 1 egg/30 g of mutton of fish and 1 tsp of extra oil and reduce 50% of pulses.
3. For females, rice can be reduced by 1 cup each during lunch and dinner.

Some Dietary Tips for the Elderly

Some of the age-old food habits of the elderly people which are carried over from childhood are difficult to change. However, some dietary modifications are inevitable considering both quality and quantity of the diet, physical activity and general health condition of the elderly. Following are some of the simple dietary tips which help the elderly to maintain normal health and stay fit.

1. Eat simple but nutritious diet.
2. Take frequent but small meals/mini supplements.
3. Use liberal amounts of green leafy vegetables, other vegetables, fruits and whole grains to improve the quality of the diet.
4. Take a handful of sprouted grams/salads.
5. Take plenty of fluids (including water) and semi-solids.
6. Avoid fried foods.
7. Reduce total fat and refined carbohydrates.
8. Reduce salt intake.
9. Avoid fasting.

Non-Dietary Life Style Tips

1. Try to lead a harmonious way of life by maintaining good social and psychological environment.
2. Do regular exercises like bending/brisk walk.
3. Avoid solitary life/social isolation and inactivity.

Recipes for the Elderly

During old age, considering the problems of chewing food and digestion, there is a need to provide soft cooked nutritious recipes for the old people. Another important factor that has to be remembered is that, quite often, the elderly get disinterested in cooking food every day, and eating a variety food, especially if they are left alone. Some do not like to cook food which involved elaborate cooking procedures. There is also another group of elderly who try to skip meals, while others try to overeat, which results in under/overnutrition (obesity). It is, therefore, necessary, to formulate simple, but nutritious recipes which help the elderly was therefore undertaken with the following criteria:

1. Recipes should be nutritious supplements/mini meals.
2. Recipes can be easily prepared using a variety of nutritious foods.
3. Recipes should be easy-to-cook involving minimal time for cooking/no cooking.
4. Recipes should be ready-to-eat as and when necessary; and
5. Recipes can be easily stored for at least a fortnight without any spoilage.

Two types of recipes were prepared, i.e.:

1. Easy-to-cook; and
2. Ready-to-eat.

These recipes included the following as given below:

List of easy to and ready to cook recipes

Easy-to-cook	*Ready-to-cook*
Dalia	Black gram dhal laddu
Ragi ambali	Coconum laddu
Ragina	Groundnut laddu
Khichidi	Sesame laddu
Perugu atukulu (pressed rice with curd)	Cheera
	Groundnut chikki
Savia upma	Mixture (chidwa)
Suji upma	Mathi
Poha (pressed rice upma)	Namakpara
Methi paratha	
Curd salad	
Sprouted green gram/bengal gram whole (cooked)	
Suji or rice kheer	

The above recipes were prepared using a variety of locally available nutritious foods. The average calories per serving provided by these recipes ranged between 150-300.

Example dalia

Ingredients	*Weight*	*Measure/No*
Broken wheat	100	2/3 K
Green gram dhal	100	2/3 K
Cumin seeds	5	1 tsp
Grated carrot	100	Four
Black pepper powder	2	½ tsp
Oil	15	4 tsp
Salt	To taste	1 tsp
Water	450 ml	3 K

K = Katori (Volume = 150 ml).

Method

Heat the oil in pressure cooker. Add broken wheat and cumin and fry till they turn golden brown. Add the rest of the ingredients and cook at 15 lbs pressure for 2 minutes.

Total weight of cooked dalia = 750 g, Measures = 7 K.

Nutritive value

Calories	900
Protein (g)	42
Fat (g)	19
Calcium (mg)	390
Iron (mg)	17

Ready-to-eat recipes–Black gram dhal laddu

Ingredient	*Weight (g)*	*Measure/No.*
Black gram dhal	100	2/3 K
Jaggery	100	2/3 K
Onions (medium size)	50	1
Cashewnuts	20	18
Cardamom	2	2
Ghee	40	1/3 K

Method

Roast black gram dhal on slow fire till golden brown and powder it. Heat ghee, fry cashewnut pieces and remove them. Melt jaggery, add dal powder, ghee, powdered cardamom and cashewnuts. Mix well and make balls just after a minute.

Total weight of laddu = 125 g, Number of laddus = 10.

Nutritive value

Calories	1300
Protein (g)	28
Fat (g)	61
Calcium (mg)	244
Iron (mg)	22

STUDY QUESTIONS

1. How do you differentiate between chronological and physiological ageing? What are the different scientific disciplines that deal with the health and well being of the aged and how do they do it?
2. Give a brief account of the biological aspects of ageing?
3. How does the modern society with rapidly changing values is not proving itself upto task to take care of its elderly? Explain briefly.
4. Give a comprehensive view of the role of nutrition in slowing down the pace of ageing and decreasing the incidence of disease in elderly.
5. Write a short note on dietary management of the elderly.

CHAPTER 32

Nutrient Drug Interactions

Chapter Outlines

- Terms related with drug action
- Effects of drugs on nutritional status
- Effects of drugs on nutrient metabolism
- Interference with reabsorption by kidney
- Effects of foods and nutrients on drugs
- Body's homeostatic mechanisms affect drug excretion
- Study questions

TERMS RELATED WITH DRUG ACTION

To make the scenario become familiar, it is worthwhile to understand a few terms relate with drug action.

A drug is a substance other than food intended to affect the structure or function of the body. The term drug includes alcohol and both perspiration and over the counter drugs. Food drug interaction is a broad term that includes drug nutrient interactions and the effect of a medication on nutritional status. For example, a drug that causes chronic nausea or mouth pain may result in poor intake and weight loss. Likewise, the term drug nutrient interactions refers to the result of the action between a drug and a nutrient that would not happen with the nutrient or the drug alone. Besides, drug action is directly related to bioavailability of a drug which the degree to which a drug or other substance reaches the circulation and becomes available to the target organ or tissue associated with bioavailability is another term half life which is amount of time it takes for the blood concentration of a drug to decrease by one half of its steady state level. Apart from healing effects, drugs are often talked about their side effects.

Side effects of the drug means adverse effect/reactions that cause discomfiture or disease symptom in the body. Pharmacokinetics of a drug refers to the drug taking its course through the body by absorption, distribution, metabolism and excretion. Absorption of the drug from the site of administration to the bloodstream; depends on route of administration, chemistry of the drug and its ability to cross membranes, rate of gastric emptying (for oral drugs) and GI movement and the quality of the product formulation. Food components and nutritional supplements can interfere with absorption, especially if the drug is taken orally. The next step or distribution occurs when the drug leaves the systemic circulation and moves to various parts of the body. Infact, drug in the blood stream are often bound to plasma proteins. They become unbound to leave the blood and affect target organs. Thus, low serum albumin can increase availability of drugs and potentiates their effects. Finally, metabolism or biotransformation takes place primarily in the liver; cytochrome P-450 enzyme system facilitates drug metabolism; metabolism generally changes fat soluble compounds to water soluble that can be excreted. Foods or dietary supplements that increase or inhibit these enzyme systems can change the rate or extent of drug metabolism. Finally, drug is eliminated from the body as an unchanged drug or metabolite. Renal excretion the major route of elimination; affected by renal function and urinary pH. Besides some drugs eliminated in bile and other body fluids. Pharmacodynamics is another term which connotes the physiologic and biochemical effects of a drug, as well as the mechanism of action, e.g., how a drug works, often the drug molecule binds to a receptor, enzyme; or ion channel, producing a physiological response. Likewise, pharmacogenomics is a recent term which genetically determined variations that are revealed solely by the effects of drugs and they pertain only to a subset of people. Examples include G6PD (glucose-6-phosphate dehydrogenase) enzyme deficiency, warfarin resistance, and slow inactivation of isoniazid (IHN), an anti-tuberculosis drug.

All in all, the effects of food drug interactions and benefits of minimizing food drug interactions can be summed up as follows:

EFFECTS OF DRUGS ON NUTRITIONAL STATUS

Any person taking a drug risks potentially harmful effects from food and drug interactions. Nutritional status can be affected because these interactions can alter (1) food intake, (2) the absorption of nutrients or drugs, (3) the metabolism of nutrients or drugs, and (4) the excretion of nutrients or drugs. Some known interactions are considered clinically desirable and result in the control of a disease process. For example, by restricting a patient's dietary vitamin K, the effect of warfare (an anticoagulant) is prolonged. However, many effects resulting from food and drug interactions are undesirable. These include nutritional deficiencies, growth retardation in children, loss of disease control and acute toxic reactions. Some persons, especially the elderly, are at higher risk than others for suffering unwanted effects.

Factors Increasing the Risk of Drug Nutrient Interactions

The risk of a drug nutrient interaction is increased if a patient:

- Is malnourished.
- Consumes alcohol.
- Takes a high potency vitamin or mineral supplement.
- Is receiving many drugs.
- Patient with chronic disease.
- Elderly.
- Foetus.
- Infant.
- Pregnant woman.

Bioavailability of a drug is the degree to which a drug or other substance reaches the circulation and becomes available to the target organ or tissue and half life is amount of time intakes for the blood concentration of a drug to decrease by one half of its steady state level.

Side effects of the drug means adverse effect/reactions or any undesirable effect or disease symptom in the body that cause discomfit.

Depending on the desired therapeutic effect, dietary intake of protein and/or carbohydrate may be modified.

Food and drug interactions can be complex, especially if the patient is on multiple drug regimens or is high risks for other reasons. Having a sound knowledge of potential food and drug interaction is an important function of health care professionals. Physicians, dietitians, pharmacists, and nurses have a joint responsibility in being aware of and controlling such interactions. The clinical pharmacist can be of help to the nurse when scheduling medications for optimal effect. Likewise, the clinical dietitian may be asked to assess a patient's risk for food drug interaction.

Number of drugs has a variety of effects on foods and nutrients:

1. Drugs can affect food intake.
2. Drugs can alter the absorption of nutrients through luminal and mucosal effects.
3. The metabolism of nutrients can be affected by drugs; and
4. Drugs can increase or decrease the excretion of certain nutrients.

Effect of Drugs on Food Intake

Even before food is ingested, drugs can affect food intake. Several drugs increase or decrease appetite interferes with the senses of taste and smell and gastric irritation. Food is sometimes used to these and other side effects of drugs.

Changing Appetite

As stimulants, including dextroamphetamine and thylphenidate, both used in the treatment of narpesy (ADD), have the effect of depressing the desire for food. One of the side effects of these stimulants in children is slowed growth.

Anti-neoplastic drugs or agents that prevent the development, growth, or proliferation of malignant are notorious for causing a loss of appetite (anorexia). Examples of such antineoplastic drugs are plicamycin and vincristine.

Many antihistamines, including output: Other side effects including severe nausea, vomiting and stomatitis exacerbate the anorexia. These side effects follow pheniramine and diphenhydramine use eventually, causing anorexia.

Medroxyprogestrone, a female hormone used as an oral contraceptive and in cyclic hormone therapy after menopause, also increases appetite. This hormone occurs naturally in the second half of the menstrual cycle as in pregnancy (to support the growth requirements of the mother and foetus). To minimize its effects, several nursing interventions might be appropriate: increasing the fibre content of the patient's diet and encouraging the person to drink 6 to 8 glasses of water daily, to eat slowly and to chew food thoroughly.

Changes in Taste and Smell

The senses of taste and smell influence the response of the foods. Some drugs after the perception of these senses making foods and beverages taste bitter, metallic or unpleasant. Although this usually leads to a decreased appetite, some individuals will try to rid themselves of the sensation by eating constantly.

Acetylsalicyclic acid (ASA), more commonly known as aspirin, is a drug used to control pain or to reduce fever. It also is taken in small daily doses to decrease the risks of heart attacks. One gram of ASA about three adult dose tablets increases the taste perception of bitterness.

An anti-infective used for tuberculosis and other serious infections, streptomycin is excreted in the saliva. One result is a metallic or bitter taste even when the drug is administered by intramuscular injection.

Gastric Irritation

Drugs that cause gastric irritation are often taken with food to reduce this side effect. Chronic use of aspirin can lead to gastric bleeding and anemia. Taking aspirin with food, milk, biscuits, or a full glass of water reduces of stomach irritation. Others non-steroidal anti-inflammatory drugs (NSAIDs) and potassium chloride are also associated with gastric irritation.

Effect of Drugs on Nutrient Aabsorption

Drugs can affect the absorption of nutrients in several ways. Drug induced alterations in absorption are categorised according to two general mechanisms of action: the luminal or the mucosal effects.

Luminal Effects

The luminal effect refers to drug induced changes within the intestine that affect the absorption of nutrients or drugs without altering the intestine itself. These drug induced changes may affect peristalsis, pH, or the formation of complexes. Laxatives may interfere with the absorption of nutrients and other drugs because they stimulate peristalsis and thus cause a rapid transit time of intestinal contents.

The absorption of weakly acidic drugs takes place in the stomach whereas the absorption of neutral an alkaline drugs takes place in the small intestine. Drug induced changes in the pH of these sites influence the absorption of both nutrients and drugs. For example, an acid pH is necessary for folic acid absorption. It is also required for intrinsic factor to combine with vitamin B_{12} (extrinsic factor) for the absorption of vitamin B_{12}. Because long term antacid or potassium chloride therapy neutralizes gastric acidity, the result is a decrease in the absorption of both folic acid and vitamin B_{12}. Antacids and potassium also decrease the absorption of iron because an acid medium is necessary to convert ferric iron ($Fe3+$) to ferrous iron ($2+$), the ore absorbable form.

Sometimes, foods or nutrients bind with or form complexes with drugs. This combining can increase, decrease, or prevent the absorption of one or the other.

Cholestyramine, a lipid lowering agent, binds with bile salts, which increases the excretion of cholesterol. Unfortunately, it may also bind with the fat soluble vitamins A, D, E and K. These vitamins are then excreted along with the cholesterol. Because vitamin K is not stored in the body in significant amounts, cholestyramine therapy can lead to a deficiency of prothrombin and haemorrhage.

Mucosal Effects

The luminal effects do not affect the tissues or organs. In contrast, mucosal effects are drug induced changes that affect the absorption of nutrients or drugs by damaging or altering tissue structures. Mucosal effects include decreased digestive enzymes, damaged intestinal mucosa, and inhibited transport mechanism.

Long-term alcohol consumption damages the pancreas, decreasing enzyme production. Thus the breakdown of amino acids and fats, chiefly governed by the cation of pancreatic enzymes, is slowed or insufficiently completed. The result is reduced to poor absorption of amino acids and fats.

Inhibited Transport Mechanisms

Several nutrients have to be helped across the intestinal membrane to the bloodstream. A number of drugs impair the absorption of nutrients through their effects on the transport mechanisms. Para-aminosalicylate (PAS), an anti-tubercular drug, is administered for a prolonged period (1 to 2 years) to be effective. This drug interferes with the uptake and transport of vitamin B_{12} across the mucosal wall.

EFFECTS OF DRUGS ON NUTRIENT METABOLISM

Many drugs alter the metabolism of nutrients. Two commonly prescribed classes of drugs, corticosteroids and beta-adrenergic blocking agents, change the way the body uses energy nutrients. Drugs also disrupt vitamin metabolism by a variety of mechanisms.

On Nutrient Excretion

Drugs usually cause excessive excretion, rather than retention, of nutrients. (1) Drugs can act on the excretion of nutrients for binding sites, (2) form chemical bonds with the nutrient, (3) deplete the nutrient supply in the body's tissues, and (4) interfere with the kidney's reabsorption of the nutrient back into the bloodstream.

INTERFERENCE WITH REABSORPTION BY KIDNEY

Many diuretic agents prevent normal reabsorption of sodium into the blood stream within the kidney. This increases the amount of sodium excreted by the kidney into the urine. Along with the sodium, water is also excreted. Often the drug is not specific enough to dispose of sodium alone. Many diuretics also cause loss of potassium. Sometimes the client must take pharmacologic doses of potassium chloride to prevent hypokalemia. One diuretic, furosemide, produces calcium loss in addition to potassium-sparing, eliminating the need for supplementation. In a study of drug nutrient interaction, between 11 and 36 percent of long-term care facility patients were shown to be at risk for hyper or hypokalemia, serum potassium outside the normal ranges.

EFFECTS OF FOODS AND NUTRIENTS ON DRUGS

Foods and nutrients can decrease, delay or increase the absorption of drugs. They can also cause alterations in drug metabolism.

Effects of Foods on Drug Metabolism

Foods can alter the metabolism of drugs. One metabolic food drug interaction can be life threatening.

Monoamine Oxidase Inhibitors

The usual abbreviation for this group of drug is MAO inhibitor. Several antidepressants are MAO inhibitors and some other drugs produce similar reactions.

Mechanism of Drug Action

These drugs prevent the breakdown of tyramine and dopamine, chemicals necessary for proper functioning of the nervous system. The drugs' therapeutic effect is to increase the concentration of epinephrine, norepinephrine, serotonin and dopamine in the central nervous system. thus counteracting depression.

In the peripheral nervous system the MAO inhibitors also prevent the release of norepinephrine that builds up in the nerves. The stores of norepinephrine become specially high in the nerves that regulate the size of blood vessels. The result is a decreased ability to constrict peripheral blood vessels. The vasodilation ths produced leads to hypotension. To compound the situation, the drugs also inhibit the body's normal response to a low blood pressure, an increased heart rate. Thus the individual displays the unusual combination of hypotension and bradycardia.

Effect of Foods on MAO Inhibitors

Some foods contain tyramine, a metabolic intermediate product in the conversion of the amino acid tyrosine to epinephrine. Foods containing degraded protein such as aged cheese are high in tyramine. When a patient on MAO inhibitors consumes foods or beverages high in tyramine, the drugs prevent the normal breakdown of tyramine. A consequence, the tyramine oversupply leads to excessive epinephrine producing hypertension. Sometimes the blood pressure is severely elevated, which can cause intracranial haemorrhage.

Effects of Other Nutrients

Certain nutrients increase the amount of a drug in the bloodstream, thus increasing or decreasing the risk of toxicity. For example, fat displaces the antianxiety drug diazepam from protein binding sites, thus increasing the amount of unbound drug circulating in the bloodstream. This increased serum concentration leads to increased activity of the drug.

Warfarin achieves anti-coagulation by fooling the liver into accepting it as vitamin K. For maximum therapeutic effect, the amount of foods high in vitamin K consumed should be consistent, not excessive one day and scanty the next.

BODY'S HOMEOSTATIC MECHANISMS AFFECT DRUG EXCRETION

In addition to nutritional status, the status of acid base balance and fluid and electrolyte balance affect the excretion of drugs. To consider either acid base balance or fluid and electrolyte balance in isolation risks oversimplifying the body's functions. The functions of these regulatory systems are interwoven.

Acid Base Balance

The kidney is the gatekeeper of the bloodstream. The contents of urine reflect the metabolic state of the body. The end products of the foods consumed and the drugs taken make the urine either more acid or more alkaline. Freshly voided urine usually has an acid pH, averaging about 6.0.

Alkaline Urine

Large amounts of citrus juices or a vegetarian diet cause the urine to become alkaline. When the body is producing alkaline urine, the kidney will take loner to excrete alkaline drugs. Higher levels of the drugs will remain in the blood stream for a longer period. Examples of alkaline drugs are the cardiac anti-dysrhythmic quinidine; and the amphetamine stimulant. If the patients metabolism causes alkaline urine these drugs will give more pronounced and prolonged effects. Patients treated with these drugs should neither change the amounts of citrus juice they consume nor become vegetarians without consulting the physician.

The opposite effect occurs when a person's metabolism produces alkaline urine and the drugs are acidic. The kidney excretes acidic drugs faster than usual if the urine is alkaline. One acidic drug that should spring to mind immediately is acetylsalicylic acid. Another acidic drug is the barbiturate commonly used as an anti-convulsant, phenobarbital. The kidney will discard either of these drugs faster than normal if the patient is producing alkaline urine.

Acid Urine

Large doses of ascorbic acid (vitamin C) make the urine more acidic. Vitamin C is sometimes given specifically for the purpose of acidifying the urine. For example, a urinary pH of 5.5 or less is necessary for the urinary anti-infective drug methanamine to be effective.

Optimal nutritional status is preserved. Accidents and injuries are avoided. Disease complications are minimized. The cost of health care services is reduced. There is less professional liability. Licensing agency requirements are met.

Benefits of minimizing food drug interactions lead to medications achieve their intended effects, cause improved compliance with medications call from, less need for additional medication or higher dosages as well as fewer caloric or nutrient supplements are required. Further, it helps in minimizing disease complications and gives a long way in preserving nutritional status and reducing health care services.

STUDY QUESTIONS

1. Explain the terms:

   (i) Drug action, (ii) Side effects of drug, (iii) Biotransformation of drug, (iv) Pharmacodynamics of drug.

2. Discuss briefly the effects of drugs on nutritional status.
3. Explain the effects of drugs on nutrient metabolism.

CHAPTER 33

Eating Disorders: Causes, Diagnosis and Treatment

Chapter Outlines

- Eating sans order
- Anorexia nervosa
- Bulimia nervosa
- Eating disorders not otherwise specified (EDNOS)
- Fallouts triggered by eating disorder behaviours
- Causes of eating disorders
- Diagnosis criteria of eating disorders
- Study questions

EATING SANS ORDER

Consumption of food serves a number of psychological, social and cultural purposes for human beings, apart from serving the basic nourishing objective. Likewise, preparing, providing and distributing food may become a means of expressing love or indifference in family relationships. In our social set ups we repeatedly come across with images of pleasing, attractive bodies and more often than not one cannot help going for dieting to achieve slimness and ability one finds in TV programme, movies and advertisements. Some people are more receptive and vulnerable to progress from normal responses to hunger and satiety sensations to abnormal, obsessive eating behaviours, at times, for genetic, psychological and physical reason.

As a matter of fact, fasting and feeding are not always imposed upon people by nature. More often than not, human psyche or circumstances make them impose these conditions upon themselves. An eating disorder is to eat, or avoid eating, which negatively affects both, one's physical and mental health. It is marked by extremes. It is present when a person experiences severe disturbances in eating behaviuor, such as extreme reduction of food intake or extreme overeating, or feelings of extreme distress or concern about body weight, size or shape. As a matter of fact, an eating disorder involves a distorted pattern of thinking about food / snacking and size/weight. There is a preoccupation and obsession with food, as well as an issue of control or lack of control around food and its consumption. Eating disorders frequently appear during adolescence or young adulthood, but they can also develop during childhood or even later in life. Although eating disorders primarily affect women and girls, boys and men are also vulnerable, albeit to a smaller extent. Like females who have eating disorders, males with the illness have a warped sense of body image. Anorexia nervosa and bulimia nervosa have conditions similarities and people similarities. These conditions generally develop during the teens and early adult years or youth. Primarily, these disorders afflict females from middle and upper class families. Interestingly, people with either anorexia nervosa or bulimia nervosa are obsessed with the appearance of their bodies and are preoccupied by thoughts of food, eating and dieting.

Thus an eating disorder is a severe change in eating pattern linked to psychological changes. The change is associated with food restricting, binge eating pursuing and fluctuation in weight. These disorders often are long-term illnesses that may require long-term treatment. In addition, they frequently occur with other mental disorders such as depression, substance abuse, and anxiety disorders. The earlier these disorders are diagnosed and treated, better the chances are for full recovery. This article identifies the basic facts including common signs, symptoms, and treatment for the most common eating disorders: anorexia nervosa, bulimia nervosa and binge-eating disorder.

If one looks intensively, one finds that eating disorders are often described as an outward expression of internal emotional pain and confusion. Obsessive thoughts about, and the behaviour associated with, food are maladaptive means of dealing with emotional distress through food denial or binging which cannot be expressed in any other satisfactory way. The emotional distress is often to do with a negative perception of self, a feeling of being unable to change "bad" things about one self and in using food as an inappropriate way of taking control. These complex conditions can arise from a variety of potential causes in females, and at times, even in boys and men. Once started, however, they can create a self-perpetuating cycle of physical and emotional destruction. When low body weight becomes an important goal, people begin to view normal healthy body weight as being too fat, and they take unhealthy actions to loose weight. Further, any severe restriction of energy intake may lead to binging, and set in motion a see-saw swing of repeated weight losses and gains called weight cycling. The reason for this seems obscure as it is not easy to seek. However, the disorders do seem to be the multifactorial; myriad combinations of socio-cultural, neurochemical and psychological factors.

Apart from the two main types of eating disorders, viz anorexia nervosa and bulimia nervosa, a third category is "eating disorders not otherwise specified (EDNOS)", which includes several variations. Most of the disorders falling into the latter category are similar to anorexia or bulimia but with slightly different characteristics. Binge-eating disorder can also be taken as one type of EDNOS

Pointwise description of the eating disorders can be as follows:

ANOREXIA NERVOSA

Anorexic people starve themselves with the aim of losing weight to a point which others would consider to be very thin, although the sufferer is unlikely to perceive themselves as such. The longer the condition continues, the more difficult it can be to tackle, and in severe cases, can necessitate hospitalization or can even prove fatal. Sufferers are typically in their teens or twenties and most of them are girls and women, although around 5-10% males, have also been found to suffer from it. The following are symptoms of anorexia nervosa:

- Distorted perceptions of one's weight, size and shape.
- Behaviour which results in a marked weight loss.
- A morbid fear of gaining weight or becoming fat.
- Excessive exercising (while starving).
- Cessation of periods in women.

BULIMIA NERVOSA

Bulimic people may well maintain their normal weight. The condition is characterized by:

- Bouts of eating followed by purging.
- Distorted perception of own weight, size and shape.
- A powerful urge to overeat, leading to binge eating and a resultant feeling of being out of control. Purging comes as a rearguard action of gaining control sort of clutching at the straws.

Anorexia nervosa	Bulimia nervosa
• Rigid dieting causing dramatic weight loss.	• Secretive binge eating, never overeating before people.
• Obsession with leanness and body image associated with it. Always in relentless pursuit of thinness.	• Eating when depressed or under stress.
• Indulging in rituals involving food and excessive exercise.	• Binging followed by fasting or exercises; purging through laxative and diuretic use as well as through self induced vomiting.
• Maintenance of rigid control over eating and life style.	• Low self esteem embarrassment and depression; especially after binging.
• Intense phobia about gaining weight.	• Fluctuating weight as a consequence of binging and fasting.
• Feeling of purity, power and superiority through maintenance of strict regimen of self denial.	• Loss of control, fear of not being able to stop eating.
• Preoccupation with food, its preparation and with observing another person eats.	• Food is the only comfort/escape, that too in enormity, both in terms of quality and quantity. Tend to be impulsive about food binging.
• Erratic or no menses even after puberty.	• Normally no menstrual irregularities.

- Compensatory behaviour such as self-induced vomiting; misuse of laxatives, diuretics, anemia or other medication; fasting; or excessive exercise.
- A morbid fear of gaining weight or becoming fat.

Given hereunder are the salient features of the two major disorders; anorexia nervosa and bulimia nervosa, juxtaposed with each other for use in the awareness campaigns to help the adolescents and youth, especially of the fairer sex, to discover their risks and to reflect upon their personality concerns and eating habits, in a prelude to modifying it.

EATING DISORDERS NOT OTHERWISE SPECIFIED (EDNOS)

The large group of women patients with presence of EDNOS consists of sub acute cases of anorexia nervosa or bulimia nervosa.The nature and intensity of the medical and nutritional problems and the most effective treatment modality will depend on the severity of impairment and the symptoms. These patients may have met all criteria for anorexia except that they have not missed three consecutive menstrual periods. Or, they may be of normal weight and purge without binging. Although the patients are otherwise free from medical complications, yet in some cases such problems may also occur.

EDNOS also include Binge Eating Disorder (BED) in which the patient has binging behaviour without the compensatory purging seen in bulimia nervosa. It is estimated that prevalence of this disorder is 1 to 2% of the population. Binge episodes must occur at least twice a week and have occurred for at least 6 months. EDNOS have mostly been found to be of the following kinds:

Compulsive Eating

- Recurrent episodes of binge eating and consequent feeling of being out of control.
- Marked distress about binge eating and the attempts to control it.
- During a binge the person may eat more quickly than normal; eat until uncomfortably over-full; eat large amounts even when not hungry; tend to "graze" rather than eat meals; eat alone in secret; feel disgusted and guilty with oneself.

Food Deprivation

- Weight-loss accomplished primarily through extreme dieting, fasting or excessive exercise, mostly by one or other means singly.

Non-Specified

Other, but related difficulties with food include:

- Anorexic behaviour though still menstruating.
- Someone of normal weight inducing vomiting or purging after small amounts of food.
- Chewing and spitting food rather than swallowing.

FALLOUTS TRIGGERED BY EATING DISORDER BEHAVIOURS

There are many men and women suffering with all types of eating disorders that do not appear in any specific weight range. Interestingly, some of those with anorexia can be slightly overweight while some of those with compulsive eating can be slightly underweight. Variations for all who suffer can be anywhere from extremely underweight to extremely overweight to anywhere in between. The outward appearance of anyone with an eating disorder does not dictate the amount of physical danger they are in, nor does it determine the emotional conflict they feel inside. Most common fallouts that accompany eating disorder behaviour are:

Malnutrition: It is caused by undereating or overeating. The word malnutrition indicates deficiency for energy, protein and micronutrients (e.g., vitamin A, iodine and iron) either singularly or in combination. It can cause severe health risks including (but not limited to) respiratory infections, kidney and vision problems.

Dehydration: It is caused by the depletion or lack of intake of fluids in the body, or by restriction of carbohydrates and fat. Restriction/Starvation, vomiting and laxative abuse are the primary causes of dehydration. Symptoms include dizziness, weakness, or darkening of urine.

Electrolyte imbalances: Electrolyte balance is essential to the production of the body's "natural electricity" that ensures healthy teeth, joints and bones, nerve and muscle impulses, kidneys and heart functioning, blood sugar levels and the delivery of oxygen to the cells. Situations of electrolyte imbalance affect these functions in subtle or serious ways.

Hyponatremia (related to "water-loading"): Electrolytes are essential to proper body functioning. Drinking too much water (more than eight, eight-ounce glasses in less than twelve hours), can cause hyponatremia (not enough sodium in the blood), especially in someone already malnourished or dehydrated. Hyponatremia can cause nausea, vomiting and even fluid in the lungs and brain.

CAUSES OF EATING DISORDERS

People with eating disorders struggle with issues of identity and self-control. They deal with food as a means to cope with stress, low self-esteem and apprehensions of the plight in coming times. In the causation of eating disorders; genetics and neurochemical upheavals in the brain may have a role with definite contributors from emotional and societal pressures, family troubles, loneliness, anger, depression and fear of making a laughing stock of oneself before others due to body weight, shape or size. This all makes the sufferers take to distorted eating behavior.

People get into these complex conditions that arise from a combination of long-standing behavioral, biological, emotional, psychological, interpersonal and social factors. While eating disorders may begin with preoccupations with food and weight, they are most often about much more than food. In fact, such people often use food and the control of food as an attempt to compensate for feelings and emotions that may otherwise seem over-whelming. For some, dieting, bingeing, and purging may begin as a way to cope with painful emotions and to feel in control of their lives, but these behaviours eventually damage their physical and emotional health, self-esteem, and sense of competence and control.

Psychological Factors that Contribute to Eating Disorders

- Low self-esteem.
- Feelings of inadequacy or lack of control in life.
- Depression, anxiety, anger, or loneliness.

Interpersonal Factors that Contribute to Eating Disorders

- Troubled family and personal relationships.
- Difficulty in expressing emotions and feelings.
- History of being teased or ridiculed based on size or weight.
- History of physical or sexual abuse.

Social Factors that Contribute to Eating Disorders

- Cultural pressures that glorify "thinness" and place value on obtaining the "perfect body" especially in females.
- Narrow definitions of beauty that include only women and men of specific body weights and shapes.
- Cultural norms that value people, especially women, on the basis of physical appearance and not inner qualities and strengths.

Biological Factors that Can Contribute to Eating Disorders

Scientists are still researching possible biochemical or biological causes of eating disorders. In some individuals with eating disorders, certain chemicals in the brain that control hunger, appetite and digestion have been found to be unbalanced.Through exact meaning and implications of these imbalances have not become clear yet, the implication of genetics seems to obvious in some cases because:

- Eating disorders often run in families. Current research indicates that there are significant genetic contributions to eating disorders. Since some aberrations caused by nature can be redressed by nurture thus professional help and counselling are recommended in the treatment of eating disorders.

DIAGNOSIS CRITERIA OF EATING DISORDERS

Anorexia Nervosa

A. Refusal to maintain body weight at or above a minimally normal weight for age and height (e.g., weight loss leading to maintenance of body weight less than 85% of that expected; or failure to make expected weight gain during period of growth, leading to body weight less than 85% of that expected).

B. Intense fear of gaining weight or becoming fat, even though underweight.

C. Disturbance in the way in which one's body weight or shape is experienced, undue influence of body weight or shape on self-evaluation, or denial of the seriousness of the current low body weight.

D. In postmenarcheal females, amenorrhea, i.e., the absence of at least three consecutive menstrual cycles. [A woman is considered to have amenorrhea if her periods occur only following hormone (estrogen) administration].

Specific Types of Anorexia Nervosa

Restricting type: During the current episode of anorexia nervosa, the person has not regularly engaged in binge-eating or purging behaviour (i.e., self-induced vomiting or the misuse of laxatives, diuretics or enemas).

Binge-eating/purging type: During the current episode of anorexia nervosa, the person has regularly engaged in binge-eating or purging behaviour (i.e., self-induced vomiting or the misuse of laxatives, diuretics or enemas).

Bulimia Nervosa

A. Recurrent episodes of binge-eating: An episode of binge-eating is characterized by both of the following:
   1. Eating in a discrete period of time (e.g., within any 2-hour period), an amount of food that is definitely larger than most people would eat during a similar period of time and under similar circumstances.
   2. A sense of lack of control overeating during the episode (e.g., a feeling that one cannot stop eating or control what or how much one is eating).

B. Recurrent inappropriate compensatory behaviour in order to prevent weight gain, such as self-induced vomiting; misuse of laxatives, diuretics, enemas, or other medications; fasting; or excessive exercise.

C. The binge-eating and inappropriate compensatory behaviours both occur, on average, at least twice a week for three months.

D. Self-evaluation is unduly influenced by body shape and weight.

E. The disturbance does not occur exclusively during episodes of anorexia nervosa.

Specific Types of Bulimia Nervosa

Purging type: During the current episode of bulimia nervosa, the person has regularly engaged in self-induced vomiting or the misuse of laxatives, diuretics or enemas.

Non-purging type: During the current episode of bulimia nervosa, the person has used other inappropriate compensatory behaviours, such as fasting or excessive exercise, but has not regularly engaged in self-induced vomiting or the misuse of laxatives, diuretics or enemas.

Eating disorders not otherwise specified: The eating disorders not otherwise specified category is for disorders of eating that do not meet the criteria for any specific eating disorder. Examples include:

1. For females, all of the criteria for anorexia nervosa are met except that the individual has regular menses.
2. All of the criteria for anorexia nervosa are met except that, despite significant weight loss, the individual's current weight is in the normal range.
3. All of the criteria for bulimia nervosa are met except that the binge-eating inappropriate compensatory mechanisms occur at a frequency of less than twice a week or for duration of less than 3 months.
4. The regular use of inappropriate compensatory behaviour by an individual of normal body weight after eating small amounts of food (e.g., self-induced vomiting after the consumption of two cookies).
5. Repeatedly chewing and spitting out, but not swallowing, large amounts of food.
6. Binge-eating disorder; recurrent episodes of binge-eating in the absence of the regular use of inappropriate compensatory behaviours characteristic of bulimia nervosa (Milos, *et al.*, 2005).

Treating anorexia nervosa and bulimia nervosa: It needs to involve three components:

- Restoring the person to a healthy weight.
- Treating the psychological issues related to the eating disorder.
- Reducing or eliminating behaviours or thoughts that lead to disordered eating and preventing relapse.

Some research suggests that the use of medications, such as anti-depressants, antipsychotics or mood stabilizers, may be modestly effective in treating patients with anorexia by helping to resolve mood and anxiety symptoms that often co-exist with anorexia. Recent studies, however, have suggested that anti-depressants may not be effective in preventing some patients with anorexia from relapsing. In addition, no medication has shown to be effective during the critical first phase of restoring a patient to healthy weight. Overall, it is unclear if and how medications can help patients conquer anorexia, but research is ongoing. Different forms of psychotherapy, including individual, group and family-based, can help address the psychological reasons for the illness. Some studies suggest that family-based therapies in which parents assume responsibility for feeding their afflicted adolescents are the most effective in helping a person with anorexia gain weight and improve eating habits and moods.

A combined approach of medical attention and supportive psychotherapy designed specifically for anorexia patients is more effective than just psychotherapy. But the effectiveness of a treatment depends on the person involved and his or her situation. As with anorexia, treatment for bulimia often involves a combination of options and depends on the needs of the individual.To reduce or eliminate binge and purge behaviour, a patient may undergo nutritional counselling and psychotherapy, especially cognitive behavioural therapy (CBT), or be prescribed medication. Some anti-depressants, such as fluoxetine (Prozac), may help patients who also have depression and/or anxiety. It also appears to help reduce binge-eating and purging behaviour, reduces the chance of relapse, and improves eating attitudes. CBT that has been tailored to treat bulimia also has shown to be effective in changing binging and purging behaviour as in EDNOS, and in positively modifying eating attitudes. Therapy may be individually oriented or group-based.

In the present materialistic era, of cut throat competitions, conflicts and costly life-styles; the urge and yearning for pleasure, physical appearance and popularity makes one tread the path of faulty eatings. Eating disorders are also a manifestation of an ostrich like behaviour where the person makes eating as the scapegoat for hiding problems whose answers have become elusive for him/her. A girl or woman, or occasionally a boy or adult, use self-starvation or binging as a means of exercising some control direction over his/her environment in a bid to deal with the problem of self-image and inadequacy. In this age of literacy and enlightenment, it is important to gain awareness about these disorders so as to stear either clear without falling prey to them or to drive them out taking them as stumbling blocks in the pursuit of real accomplishment, progress and actualization.

In a nutshell, to prevent eating disorders, parents, peers and professionals should counsel the adolescents and youth focussing on following points:

- On discouraging and restricting dieting, meal skipping and fasting.
- On informing the adolescents and the youth about the changes that occur during puberty, reassuring them that they all are normal and natural.
- On eradicating misconceptions about nutrition, normal body weight and approaches to weight loss.
- On emphasising positive nutrition and healthful food properties free from obsessions and hypocrisies.

Thus there are no simple causes or solutions to the eating disorders as they are rooted in biological, psychological and social facets of human persona. Imparting awareness to the individuals, especially girls and women, through counselling; as they reach adolescence and puberty and orienting them towards appropriate preventive measures and coping strategies can save the youth from the vagaries of eating disorders.

STUDY QUESTIONS

1. Explain the term 'eating disorder' and discuss its major types.
2. Write clearly about the causes of eating disorders.
3. What impairment in body functioning takes place due to eating disorders? Explain.
4. Discuss the various components in the treatment of eating disorder.

CHAPTER 34

Nutritional Management of 'Inborn Errors of Metabolism'

Chapter Outlines

- Meaning of the term
- Genetic basis
- Defects in one or more genes cause inborn errors of metabolism
- Inborn errors of amino acid metabolism
- Inborn errors of carbohydrate metabolism
- Inborn errors of lipid metabolism
- Study questions

MEANING OF THE TERM

The term inborn error of metabolism, also known as inherited disorder of metabolism, was coined more than a hundred years ago by Sir Archibald E. Garrod in which he pointed towards four diseases of hereditary nature. These were alkaptonuria, a defect of phenylalanine metabolism in which a metabolite excreted into the urine becomes dark upon standing; albinism, also a defect of phenylalanine metabolism characterized by lack of pigmentation; cystinuria, or an excessive excretion of cystine because of a defect in the renal tubules that prevents the reabsorption of the amino acid cystine; and pentosuria, characterized by the presence of pentose sugar in the urine owing to the lack of an enzyme needed for the metabolism.

As the facts became more clear in the later years, it was found that there are more than 100 disorders that originate as a result of one or more mutations of the genes so as to hamper the specific metabolic functions leading to an amino acid, sugar or lipid deposition. The aberration may affect the bio-synthesis of a cellular product, interfere with the transport of substances across cell membrane, or produce rank toxic effects on tissues, brain being most vulnerable of all because of the accumulated intermediate products.

Whereas some inborn errors cause no serious limitations on the individual; others lead to changes in the central nervous system due to the presence and deposition of abnormal metabolites causing severe mental retardation; still others may become lethal shortly after birth. Likewise, some of them become evident a few days after birth, others, like gout, may show signs slowly at a later stage. Further, dietary management becomes effective in the control of some disorders, no known therapy gives respite in others.

Since the damage begins at birth, the inborn errors of metabolism are characterized by serious mental retardation if the condition is not managed promptly. During the infant years of life, brain grows and develops very rapidly and any interference with its growth cannot be fully corrected at a later time as the growth of brain becomes more or less complete in the initial 3-4 years. Thus, diagnosis during infancy is all important, lest the damage becomes too serious to make the effective treatment take its course. Inexpensive screening tests like urine test for abnormal metabolites may be applied to some conditions during the first few weeks of life.

Conditions for which dietary management has been tenable are discussed. In many disorders, the diet is planned around specialized formulae that supply the energy, protein, and micro nutrients needed, but are made to be low in specific amino acids or sugars as may be the case, in keeping with the metabolic defect. Some amounts of natural foods too are used to provide a regulated intake of protein and certain amino acids, besides other required nutrients. The diet for phenylketonuria becomes an illustrated example for the considerations that must be kept in mind when planning highly specialized diets for other inherited disorders of metabolism.

Nutritional management of children with inborn errors of metabolism is no less than a challenge. They are treated primarily in specialty clinics of major hospitals being looked after by a team of skilled specialists who monitor the child's progress on a regular systematic basis. Since the number of patients are small, medical and nutritional team members familiarize with the child and parents and optimize on their ability to cope with the problems involved in the management of disorder. As a matter of fact, dietary management is a special challenge for both, the dietitian and the family. The importance of quantitative and qualitative inclusion of various foods permitted cannot be overemphasized for, in many cases, high amounts can lead to neurological damage. Likewise, insufficient amounts of specific foodstuffs can impair normal growth and development. It is really walking the tight rope. Further, the child's progress needs to be monitored closely and the diet adjusted in consonance with physical and bio-chemical changes. The diet must be nutritionally adequate for all nutrients except for the limiting one(s). The dietitian must familiarize with new food products coming into the market and their nutrient composition in order to adequately counsel patients and their families regarding their partaking and usage. The nurse, being not directly involved in the planning of highly specialized diets, needs to be aware of the child's thriving and growth on the specified diet, as also of problems that become apparent due to over/under consumption of the prescribed diets. The nurse must also understand the general principles of diet planning and should be aware of food sources of the nutrients that are limited, in order to be able to answer concerns and evaluate information conveyed by family concerning the diet. Day-to-day dietary manoeuvring is as much challenging for the parents and family as the scientific aspects of disease management are for the health professional. The family must not slacken the strict adherence to the diet by the child, plan thoughtful menus, and encourage the child to eat products prepared for the purpose.

The information presented here in this chapter is insufficient, even illustrative, to enable the dietitian to efficiently plan nutritional care for children suffering from inborn errors of metabolism. To be sincere, the information presented here is aimed at giving an overview of some conditions along with prudent dietary planning to overcome these, emphasizing the necessity for continuous counselling of parents for the child's nutritional management.

GENETIC BASIS

The genetic code itself consists of the sequences of nucleotides within the DNA molecule, which act by programming the synthesis of the specific proteins that make up each species including human. The DNA and its nucleotide sequences are located in the nucleus of the cell, but the protein synthesis occurs in the cytoplasm. The genetic information, therefore, must be carried from the DNA, which never leaves the cell nucleus, to the site of action in the cyotosol. This is accomplished by another macromolecule, ribonucleic acid (RNA), which exists in both the nucleus and the cytoplasm of the cell. RNA is very similar to DNA except that it consists of a single strand of nucleotides instead of a double strand, its 5 carbon sugar is ribose instead of deoxyribose (from which the names of the two molecules are derived), and it contains uracil (U) as pyrimidine nitrogenous base, instead of thymine.

Actually, several kinds of RNAs are required to carry out the instructions of DNA. Messenger ribonucleic acid (mRNA) is produced in the nucleus of the cell modeled by a single strand of DNA which partially separates from its complementary strand for this purpose. The completed mRNA molecule then moves through nuclear membrane and enters cytoplasm of the cell. Here it encounters the ribosomes, the parts of the cell that actually synthesize proteins.

Ribosomes are able to synthesize every protein but must be given specific 'instructions' in order to 'know' which proteins to produce in a given cell.

Codon–the functional unit of protein synthesis, and thus of heredity, is a sequence of three nucleotides celled a codon. Each codon is identified by the three letters standing for its component nucleotides. There are 64 different nucleotides. Each of 61 of them codes for only one specific amino acid; for example UUU for phenyl alanine, AAG for lysine, AGA for arginine and GAA for glutamic acid. But there are only 22 amino acids, and so some may be called for or coded by more than one codon. L-lysine, for example, is coded either AAG or AAA, and serine by UCU, UCC, UCA or UCG. The remaining three codons, UAG,

UGA, UAA; are chain-terminating (or 'nonsense') codons which signal the end of a particular message sequence.

Making of Polypeptide

In the bloodstream, ready to enter the cell cytoplasm at an instant's notice, is a supply of amino acids that have resulted both from digestion of dietary protein and from breakdown of cellular protein. Waiting in the cytoplasm are molecules of transfer ribonucleic acid (tRNA). Each tRNA molecule contains a 3-nucleotide sequence that 'fits' or complements a similar sequence on the mRNA strand, and each tRNA molecule is also able to attach to a particular amino acid from the cellular amino acid pool.

Once the mRNA enters the cytoplasm, ribosomes cluster along its length. The mRNA and its attached ribosomes are known as polyribosome complex. Each ribosome moved along the strand of mRNA, touching two codons at a time. Codon by codon, a tRNA molecule and an amino acid arrive on the scene. Enzymes in the ribosome form a peptide bond which attaches the new amino acid to the growing peptide chain. The tRNA molecule is released and the ribosome moves along the mRNA to the next codon, where instructions for the next amino acid in the sequence are received in the form of next codon. As each appropriate tRNA molecule carrying its amino acid responds, the polypeptide chain grows longer.

DEFECTS IN ONE OR MORE GENES CAUSE INBORN ERRORS OF METABOLISM

Despite its amazing complexity, the protein synthesizing process functions almost to perfection in virtually every individual. But in some conditions, a key component of the mechanism fails to work. These inborn errors of metabolism are due to inherited defects that result in biochemical abnormalities, often with serious clinical symptoms. To illustrate, consider here one of the most familiar of such diseases, phenylketonuria or PKU.

Usually, defects are the result of damage to a single gene, the unit by which hereditary traits are transmitted. Genes can be described as the set of nucleotide codons on a DNA molecule that direct the formation of a particular protein from its component amino acids. However, it is convenient to refer to genes in terms of their net effect in imparting traits, as has been traditional since Gregor Mendal first suggested their existence a centuary ago.

A damaged gene is known as mutant. Mutation result from factors, such as exposure to radiation, that interfere with the replication of the DNA molecule. Even if a single nucleotide was missing, or if an incorrect nucleotide were to replace a correct one, the mRNA strand would be transmitting the 'wrong' information leading to the addition of an incorrect amino acid. If the resulting protein were a metabolic enzyme, the metabolic process for which it was necessary could not take place.

This is precisely what happens in PKU. For some reason, some incorrect nucleotide is present in the DNA strand that codes for the structure of the enzyme necessary for metabolizing phenylalalanine. Since phenylalalanine is an essential amino acid, its specific amount must be obtained from dietary sources. The genetic defect does not interfere with the utilization of this necessary amount. But excess phenylalalanine is normally converted by the enzyme into the non-essential amino acid tyrosine, which is used for growth and other functions. If this pathway is blocked because the enzyme is missing, phenylalanine is metabolized by alternate pathways and accumulates along with its abnormal metabolites, in body fluids. At the same time, there results an inadequate amount of tyrosine. The combination of excessive phenylalanine and its by-products and an inadequate tyrosine, result in the symptoms found in untreated phenyl ketoneuric patients. The condition of PKU can be diagrammed as follows:

Main pathway

Normal individual: Phenylalanine   Tyrosine   (Large amounts)

Minor pathway

Phenylalanine   Phenylketones   (Trace amounts)

PKU Patients

Minor pathway

Phenylalanine ⟶ Tyrosine   (Trace amounts)

Main pathway

Phenylketones   (Large amounts)

The symptoms, which appear in infants between 6 and 18 months of age, include irritability, hyperactivity, convulsions, seizures, lighter skin and hair colour than other family members, moderate to severe mental retardation, and a general slowdown of physical growth and development. Untreated individuals have a short life expectancy, with only a 25% chance of surviving past the third decade.

INBORN ERRORS OF AMINO ACID METABOLISM

Amino acids are the building blocks of proteins and have many functions in the body. Hereditary disorders of amino acids can result from defects in the catalytic breakdown of amino acids. Because these disorders cause symptoms early in life, newborns need to be routinely screened for phenylketonuria, maple syrup urine disease, homocystinuria, tyrosinemia, and a number of other, lesser known, inherited disorders.

Disorders of Phenylalanine Metabolism

Phenylketonuria

Phenylketonuria (PKU) is the most common disease caused by a deficiency of an enzyme of amino acid metabolism. The name comes from the excretion of phenylpyruvic acid, a phenylketone, in the urine. Phenyl pyruvate is also excreted as an oxidation product. Besides, phenylacetate, which gives the urine a "mousey" odor. These three metabolites are found only in trace amounts in urine in the healthy person. The symptoms of mental retardation associated with this disease can only be prevented by a phenylalanine free diet. Classical PKU is an autosomal recessive deficiency of phenylalanine hydroxylase. Phenylketonuria occurs in infants born without the ability to normally break down phenylalanine and enzyme, phenyl alanine hydroxylase, is needed to convert phenylalanine to tyrosine. Its symptoms of phenylketonuria include intellectual disability, seizures, nausea, vomiting, an eczema-like rash, and a mousy body odor. A strict phenylalanine-restricted diet allows for normal growth and development. In fact, phenylalanine is an essential amino acid that cannot be synthesized in the body but is present in food. Excess phenylalanine is normally converted to tyrosine, another amino acid, and eliminated from the body. Without the enzyme that converts it to tyrosine, phenylalanine builds up in the blood and is toxic to the brain, causing intellectual disability.

In some cases there are severe neurological symptoms and very low IQ. These are generally attributed to toxic effects of phenylalanine, possibly because of reduced transport and metabolism of other aromatic amino acids in the brain due to competition from the high phenylalanine concentration. Another characteristic is light color of skin and eyes, due to under pigmentation because of tyrosine deficiency. Basis of treatment is to feed affected infants a synthetic diet low in phenylalanine, but including tyrosine, for about four to five years and impose dietary protein restriction for several more years or for life.

The behaviour of untreated children is that they are considerably hyperactive, exhibit poor coordination, irritability, and at times they have seizures. Good management of PKU involves (1) An early diagnosis after birth. (2) A nutritionally adequate diet adjusted to meet the requirements for normal growth and development. (3) Keeping restriction on phenylalanine intake in order to have an acceptable range of serum phenylalanine. (4) Continuous monitoring of biochemical and clinical parameters related with the disease. (5) An elaborate programme of imparting awareness to the parents about the disease, its repercussion and management.

In cases where the treatment begins within the first few weeks of life, there remains more or less normal mental and physical development. Best way of management of the disease is team approach which should include the physician, nurse, biochemist, social worker, nutritionist and parents.

There is no need to give low phenylalanine diet if the serum phenylalanine level is below 15 mg/100 ml. Such a diet is prescribed when serum phenylalanine level is more than 30 mg/100 ml. Infants, where phenylalanine intake is adjusted to keep serum levels below 15 mg/100 ml during the first years of life and thereafter, can have satisfactory development of brain. Commercial preparation named Lofenalac has 95% of phenylalanine removed to serve as the chief source of proteins sans phenylalaninefor infants. Use of Lofenalac also permits the intake of some natural foods containing phenylalanine to ensure hassle-free normal growth.

Disorders of Tyrosine Metabolism

Tyrosinemia

Tyrosinemia (Tyrosinosis) is caused by lack of the enzyme needed to metabolize tyrosine. The most common form of this disorder mostly affects the liver and the kidneys. Children with tyrosinemia are unable to completely metabolize the amino acid tyrosine. The absence or deficiency of tyrosine aminotransferase produces accumulation and excretion of tyrosine and its metabolites causing a variety of symptoms.

There are two main types of tyrosinemia: type I and type II. Type I, hepatorenal tyrosinemia is more serious, involving liver failure, renal tubular dysfunction, rickets and polyneuropathy caused by a deficiency of fumarylacetoacetate hydroxylase. Accumulation of fumarylacetoacetate and malylacetate, both of which are alkylating agents, can lead to DNA alkylation and tumorigenesis. The disease, oculocutaneous or type II tyrosinemia results in eye and skin lesions and mental retardation. Both the types of tyrosinemia are autosomal recessive disorders and thus very rare in occurrence.

To begin with, a protein hydrolysate low in phenylalanine and tyrosine is used along with some milk to provide essential and other amino acids. If blood methionine levels are elevated, a synthetic mixture of amino acids without tyrosine, phenylalanine, and methionine is used together with a protein-free supplement to provide energy (carbohydrate, fat) and micronutrients (vitamins and minerals). A diet low in phenylalanine, tyrosine, and methionine becomes the basis of nutritional management.

Albinism

Skin and hair color are controlled by an unknown number of genetic loci in humans and exist in infinite variation in mice. Many conditions have been described in which the skin has little or no pigment. However, the chemical basis is not established for any except classical albinism, which results from a lack of tyrosinase. Tyrosinase enzyme is essential for the conversion of tyrosine to melanine, the characteristic skin pigment. Lack of pigment in the skin makes albinos sensitive to sunlight, making them vulnerable to carcinoma of the skin in addition to burns. Further, lack of pigment in the eyes may contribute to photophobia. As such there is no dietary therapy known for albinism.

Disorder of Branched Chain Amino Acid (Valine, Leucine, Isoleucine) Metabolism

Maple Syrup Urine Disease

Maple syrup urine disease is commonly caused by lack of the enzyme (branched chain alpha keto dehydrogenase complex) needed to metabolize branched chain amino acids (leucine, isoleucine and valine). By-products of these amino acids cause the urine to smell like maple syrup.

Children with maple syrup urine disease are unable to metabolize certain amino acids. By-products of these amino acids build up, causing neurologic changes, including seizures and intellectual disability. These by-products also cause body fluids, such as urine and sweat, to smell like maple syrup.

Conceptually, a diet restricted in leucine, isoleucine, and valine is used. A formula diet consisting of commercially available mixture of amino acids without the branched-chain amino acids, some milk, and a protein-free supplement have been prescribed. Fruits, vegetables, and cereals low in protein are added in controlled amounts as the child grows.

Disorder of Methionine Metabolism

Homocystinuria

Homocystinuria is caused by lack of the enzyme (cystathionine synthase) needed to metabolize homocysteine. This disorder can cause a number of symptoms, including decreased vision and skeletal abnormalities. Children with homocystinuria are unable to metabolize the amino acid intermediate homocysteine, which, along with certain toxic by-products, builts up to cause a variety of symptoms. Symptoms may be mild or severe, depending on the particular enzyme defect.

Infants with this disorder are normal at birth. The first symptoms, including dislocation of the lens of the eye, causing severely decreased vision, usually begin after 3 years of age. Most children have skeletal abnormalities, including osteoporosis. Children are usually tall and thin with a curved spine, chest deformities, elongated limbs and long, spiderlike fingers. Without early diagnosis and treatment, mental (psychiatric) and behavioural disorders and intellectual disability are common. Homocystinuria makes the blood more likely to clot spontaneously, resulting in strokes, high blood pressure, and many other serious problems.

Patients of classic homocystinuria respond to pharmacologic doses of pyridoxine (B6), a coenzyme for cystathionine synthetase. For others, a regimen of pyridoxine, folic acid, and betaine or choline is associated with improved clinical response and decrease in plasma homocysteine levels. Folic acid and betaine have also been used in homocystinuria due to defects in the folate remethylating pathway.

To patients who respond to pyridoxine therapy, a normal, but not excessive, protein intake is given. For those unresponsive to pyridoxine, a low-methionine diet supplemented with cystine is recommended. A special formula, low in methionine, is also used. Considerations in the diet planning are similar to those in phenylketonuria—calculating the amount of formula needed to meet protein and calorie requirements, and finding amounts of other foods permitted.

Disorder of Tryptophan Metabolism

Alkaptonuria

The first condition identified as an "inborn error of metabolism" was alkaptonuria. Individuals deficient in liver and kidney homogentisate oxidase, an enzyme of tryptophan metabolism which causes oxidation of homogentisic acid, excrete almost all ingested typtophan as the colourless homogentisic acid in their urine due to the metabolic block occurring at the oxidation of intermediate homogentisic acid. This auto-oxidizes to the corresponding quinine, which polymerizes to form an intensely dark colour. Concern about the dark urine is the only the sequence of this condition early in the life. Homogentisic acid is slowly oxidized to pigments that are deposited in bones, connective tissues and other organs, a condition called ochronosis because of the ochre colour of the deposits. This is thought to be responsible for the associated arthritis.

It is a very rare disorder, and more often than not, does not appear life threatening. Essential precautions involve avoiding a high protein diet. Protein content of the diet is maintained marginally adequate with a fair representation of plant based protein foodstuffs and the overall diet is kept balanced in terms of other nutrients. Thus as such there is no specific therapy known for alkaptonuria. Intake of vitamin C is recommended to prevent the oxidation of homogentisic acid to prevent the deposition of ochronotic material in the cartilage to relieve the patient from arthritis like symptoms.

INBORN ERRORS OF CARBOHYDRATE METABOLISM

Galactosemia

The disease, galactosemia, is caused by the absence of enzyme galactose-1-phosphate uridyl transferase abbreviated as P-Gal-transferase. It is needed in the liver for the conversion of galactose to glucose. Galactose is derived from the hydrolysis of lactose, the milk sugar, in the intestine. It is absorbed normally in the patient, but in the absence of P-Gal-transferase, galactose, galactose-1-phosphate, and galactitol accumulate in the blood and tissues. Urine tests show the presence of galactose, albumin, and amino acids in the urine sample. A galactose tolerance test establishes the diagnosis.

The disease becomes manifest within a few days after birth by symptoms like anorexia, vomiting, diarrhea, drowsiness, jaundice, puffiness of the face, edema of the lower extremities and weight loss. The spleen and liver enlargement, and in some there may be evidence of liver failure within a short time leading to early death. Mental retardation becomes apparent very early in the course of the disease, and cataracts develop within the first year.

Milk is the important dietary source of lactose, which in turn yields galactose. Human milk is especially high in lactose, and thus the breast-fed infant who lacks the necessary enzyme show symptoms very early. Obviously, Its replacement by non-milk formula leads to rapid improvement as a rule. All the symptoms disappear except the mental retardation that has already occurred which is not reversible. Damage to the central nervous system is the greatest during the first few months of life, when growth is rapid. Therefore, the promptness in initiation of therapy is essential.

Hereditary Fructose Intolerance

In this inborn error there is a deficiency of liver type fructose-1-phosphate aldolase, which splits fructose-1-phosphate into glyceraldehydes and dihydroxyacetone phosphate. The accumulation of fructose-1-phosphate prevents replenishment of cellular inorganic phosphate needed for regeneration of ATP. Introduction of table sugar sucrose or fructose in the infant's diet before 6 months of age results in anorexia, vomiting, failure to thrive, hypoglycemic convulsions, and dysfunction of the liver and kidney. Older children with the defect are often asymptomatic or they may have spontaneous hypoglycemia. When an oral dose of fructose is given, the blood fructose and magnesium levels rise, but the levels of glucose and phosphate fall. The hypoglycemia that occurs on partaking sucrose or fructose is believed to be caused by reduced glycogenolysis and gluconeogenesis due to the inhibition of key enzyme of these pathways, the phosphoglucomutase, by accumulated fructose - 1 - phosphate. In this condition, glucose cannot be made from either glycogenolysis or gluconeogenesis. The patients kept on sucrose and fructose free diets remain symptoms free. The patients are also prohibited to consume fruit and foods with rich levels of fructose.

INBORN ERRORS OF LIPID METABOLISM

Numerous inherited are caused by errors in fatty acid metabolism. They may be described as fatty acid oxidation disorders or as a lipid storage disorders, and result from enzyme defects affecting the ability of the body to oxidize fatty acids in order to produce energy within muscles, liver, and other cell types.

As such there are no known nutritional management strategies for these disorders. Certain measures are taken on case to case basis, by affecting quantitative and/or qualitative alterations in dietary fat intake for patients suffering from one or the other disorders of this type.

STUDY QUESTIONS

1. Explain the term inborn errors of metabolism giving the suitable examples.
2. Explain the genetic basis of inborn errors of metabolism.
3. Why nutritional management of inborn errors of metabolism is a challenge? Explain giving the example of phenylketonuria.
4. Discuss galactosemia and hereditary fructose intolerance along with their nutritional management.
5. Explain the inborn errors of metabolism—Tyrosenemia, homocysteinuria and alkaptonuria, giving tips about their nutritional management.

Nutritional Glossary

Absorption: The movement of digested food substances from the lumen of the intestine into intestinal cells and from there into the blood stream for distribution to other parts of the body.

Absorption cells: A class of cells that line the villi (finger like projections in the small intestine) and participate in nutrient absorption.

Acesulfame-K: An artificial sweetener that yields no energy to the body: it is as much as 200 times sweeter than sucrose.

Achlorhydria: A state of reduced acid production by the stomach, primarily resulting from loss of the acid-producing cells in the stomach, a condition associated with ageing.

Acid: Any substance that releases hydrogen ions in solution.

Acquired immunodeficiency syndrome (AIDS): A disease characterized by poor function of one class of white blood cells (called helper T cells). The resulting poor immune function leaves the person quite susceptible to infection, which can, in turn, result in rapidly failing health and death.

Active absorption: Absorption using a carrier and expending energy. In this way the absorptive process can absorb nutrients, such as glucose, against a high concentration in the absorptive cells.

Ad libitum: At one's desire or pleasure.

Adenosine triphosphate (ATP): The main energy currency for cells. ATP energy is used to promote ion pumping enzyme activity, and muscular contraction.

Adipose (fat) cells: A group of fat-storage cells.

Adult onset obesity: Obesity that develops in adulthood: characteristically, the individual has a normal of adipose cells but each cell is enlarged because of fat storage. May lead to non-insulin dependent diabetes mellitus, or type II diabetes.

Aerobic: Requiring oxygen.

Alcohol: Ethyl alcohol or ethanol. An energy-yielding substance found in beer, wine and distilled spirits as also in fermented foods.

Aldosterone: A powerful hormone produced by the adrenal glands that acts on the kidneys to cause sodium reabsorption, and in turn, water conservation.

Alkaline (basic) pH: A pH greater than 7.

Alkalosis: Life threatening state in which the pH of body fluids rises above 7.4 may be caused by disorders of respiration (breathing) or metabolism.

Allergen: An antigen whose presence in the blood causes an allergic reaction. Most allergenic substances are normal plants or foods to which an individual has developed sensitivity.

Allergy: An immune response that occurs when immune bodies (antibodies) react with a foreign substance (antigen) in an unusual way to produce histamine.

Alpha-linolenic acid: A fatty acid with 18 carbon atoms and three double bonds; omega-3.

Alveoli: The small air sacs of the lungs.

Amino acid: The building block for proteins: amino acids have a carbon in the center with a nitrogen and other atoms attached.

Amniotic fluid: The fluid that surrounds and protects the foetus in the uterus.

Amylase: Starch–digesting enzymes from the salivary glands or pancreas.

Amylopectin: The branched-chain digestible polysaccharide made of glucose units.

Amylase: Straight-chain digestible polysaccharide made of glucose units.

Anabolism: The process of building compounds.

Anaerobic: Not requiring oxygen.

Anaphylactic shock: A severe allergic response that results in greatly lowered blood pressure as well as in respiratory and gastrointestinal distress.

Androgen: A general term for hormones that stimulate development of male sex organs; testosterone is an example.

Anaemia: Poor oxygen-carrying ability of the blood, caused by a reduction in the number of healthy red blood cells.

Anergy: Lack of an immune response to foreign compounds entering the body.

Animal model: A disease in animals that duplicates human disease and thus can be used to further understand human diseases.

Anorexia nervosa: An eating disorder involving a psychological loss of appetite and self-starvation, resulting in part from a distorted body image in various social pressures associated with puberty.

Anthropometry: The measurement of weight, heights, circumferences, and skin fold thicknesses of the body.

Antibody: Blood proteins that inactivate foreign proteins found in the body, thus preventing infection.

Anticarcinogens: Compounds that potentially inhibit the development of cancer.

Antidiuretic hormone (ADH): A hormone secreted by the pituitary gland that acts on the kidneys to decrease water excretion.

Antioxidant: A compound that can donate electrons to electron-seeking (oxidizing) compounds.

Apolipoproteins: Proteins embedded in the outer shell of lipoproteins.

Appetite: The psychological drive to fond and eat food, often in the absence of hunger.

Arachidonic acid: A fatty acid with 20 carbon atoms and four double bonds; omega-6.

Areola: The circular dark area of skin at the center of the breast.

Arthritis: Inflammation at a point where bones join; the disease has many possible causes.

Aseptic processing: A method by which food and its contents are sterilized simultaneously; this process allows manufacturers to produce boxes of milk that can be stored at room temperatures.

Aspartame: An alternate sweetener made of two amino acids (part of protein).

Atherosclerosis: A buildup of fatty material (plaque) majorly cholesterol in the arteries, including those surrounding the heart.

Atom: The smallest combining unit of an element.

Autodigestion: Literally, self-digestion. The stomach limits autodigestion by covering itself with a thick layer of mucous and by producing enzymes and acid only when needed for digestion of food.

Autoimmune: Immune reaction against normal body cells; self against self.

Avidin: A protein found in raw egg white that can bind vitamin biotin and inhibits its absorption. Cooking destroys avidin.

Baryophobia: A poor rate of growth in children associated with parents underfeeding them in an attempt to prevent obesity and heart disease.

Basal metabolism: The minimum energy the body requires supporting itself when resting and awaking. It amounts to roughly 1 kilocalorie per minute, or about 1400 kilocalories per day.

Base: Any substance that releases hydroxyl ions.

Basic four: General division of all foods grouped on the basis of necessary nutrients (other than energy and fat). Four groups include dairy, meat and meat substitutes, fruits and vegetables, and grains and cereals.

Behavior chains: Activities linked in a person's lifestyle, such as snacking while watching television.

Benign: Harmless.

Beriberi: A thiamin-deficiency disorder characterized by muscle weakness, loss of appetite, nerve degeneration, and sometimes edema.

BHA and BHT: Butylated hydroxyl anisole and toluene; two common synthetic antioxidants that are added to foods.

Bile: A substance made in the liver and stored in the gallbladder; it is released in the small intestine to aid fat absorption.

Bioavailability: The degree to which an ingested nutrient is absorbed and so is available to the body.

Biochemical changes: Nutritional deficiency symptoms as reflected in the blood or urine, such as low levels of nutrient by-products or low enzyme activities. These indicate reduced biochemical functioning in the body.

Bioelectrical impedance: A method of estimating total body fat by measuring the impedance (resistance) of a low-energy electrical current by the body.

Biological value of the protein: The body's ability to retain protein (nitrogen) absorbed from a food.

Biotechnology: The use of advanced scientific techniques to alter, and ideally, improve characteristics of animal and use of biological organisms and processes for human benefit.

Blood doping: A technique by which an athlete's red blood cells are concentrated and then later reintroduced into the athlete.

Body mass index: Weight (in kilograms) divided by height squared (in meters); a value of 30 or higher indicates obesity.

Bomb calorimeter: An instrument used to determine the caloric content of foods.

Bonds: A sharing of electrons, charges or attraction, used to link two atoms.

Brown adipose tissue: A specialized form of fat storage that produces large amounts of heat by metabolizing energy-yielding nutrients without synthesizing much usable energy for the body. Much of the energy is released as heat.

Buffer: Compound that can cause a solution to resist change in its pH on the addition of an acid or base.

Bulimia: An eating disorder in which large quantities of food are eaten at one time and then purged from the body by vomiting, use of laxatives, or other means.

Beta-carotene: An orange pigment found in many fruits and vegetable, such as peaches and carrots. The body can use beta-carotene to make vitamin A.

Cachexia: Extreme emaciation, malnutrition and weakness following some disease, trauma or starvation syndrome. Common in some cancers.

Cancer: A condition characterized by uncontrolled growth of body cells.

Carbohydrates loading: The process of consuming a very high carbohydrate diet for 6 before an athletic event to try to increase muscle glycogen stores.

Carbohydrates: Compounds containing carbon, hydrogen and oxygen atoms; known as sugars, starches. hydrates of carbon.

Carcinogens: Compound that have the potential to cancer.

Cardiac output: The amount of blood pumped by the heart.

Cardiovascular: Pertaining to the heart and blood vessels.

Cariogenic: A substance, often rich in carbohydrates, that promotes dental caries (e.g. caramels and raisins).

Carnitine: A compound used to shuttle fatty acids into the cell mitochondria, allowing the fatty acids to burn for energy.

Carotenoids: Pigment substances in plants that often can form vitamin A. B-carotene is the most active form.

Casein: A protein found in milk that forms curds; a major protein of milk.

Cash crops: Crops grown by a country specifically for export rather than to feed the country's citizens (e.g., coffee, tea and bananas).

Catabolic: Breaking downs compounds.

Catalyst: A compound that speeds up reaction rates but is not altered by the reaction.

Cell: A minute structure; the living basis of all plant and animal organization. Cells can both take up compounds from their environment and excrete compounds into it.

Cellulose: A straight chain polysaccharide of glucose molecules that is indigestible; part insoluble fiber.

Celsius: A centigrade measure of temperature.

Centimeter: A measure of length in the metric system; 100 centimeters equal 1 meter.

Cerebrovascular accident (CVA): Death of part of the brain tissue as a result of a blood clot.

Chain breaking: Breaking the link between two or more behaviors that encourage overeating, such as snacking while watching television.

Chemical score: A ratio comparing the essential amino acid content of the protein in food with the essential amino acid content in an ideal protein; lowest ratio for an essential amino acid becomes its chemical score.

Chemical reaction: An interaction between two chemicals that changes both participants.

Chinese restaurant syndrome: A sensitivity or allergic reaction to monosodium glutamate.

Cholesterol: A waxy fat, made only by animals, that is found in all body cells, its structure contains multiple chemical rings.

Chronic: Long standing, developing overtime; slow to develop or resolve. When referring to disease, this indicates that the disease, progress is slow and tends to remain for a long time if once developed, as with heart disease.

Chylomicrons: Dietary fats that are surrounded by a shell of cholesterol, phospholipids and protein. Chylomicrons are made in the intestine after fat absorption and travel through the lymphatic system to the blood-stream.

Chyme: A mixture of stomach secretions and partly digested food.

Cirrhosis: A loss of functioning liver cells, which are replaced by non-functioning connective tissue. Any substance that poisons liver cells, such as alcohol, can lead to cirrhosis.

Clinical symptom: Generally, a change in health status noted by the individual (e.g., stomach pain) or during a physical examination.

Clostridium botulinum: A bacterium that can cause a fatal type of food poisoning.

Coenzyme: The active form of many vitamins; coenzymes aid enzyme function.

Cognitive restructuring: Changing one's frame of mind regarding eating; for example, instead of using a difficult day as an excuse to overeat, substituting it with other pleasures or rewards, such as a relaxing walk with a friend.

Colic: Periodic crying in a healthy infant, apparently as a result of gas buildup.

Collagen: The major protein form found in connective tissue, cartilage and bone. Vitamin C aids in its synthesis.

Colon: Another name for the large intestine.

Colostrums: The first milk secreted during late pregnancy and the first few days after birth. This thick fluid is rich in immune factors and protein.

Complementarity of proteins: The ability of two food protein sources to make up for each other's insufficient contribution of specific amino acids, such that together they yield a high-quality protein diet.

Complete proteins: Proteins that contain ample amounts of all nine essential amino acids.

Compound: A substance composed of two or more different element (e.g., H_2O).

Constipation: A condition of infrequent bowel movements.

Control group: In an experiment, the group whose habits are not altered.

Cortical bone: Dense, compact bone that comprised the outer surface and shaft of a bone.

Cretinism: The stunting of body growth and mental development that result from inadequate maternal intake of iodine during pregnancy.

Crude fiber: The remains of dietary fiber after acid and alkali treatment; this consists primarily of cellulose and lignins.

Cystic fibrosis: A disease that, among other effects, often leads to overproduction of mucus, which can invade the pancreas and decrease the production of enzymes. The subsequent lack of lipase enzyme contributed so severe malabsorption of fat.

Daily food guide: A dietary planning tools that recommends food choice from milk and milk products; meat, fish, poultry and beans; vegetable and fruits; and breads and cereals.

Deamination: The removal of an amino group from an amino acid.

Dementia: A general loss or decrease in mental function.

Denature: Alternation of a protein's three-dimensional structure, usually as a result of treatment by heat, acid or alkaline solutions or agitation.

Dental caries: Sites of erosion on the tooth surface. Caries are caused by the acid produced when bacteria on the tooth's surface metabolize sugar.

Deoxyribonucleic acid (DNA): The site of hereditary information in cells; DNA directs the synthesis of cell proteins.

Dermatitis: Inflammation of the skin.

Diabetes, gestational: Diabetes that develops during the physical stress of pregnancy.

Diabetes mellitus: A disease characterized by high blood sugar levels that result from poor action by the hormone insulin.

Diastolic blood pressure: The pressure in the blood stream when the heart is between beats.

Dietary fibre: Substances in food (essentially all from plants) that are not digested by the processes in the stomach and small intestine.

Digestibility: The proportion of food substances eaten that can be broken down in the intestinal tract and absorbed into the bloodstream.

Digestion: The process by which food is broken into forms that can be absorbed by the GI tract.

Diphosphoglycerate: A compound used up in the red blood cells that is involved in the release of oxygen from haemoglobin.

Direct calorimetry: A method of determining energy used by the body by measuring heat produced by it.

Disaccharides: A class of sugars formed by linking two monosachharides.

Diuretic: A substance that increases the flow of urine.

Diverticula: Pouches that protrude through the wall of the large intestine. Diverticulosis is the condition of having many diverticula in the colon.

Diverticulitis: An inflammation of the diverticula caused by acids produced by bacterial metabolism inside the diverticula.

Double blind study: An experimental in which the subjects and researchers are unaware of the study assignments (placebo vs experimental) until it is completed.

Edema: The buildup of excess fluid in extracellular spaces.

Eicosanoids: Hormone like compounds synthesized from polyunsaturated fatty acids; this class of compounds includes prostaglandins, thromboxane and leukotrienes.

Eicosapenteanoic acid (EPA): An omega-3 fatty acid with 20 carbon atoms and five double bonds; present in fish oils.

Electrolytes: Compounds that break down into ion in water and thus can conduct an electrical current.

Elemental formula: Liquid formula containing nutrients in their most chemically simple, "elemental" form.

Elimination diet: A restrictive diet that systematically tests foods that may cause an allergic response by first eliminating suspected foods and then adding them back one at a time.

Embryo: The developing human life form during the second to eighth week after conception.

Emulsifier: A substance that can suspend fat in tiny droplets within a watery fluid.

Endomorph: A body type characterized by short, stubby bones, a short trunk, and very short fingers.

Endorphins: Natural body tranquillizers that may be involved in the feeding response, as well as in pain reduction.

Endosperm: The central, largest portion of grain. White flour is made from the endosperm of the wheat kernel and does not include the germ or bran.

Enriched: A term generally meaning that the vitamins thiamin, niacin and riboflavin and the mineral iron have been added to a grain product to improve nutritional quality.

Enzyme: A compound that speeds up the rate of a chemical process but is not altered by the process. Almost all enzymes are proteins.

Epidemiology: The study of how diseases rates vary between different population groups, such as the rate of lung cancer in India compared with that in Germany.

Epinephrine: A hormone also known as adrenaline; it is released by the adrenal gland (located near the kidneys) and various nerve endings in the body. Epinephrine increases glycogen breakdown in the liver, among other functions.

Epithelial cells: The surface cells that line the outside of the body and all external passages within it.

Equilibrium: In nutritional terms, a state in which nutrient intakes equals nutrient losses; this allows the body to maintain stable condition.

Essential amino acids: The amino acids that cannot be synthesized by humans in sufficient amounts and therefore must be included in the diet; there are nine essential amino acids.

Essential fatty acids: Fatty acids that must be present in the diet to maintain health; these are linoleic acid and alpha linolenic acid.

Esterification: The process of attaching fatty acids to a glycerol molecule. Removing a fatty acid is called deesterification; reattaching fatty acids is called reesterification.

Estimated safe and adequate daily intake (ESAADI): Nutrients intake recommendations that give approximate intake of some nutrients because not enough information is available to set a recommended daily allowances (RDA).

Exchange system: A grouping of foods in six lists. When the serving size for any food in a list is consumed, all foods within the list yield a similar amount of carbohydrate, fat, protein and energy.

Experiment: A test conducted to examine the validity of a hypothesis.

Failure of thrive: Inadequate gains in height and weight in infancy, often resulting from inadequate food intake.

Famine: A time of massive starvation, often associated with crop failures, war and political strife.

Fasting hypoglycemia: Low blood sugar that follow a day or so of fasting.

Fatty acid: Acids found in it; they are composed of carbon atoms linked to hydrogen atoms, with an acidic chemical group at one end.

Fat soluble vitamin: Vitamins that dissolve in substances such as ether or benzene. These vitamins include A, D, E and K.

Feeding centre: A group of cells in the hypothalamus that cause hunger when stimulated. These cells are also known as the lateral feeding centers.

Ferritin: A protein compound that serves as the storage form of iron in the blood and tissues.

Foetal alcohol syndrome (FAS): A group of physical and mental abnormalities in an infant caused by the mother's consumption of alcohol during pregnancy.

Foetus: A developing infant inside its mother from 8 weeks to birth.

Fluoroapatite: Tooth crystals containing fluoride ions that are relatively acid resistant.

Food diary: A written record of sequential food intake for a period of time. Details associated with the food intake are often recorded as well.

Food intolerance: An adverse reaction to food that does not involve the immune system.

Food sensitivity: A mild reaction to a substance in food that might be noticed as slight itching and redness of skin.

Fore milk: The first breast milk delivered in the nursing session.

Fortified: A term generally meaning that vitamins, minerals or both have been added to food product in excess of what was originally found in the products.

Fraternal twins: Infants that develop from two separate ova and sperm and therefore have separate genetic identities, although they develop simultaneously in the mother.

Fructose: A monosaccharide with six carbons found in fruits and honey.

Galactose: A six carbon monosaccharide, and isomer of glucose.

Galactosemia: A disease characterized by the build-up of the monosaccharide galactose in the bloodstream, resulting from the liver's inability to metabolize galactose. If present at birth and left untreated, galactosemia results in severe growth and mental retardation.

Gastrin: A hormone that stimulates the secretion of enzymes and acids in the stomach.

Gastrointestinal (GI) tract: The main site in the body used in digestion and absorption of nutrients. It consists of the mouth, esophagus, stomach, small intestine, large intestine, rectum and anus.

Gastroplasty: Surgery performed on the stomach to limit its volume to approximately 50 milliliters, about the size of a short glass.

Generally recognized as safe (GRAS): A group of food additives that are considered safe; the manufacturers have been allowed to use them when needed in food products.

Genes: The hereditary material on chromosomes that makes up DNA. Genes provide the blue prints for the production of cell proteins.

Genetic engineering: Alteration of genetic material in plant or animals with the intent of improving growth, disease resistance, or other characteristics.

Gestation: The time of fetal growth from conception to birth; a period of about 40 weeks after a woman's last normal menstrual period.

Gestational diabetes: A high blood glucose level that develops during pregnancy but returns to normal after birth. One cause is production of hormones by the placenta that antagonize the action of the hormone insulin.

Glucagon: A hormone made by the pancreas that stimulates the liver to break down glycogen into glucose; this raises the blood glucose level. Glucagon also performs other functions.

Glycolysis: The pathway that results in the breakdown of glucose into two-three carbon molecules.

Goiter: An enlargement of the thyroid gland (located in the neck area) often caused by a lack of iodine in the diet.

Goitrogens: Substances in food that interfere with the absorption and use of iodine; they therefore may cause goitre if consumed in large amounts.

Gram: A measure of weight in the metric system; 28 grams equal 1 ounce, and kilogram equals 2.2 pounds.

Green revolution: A period in the 1960s when much emphasis was placed on improving strains and cultivation practices of cereal grains such as rice, wheat and corn.

Growth hormone: A pituitary hormone that promotes body growth and the release of fat among other effects.

Gums: A group of soluble fibres containing chains of galactose, glucuronic acid and other monosaccharides; gums characteristically are found in matter exuded from plant stems.

Hazard: The chances that injury will result from use of a substance.

Heart attack: A rapid fall in heart function caused by reduced blood flow through the heart's blood vessels. Often part of the heart dies in the process.

Heart disease: A disease characterized by the deposition of fatty material I the blood vessels in the heart. The fatty materials reduce blood flow through the blood vessels supplying the heart.

Heart burn: A pain emanating from the oesophagus as a result of stomach acid backing up into the oesophagus and irritating the tissue in that organ.

Hematocrit: The percentage of blood that is made up of red blood cells.

Heme iron: Iron provided from animal tissues as haemoglobin and myoglobin. Approximately 50% of the iron in meat is heme iron; it is readily absorbed.

Hemicellulose: A group of insoluble fibres containing the monosaccharides xylose, galactose and glucose as well as other monosaccharide linked in an indigestible fashion.

Haemochromatosis: A disorder of iron metabolism characterized by increased iron absorption and deposition in the liver tissue; this eventually poisons the liver cells.

Haemoglobin: The iron containing protein in red blood cells that carried oxygen to the cells and carbon dioxide away from the cells. Haemoglobin also gives blood its red colour.

Haemolysis: Destruction of red blood cells. The red blood cell membrane breaks down; allowing cell contents to leak into protrude of the blood.

Haemorrhoids: Swollen veins of the rectum and anus; they often protrude into the anus.

Haemosiderin: An insoluble iron-protein compound found in the liver. Haemosiderin stores increase as the amount of iron in the liver exceeds the storage capacity of ferritin.

Herbicide: A compound that reduces the growth and reproduction of plants.

High-fructose corn syrup: A corn syrup that is 40% to 90% fructose.

High-density lipoprotein (HDL): A lipoprotein synthesized by the liver and small intestine that picks up cholesterol from dying cells and other sources and transfers it to the other lipoprotein in the bloodstream. A low HDL level increases the risk for heart disease.

Hind milk: The milk secreted at the end of a nursing session; it is higher in fat than milk.

Hormone: A compound secreted into the blood stream that acts to control the function of distant cells.

Hospice: Hospital care that emphasizes comfort and dignity in death.

Hunger: The physiological drive to find and eat food.

Hydrogenation: The addition of hydrogen atoms to the double bonds of polyunsaturated and monounsaturated fatty acids to reduce the extent of unsaturation; this process turns liquid vegetable oils into solid fats.

Hydrophilic: Attracts water (literally means "water loving").

Hydroxyapatite: A compound composed of calcium and phosphate that is deposited into the bone protein matrix to give bone strength and rigidity.

Hyperglycemia: A high blood glucose level; that is, above 140 miligrams per 100 milliliters of blood.

Hypertension: A condition also known as high blood pressure in which blood pressure remains persistently elevated, especially when the heart is between beats.

Hypoglycemia: A low blood glucose level; that is, below 40 to 50 milligrams of blood.

Hypothalamus: A grouping of cells at the base of the brain. These cells participate in many body functions, such as regulating hunger.

Identical twins: Two infants that develop from a singic ovum and sperm and consequently have the same genetic makeup.

In utero: "In the uterus". That is during pregnancy.

Incidental food additives: Additives introduced into food products indirectly from environmental contamination of ingredients or during the manufacturing process.

Incomplete protein: Dietary protein that contains less than the optimal amounts of essential amino acids.

Index of nutritional quality (INQ): A technique for identifying foods that have beneficial nutrient energy ratio.

$$\frac{\text{Amount of nutrient of food/Kcal of food}}{\text{Daily allowance for nutrient/Kcal of daily allowance}}$$

Indirect calorimetry: A method of estimating energy use by the body by measuring oxygen uptake and then using formulae to convert that gas usage into kilocalorie use.

Infectious disease: Any disease caused by invasion of the body by microorganisms, such as bacteria, fungi or viruses.

Infrastructure: The basic framework of a system or organization. For society, this includes roads, bridges, telephones, and other basic technologies.

Inoraganic: Free of carbon linked to hydrogen in the chemical structure.

Insensible: Not consciously noted by the individual.

Insoluble fibers: Fibers that mostly do not dissolve in water and are not digested even by bacteria in the large intestine. These include cellulose, some hemicelluloses and lignins.

Insulin: A hormone produced by the beta cells of the pancreas. Insulin increases the synthesis of glycogen in the liver and the movement of glucose from the bloodstream into muscle and adipose cells, among other processes.

Insulin-dependent diabetes mellitus: A form of diabetes prone to ketoses; it requires insulin therapy.

Intentional food additives: Additives knowingly (directly) incorporated into food products by manufacturers.

Intermediate density lipoprotein: The product formed after a very low density lipoprotein (VLDL) has had most of its triglyceride removed.

International unit (IU): A crude measure of vitamin activity often based on the growth rate of animals. Today these units have been replaced by more precise milligram and microgram quantities.

Intracellular fluid: Fluid contained within a cell.

Intravenous: Introduced directly into the blood-stream.

Intrinsic factor: A conjugated protein (glycoprotein) compound produced by the stomach that enhances absorption of vitamin B_{12}.

Inverted nipptesi: Nipples that contract or back up into the breast when the nipple area is squeezed, as in breast feeding. Infants cannot grasp an inverted nipple well enough to get the available milk. Inversion can usually correct.

Ion: An atom with an unequal number of electrons and protons. If the number of electrons exceeds the number of protons, the ion is negative. If the number of protons exceeds the number of electrons, the ion is positive.

Irradiation: A process whereby radiation energy is applied to foods, creating compounds within the food that destroy cell membranes, break down DNA, link proteins, limit enzyme activity and alter a variety of other proteins and cell functions that can lead to food spoilage.

Isomer: Different chemical structures for compounds that share the same chemical formula.

Kcalories or kilocalories: A measure of the energy content in foods. A kilocalorie is the heat needed to rise. 1000 grams (1 liter) of water through 1° celsius.

Ketone bodies: Incomplete breakdown products of fat containing three or four carbons. Products of acetyl-CoA (fat) metabolism containing three to four carbon atoms: acetoacetic acid, beta-hydroxybutyric acid and acetone. These contain a ketone group, hence the name. Produced in the body in diabetes mellitus and starvation conditions.

Ketosis: The condition of having high levels of ketones bodies in the bloodstream.

Kidney nephron: A unit of kidney cells that filters wastes out of the bloodstream.

Kilojoule: A measure of work in which 1 k joule equals the work needed to move 1 kilogram a distance of 1 meter with the force of 1 newton; 1 kilocalorie equals 4.8 kjoules.

Kwashiorkor: A disease of insufficient protein intake occurring primarily in young children when disease and infections also add up to high demands of protein for growth. Edema, moderate weight deficit, and weakness are common symptoms. If the child consumes insufficient protein, kwashiorkor may result.

Lactation: The period after childbirth during which milk is secreted by the mother to nurse the infant.

Lactic acid: A three-carbon acid formed during anaerobic cell metabolism; a partial breakdown of glucose; also called lactate.

Lactovegetarian: A semivegetarian food plan in which milk products are consumed as well as vegetable products.

Lacto-ovo-vegetarians: A semi-vegetarian food plan in which milk products dairy products, and eggs are included.

Lactobacillus bifidus factor: A protective factor secreted in colostrum that encourages growth of beneficial bacteria in the intestine of an infant.

Lactose: A sugar made up of glucose linked to another sugar, called lactose sugar of milk.

Lactose intolerance: Lactose is not digested as lactase production declines. Symptoms include gas and bloating after consuming dairy products.

Lanugo: The down like hair that appears after much body fat is lost as a result of semistarvation. The hair stands erect and traps air, which acts as insulation to the body, replacing that usually supplied by body fat.

Larva: One of the development stages of silk worm and other such species.

Laxative: A medication or other substance that stimulates evacuation of the intestinal tract.

Lean body mass: The part of the body that is free of all but essential body fat. About 2% of body fat is essential; the rest represents storage and so is not part of lean body mass. Lean body mass includes muscle, bone, organs, connective tissue, skin and other body parts.

Lecithin: A phospholipid containing two fatty acids, phosphate group, and a choline molecule.

Let-down reflex: A reflex stimulated by infant suckling that causes the release (ejection) of milk from milk ducts in the mother's breasts.

Life expectancy: The average length of life for a given group of people.

Life span: The potential oldest age to which a person can survive.

Lignin: A group of insoluble fibers made up of a multitringed alcohol (non-carbohydrate) structure.

Limiting amino acid: The essential amino acid in the lowest concentration in proportion to body mass.

Linoleic acid: A fatty acid with 18 carbon atoms and two double bonds; omega-6.

Lipase: Fat digesting enzymes; lipase produced by the pancreas acting in the small intestine is the most important form used in digestion.

Lipectomy: Surgical removal of body fat; also known as liposuction.

Lipids: Compounds containing carbon, hydrogen, oxygen, and sometimes other atoms. Lipids dissolve in ether or benzene and are commonly known as fats and oils.

Lipogenic: Means "creating lipid". The liver is the major lipogenic organ in the body.

Lipoprotein: A compound found in the bloodstream containing a core of lipids with a shell of protein, phospholipids and cholesterol.

Lipoprotein lipase: An enzyme attached to the outside of the cells that line the bloodstream; it breaks down triglycerides into free fatty acids and glycerol.

Liter: A measure of volume in the metric system; 1 liter equals 1.06 quarts.

Lobules: Sack like structures in the breast that store milk.

Long-chain fatty acids: Fatty acids that contain more than 12 carbon atoms.

Low birth weight (LBW): Infant weight at birth of less than 5.5 pounds (2.5 kilograms), usually because of premature birth; these infants have a higher risk of health problems.

Low density lipoprotein (LDL): The product of the intermediate density lipoprotein (LDL) containing primarily cholesterol; an elevated level of LDL is strongly linked to heart disease.

Low input sustainable agriculture (LISA): A form of farming that attempts to limit use of purchased materials such as manufactured fertilizers and pesticides, use of manure and crop rotation are typical substitutes.

Lower body obesity: The type of obesity, called gynoid, in which fat is stored primarily in the buttocks and thigh area.

Lymphatic system: The system of vessels that can accept large particles, such as products of fat absorption, and eventually pass them into the bloodstream.

Macrobiotics: A food plan that emphasizes vegetable foods over animal foods, often with heavy use of brown rice.

Macrocyte: A greatly enlarged mature red blood cell; these cells have a short life spans.

Major mineral: A mineral vital to health that is required in the diet in amounts greater than 100 milligrams per day.

Malnutrition: Falling health that results from a long-standing dietary intake fails to meet or greatly exceeds nutritional needs.

Maltose: Glucose linked to glucose a disaccharide.

Marasmus: A disease caused essentially by starvation; the person does not consume sufficient protein and kilocalories and thus has the equivalent of severe protein-energy malnutrition. The individual will be severely underweight and have little or no fat stores, little muscle mass and poor strength.

Marginal: Noticeable but not severe.

Mass movement: A peristaltic wave that simultaneously coordinates contraction over a large area of the colon. These contractions move material from one portion of the colon to another and from the colon into the rectum.

Meconium: The stool passed by an infant after birth. It has a thick, mucus like consistency.

Medium-chain fatty acids: Fatty acids that contain six to 10 carbon atoms.

Megadose: Intake of a nutrient in amounts greater than 10 times the desired RDA listed values.

Megaloblast: A large, immature red blood cell that results from the particular cell's inability to divide when it normally should.

Menarche: The onset of menses in women, which occurs usually between 10 and 13 years of age.

Menopause: The cessation of menses in women, which usually begins at about 50 years of age.

Mesomorph: A body type associated with average bone size, trunk size and finger length.

Metabolism: Sum of all such chemical reactions that occur in the body, enabling cells to release energy from foods, convert one substance into another and prepare end products of excretion.

Metastases: Cancerous tumours that begins to grow in areas of the body far from the location of the original tumor. Metastases are a sign that the original cancer has spread.

Meter: A measure of length in the metric system; 1 meter equals 39.4 inches.

Micelle: A droplet of fat surrounded by a shell of water. Emulsifiers are used to produce micelles.

Microgram: A measure of weight in the metric system; 1 million microgram equal to 1 gram.

Milligram: A measure of weight in the metric system; 1000 milligram equal to 1 gram.

Minerals: Chemical elements used in the body to promote chemical process and form body structures.

Minimum requirements for health (MRH): Nutrient intake recommendations for sodium potassium, and chloride, as set by the Food and Nutrition Board.

Miscarriage: Loss of pregnancy that occurs before 28 weeks of gestation; also called spontaneous abortion.

Molecule: A group of like or unlike atoms that are chemically linked; it is similar to a compound, which is a group of different types of atoms bonded together in definite proportion.

Monoglycerides: A breakdown product of triglycerides, consisting of one fatty acid bonded to the carbohydrate glycerol.

Monosaccharide: A single sugar, such as glucose, that is not broken down further during digestion.

Monounsaturated fatty acid: A fatty acid containing one carbon-carbon double bond.

Mortality: Synonymous with death; rate of death.

Mottle: Discoloration or making of the surface of teeth caused by high fluoride content.

Mucilage: A group of soluble fibers consisting of chains of galactose, mannose, and other monosaccharide; characteristically found in seaweed.

Mucous: A thick fluid, secreted by glands throughout the body that contains a compound that is both carbohydrate and protein in nature. Mucous acts a lubricant and a means of protection for cells.

Myocardial infarction: During heart attack death of part of the heart muscle owing to lack of blood supply occurs.

Myoglobin: An iron-containing compound that transports oxygen and carbon dioxide in muscle tissue.

Neonatal: The first 30 days of human life after birth.

Nephrotic syndrome: Medical symptoms accompanying progressive kidney failure; often includes anorexia.

Neurotransmitter: A compound made by a nerve cell that allows communication between it and other cells.

Nitrate: A nitrogen-containing compound used to cure meats. It gives meat a pink colour and confers some resistance to bacterial growth.

No observable effect level (NOEL): The highest dose of an additive that produces no deleterious health effect in animals.

Non heme iron: Iron provided from plant sources and animal tissues other than in the form of haemoglobin and myoglobin. Non heme iron is less efficiently absorbed than heme iron.

Nonessential amino acids: Amino acids that can be synthesized by the body in sufficient amounts; there are 11 nonessential amino acids in the diet.

Non insulin-dependent diabetes mellitus: A form of diabetes in which ketosis is not common, and insulin therapy is not often required.

Nonpolar: A compound with no charges.

Nucleus: The core of an atom; it consists of protons and neutrons.

Nursing bottle syndrome: Rampant tooth decay in infants and young children usually caused by overuse of the bottle and constant sucking on energy containing liquids.

Nutrient density: The ratio formed by dividing a food's contribution to the need for a nutrient by its contribution to kilocalorie needs. When the contribution to nutrient need exceeds that of kilocalorie needs, the food has a favourable nutrient density.

Nutrients: Chemical substances in food that nourish the body by providing energy, building materials, and factors to regulate needed chemical reactions in the body. The body either can't make these substances or can't make them sufficient enough for its needs.

Nutrition: One most appropriately defines nutrition as "the sciences of food, the nutrients and the substances therein, their action, interaction, and balance in relation to health and disease, the process by which the organism (i.e., body) ingests, digests, absorbs, transports, utilizes, and excretes food substances".

Nutrition labels: A label format that must be included on foods under certain circumstances, such as when nutrients are added to foods or when a nutritional claim is made for the food.

Nutritional status: The nutritional health of a person as determined by anthropometric measures (height, weight circumferences and so on), biochemical measures of nutrients or their byproducts in blood and urine, clinical (physical) examination, and a dietary analysis; these elements can be remembered by the acronym ABCD.

Nutritionist: A person who advises about nutrition or works in the field of foods and nutrition.

Obesity: A condition characterized by excess body fat, usually defined as body weight 20% above the desirable level.

Oligosaccharides: Carbohydrates that contain 3 to 10 monosaccharide units.

Omega-6 fatty acid: A fatty acid with its first carbon-carbon double bond starting at the sixth carbon atom from the -CH_3 end.

Omega-3 fatty acid: A fatty acid with its carbon double bond starting at the third carbon atom from the CH_3 end.

Omnivore: A person who consumes foods from both plants and animals.

Opportunistic infections: Infections primarily seen in undernourished or otherwise weakened people.

Organ: A group of tissues designed to perform a specific function (e.g., the heart) an organ contains muscle tissue, nerve tissue and so on.

Organic: Contains carbon atoms linked to hydrogen in the chemical structure.

Organism: A living thing. The human body is an organism consisting of many organs that act in a coordinated manner to support life.

Osmosis: The passage of solutions across a semi permeable membrane.

Osmotic pressure: The pressure needed to prevent particles in a solution from drawing liquid across semi permeable membrane.

Osteomalacia: The adult form of rickets, osteomalacia is a weakening of the bones as a result of poor calcium content. The condition is caused by a reduction in the activity of the vitamin D hormone.

Osteopenia: Decreased bone mass stemming from cancer, hyperthyroidism or other causes.

Osteoporosis: A bone disease that develops primarily after menopause in women and is characterized by a decrease in bone density.

Ostomy: A surgically created short circuit in intestinal flow in which the end point usually opens from the abdominal cavity rather than the anus, as with a colostomy.

Outpatient: A person treated by medical personnel outside the hospital setting; for example, in a clinic or a physician's office.

Overnutrition: A state in which nutritional intake exceeds the body's needs.

Oxidize: To lose an electron or gain an oxygen atom.

Oxidizing compound: A compound capable of capturing an electron from another compound (or supplying oxygen to another compound). The word "oxidize" literally means to lose or gain an electron.

Palatable: Pleasing to the taste.

Passive absorption: Absorption that requires permeability of the substance through the wall of the small intestine, then concentration of that substance is higher in the small intestine than in the absorptive cells.

Pasteurize: The process of heating food products to kill pathogenic microorganisms and making food products infection free.

Pathway: A metabolic progression of individual steps from starting materials to ending products.

Pectin: A group of soluble fibers containing chains of galacturonic acid and other monosaccharides; characteristically found between plant cell walls.

Peer-reviewed journal: A journal that publishes research only after two or three scientists (essentially peers) who were not part of the study agree that it was well conducted and that the results are fairly represented.

Pellagra: A disease resulting from lack of the vitamin niacin in the diet; it is characterized by inflammation of the skin, diarrhea and eventually, mental incapacity.

Pepsin: A protein-digesting enzyme produced by the stomach.

Peptides: A few amino acids bonded together (often two to four).

Percent: A part of the total.when the total consists of 100 parts.

Peristalsis: A coordinated muscular contraction that is used to propel food down the GI tract.

Pernicious anemia: The anemia that results from a lack of vitamin B_{12} reabsorption; "it is pernicious" because of the associated nerve degeneration that eventually can result in paralysis.

Pesticide: A chemical substance that destroys bacteria, fungi, insects, rodents or other pests.

pH: A measure of the hydrogen ion concentration in a solution.

Phenylketonuria (PKU): A disease in which the liver cannot readily metabolize the amino acid phenylalanine. Toxic by-products of phenylalanine build up in the body, leading to mental retardation.

Phenylpropanolamine: An over-the-counter decongestant that has a mild appetite-reducing effect.

Phosphocrestine (PCR): A high-energy compound that can be used to reform adenosine triphosphate (ATP) from adenosine diphosphate (ADP).

Photosynthesis: The process by which plants use energy from the sun to produce energy yielding compounds, such as glucose.

Physiological anemia: The normal increase in blood volume that occurs during pregnancy and dilutes the concentration of red blood cells, resulting in anemia; also called haemodilution.

Phytobezoars: A pellet of fiber characteristically found in the stomach.

Pica: The practice of eating non-food items such as dirt, laundry starch or clay.

Placebo: A fake medicine used to disguise the roles of participants in an experiment.

Placenta: An organ formed only during pregnancy that secretes hormones and make possible the transfer of oxygen and nutrients from the mother's blood to the foetus and the removal of foetal wastes.

Plaque: A cholesterol-rich substance deposited in the blood vessels, it contains various white blood cells, cholesterol and other lipids and eventually calcium.

Polar: A compounds with distinct positive and negative charges, which acts like poles on a magnet.

Polysaccharides: Carbohydrates that contain upto 3000 or more glucose units; also known as complex carbohydrates.

Polyunsaturated fatty acid: A fatty acid containing two or more carbon-carbon double bonds.

Portal vein: A large vein leading to the liver. Capillary blood vessels from the intestine drain into this vein.

Positive balance: A state in which nutrient intake exceeds losses, resulting in a net gain of the nutrient in the body (e.g., when tissue protein is gained during growth). The opposite of the state is negative balance, in which losses exceed intake, as with starvation.

Pregnancy-induced hypertension: A serious disorder, also called toxemia, that can involve high blood pressure, kidney failure, convulsion and even death of the mother and the fetus. Although the exact cause is not known, good nutrition and prenatal care can prevent or limit the severity or this disorder. Mild cases are known as preeclampsia; more severe cases are called eclampsia.

Premature: An infant born before 38 weeks of gestation.

Premenstrual syndrome (PMS): A disorder found in some women in the days surrounding menstrual periods that is characterized by depression, headache, bloating and mood swings.

Preservatives: Compounds that extend the shelf life of food by inhibiting microbial growth or by minimizing the destructive effect of oxygen and metals.

Progestins: Hormones, including progesterone, that are necessary for maintaining pregnancy and lactation.

Prognosis: A forecast of a disease's course.

Prolactin: A hormone secreted by the mother that stimulates the synthesis of milk.

Protein efficiency ratio: A measure of protein quality in a food, as determined by the protein's ability to support the growth of a young rat.

Protein energy malnutrition (PEM): A condition that results when a person regularly consumes insufficient amounts of kilocalories and protein. The deficiency eventually results in body wasting and an increased susceptibility to infections.

Proteins: Compounds made up of amino acids. Proteins contain carbon, hydrogen, oxygen, nitrogen and sometimes sulphur atoms in a specific configuration. They contain the form of nitrogen most easily used by the human body.

Prothrombin: A blood protein needed for blood clotting that required vitamin K for its synthesis.

Proton: The part of an atom that is positively charged.

Psyllium: A mostly soluble type of dietary fiber found in the seeds of the plantain plant.

Quack: A person who pretends to have certain medical skills or knowledge but in reality doesn't have R protein: A protein produced by the salivary glands that enhances absorption of vitamin B_{12}.

Radiation: Literally, that which is transmitted from a centre in all directions. Various forms of radiation energy include X-rays, ultraviolet rays from the sun and microwaves.

Rancid: Having a disagreeable odour or taste, usually as a result of the breakdown of fat.

Reactive hypoglycaemia: Low blood sugar that follows meal high in simple sugars, with corresponding symptoms of irritability, headache, nervousness, swelling and confusion.

Receptive framework: The process by which a person opens and responds to learning more about a problem; it usually involves seeking more information about the issue from books and people.

Receptor pathway for cholesterol uptake: A process by which LDL molecule is taken into the cell.

Recommended dietary allowances (RDA): Recommended nutrient intakes that meet the needs of essentially all people of similar age and gender. These amounts are established by the ICMR or Food and Nutrition Board.

Reinforcement: A reaction by others in response to a person's behaviour. Positive reinforcement entails encouragement; negative reinforcement entails critics or penalty.

Renal: Referring to the kidneys where waste products are filtered out of the blood and urine is formed.

Requirement: The amount of a nutrient required by one person to maintain health; this varies from individual to individual. We don't know individual requirements for each nutrient.

Resting metabolic rate (RMR): Essentially the same as the basal metabolic rate, but the individual need not meet the strict conditions for determining a basal metabolic rate. The term often are used interchangeably.

Retinoid: Chemical forms of performed vitamin A; one source is animal foods.

Reverse transport of cholesterol: The process by which cholesterol is picked up by HDL molecules and transferred to other lipoprotein that can dispose it.

Rhodopsin: A protein involved in vision; it is made in the eye and incorporates a protein called opsin and a form of vitamin A. It is especially important to night vision.

Rickets: A deficiency disease characterized by softening of the bones because of poor calcium content. It arises from lack of vitamin D activity in the body.

Renal: Referring to the kidneys where waste products are filtered and urine formed.

Risk factor: A characteristic or behaviour that contributes to the chances of developing an illness.

Runner's anaemia: A condition found in athletes to involve a decrease in the blood's ability to carry oxygen; this may be caused by iron loss through perspiration, destruction of red blood cells from the impact of exercise, or increased blood volume.

Saccharin: An alternate sweetener that yield no energy to the body; it is 500 times sweeter than sucrose.

Safety: The relative certainty that a substance won't cause injury.

Saliva: A watery fluid produced by the salivary glands in the mouth; it contains lubricants, enzymes and other substances.

Salt: Generally refers to a mixture of sodium and chloride in a 40:60 ratio.

Satiety: A state in which there is no long a desire to eat.

Satiety centre: A group of cells in the hypothalamus that when stimulated, causes satiety. These cells are also known as the ventromedial satiety centre.

Saturated fat: A fat containing no carbon-carbon double bond in its structure.

Saturated fatty acid: A fatty acid with no carbon-carbon double bonds.

Scavenger pathway for cholesterol uptake: A process by which LDL molecules (cholesterol containing) are taken up by scavenger cell embedded in the blood vessels.

Scurvy: The deficiency disease that results after a few weeks of consuming a diet that lacks vitamin C.

Sebum: A secretion of the sebaceous glands consisting of fats, waxes an other substances.

Secrete: To produce and then release a substance from a cell in the body.

Secretin: A hormone that causes bicarbonate release from the pancreas and slow stomach emptying.

Self-monitoring: A process of tracking foods eaten and conditions affecting eating; these are usually recorded in a diary, along with the location, time and state of mind. This is a tool to help a person understand more about his or her eating habits.

Semiessential amino acids: Amino acids that when consumed, spare the need to use an essential amino acid for their synthesis.

Senile: To old age.

Seuestreants: Compounds that bind metal ions. In so doing they reduce the ion's ability to cause rancidity in compounds containing fat.

Serotonin: A neurotransmitter synthesized from the amino acid tryptophan that appears both to decrease the desire to eat carbohydrates and to induce sleep.

Set point: A term referring to the close regulation of body weight. It is known what cells control the set point nor how it actually functions in weight regulation. There is no doubt, however, that there are mechanisms that help regulate weight.

Short chain fatty acids: Fatty acids that contain fewer than six carbon atoms.

Sickle cell disease: An anemia that results from a malformation of the red blood cell protein haemoglobin, a condition cause by an incorrect amino acid composition in the haemoglobin protein chains. The disease can lead to anemia and episodes of severe bone and joint pain, abdominal pain, headache, convulsions, paralysis and eventual death.

Slough: To shed or cast off.

Small for gestational age (SGA): Infants born after normal gestation length (38 weeks) but weighing less than 2500 grams (about 5.5. pounds).

Sodium bicarbonate: An alkaline substance made basically of sodium and carbon dioxide ($NaHCO_3$).

Soluble fibres: Fibres that either dissolve or swell when in water or are metabolized by bacteria in the large intestine. Soluble fibres include pectins, gum mucilages and some hemicellulose.

Solvent: A substance in which other substance dissolve.

Sphincter: A circular, muscular valve that controls the flow of food in the GI tract.

Standard of identity: A means by which a manufacturer can avoid disclosing ingredients on a food label. If a food is produced according to a specific recipe on file with the body specifying food standard and recipes, the table need not carry a list of its ingredient. In such cases the manufacturer is using its standard of identity.

Starch: A carbohydrate made up of several units of glucose attached in a form that the body can digest; also a part of complex carbohydrates.

Steroids: A group of hormones and related compounds that are derivatives of cholesterol.

Stimulus control: Altering the environment to minimize the stimuli for eating; for example, removing foods from sight and sorting them in kitchen cabinets.

Stroke: The loss of body function that results from a blood clot in the brain, which in turn causes the death of brain tissue.

Stress: State in which nutrient needs change as a result of physical trauma, infection, disease or starvation.

Subjects: Participants in a experiment.

Symptom: A change in health status noted by the person with the problem, such as a stomach pain.

Synapse: Spaces between nerve cells. One nerve stimulates other nearby cell, including other nerve cells, by releasing chemicals that cross the synapses. These chemicals excite neighboring cells through synapses.

Systolic blood pressure: The pressure in the bloodstream associated with the pumping of blood from the heart.

Tetany: A body condition marked by sharp contraction of muscles and failure to relax afterward; usually caused by abnormal calcium metabolism.

Theory: An explanation for a phenomenon that has numerous lines of evidence to support it.

Thermic effect of food: The increase in metabolism occurring during the digestion, absorption and metabolism of energy yielding nutrients. This effect represents 5% to 10% to kilocalories consumed. Also known as specific Dynamic Action (SDA) of food.

Tissue: A group of cells designed to perform a specific function; muscle tissue is an example.

Tocopherols: The chemical name for some forms of vitamin E.

Toxic: Poisonous, caused by a poison.

Toxicity: The capacity of a substance to produce injury at some level of intake.

Toxicology: The scientific study of harmful substances.

Trabecular bone: The spongy, inner matrix of bone, found primarily in the spine, pelvis and ends of bones.

Trace minerals: A mineral vital to health that is required in the diet in amounts less than 100 milligrams per day; usually not more than a few milligrams.

Transamination: The transfer of an amino group from an amino acid to a carbon skeleton to form a new amino acid.

Triglyceride: The major form of lipid in food. It is composed of three fatty acid bonded to the carbohydrate glycerol.

Trimester: One of the three 13-14 week periods that make up a normal pregnancy.

Trypsin: A protein digesting enzyme secreted by the pancreas to act in the small intestine.

Tumor: An abnormal growth or mass of cells in some part of the body, may be harmless or cancerous.

Ulcer: Erosion of the tissue lining in either the stomach or the upper small intestine; usually referred to as a peptic ulcer.

Undernutrition: Falling health results from a long standing dietary intake that does not meet nutritional needs.

Unsaturated fat: A fatty acid containing one or more carbon-carbon double bonds in its structure.

Urea: A nitrogen containing waste product found in urine. Most nitrogen excreted from the body leaves in this form.

Vegan: A person who consumes no animal products.

Vegetarian: A person who avoids eating animals products to a varying degree, ranging from eating no animal foods to simply not eating food from four footed animals.

Very low density lipoprotein (VLDL): The lipoprotein that initially leaves the liver it carries both type cholesterol and lipid newly synthesized by the liver.

Very low calorie diet (VLCD): Also known as protein sparing modified fast (PSMF), this diet allows the consumption of 400-700 kilocalories per day in liquid form. Of this about 30 grams or so are carbohydrate; the rest is protein.

Villi: Finger like protrusions into the small intestine that participate in digesting and absorption of food.

Visual cycle: A chemical process in the eye that contributes to vision. A form of vitamin A retinol is used in process.

Vitamins: Carbon containing compounds needed in very small amounts in the diet to help promote and regulate chemical reactions and processes in the body.

Water soluble vitamin: Vitamins that dissolve in water; these include the B vitamins and vitamin C.

Whey protein: Such as lactalbumin, found in great amounts in human milk. These are easy to digest.

Whole grains: Grains containing the entire seed of the plant, including the bran, germ and endosperm (starchy interior).

Xerophthalmia: Literally "dry eye". A cause of blindness that results from vitamin A deficiency. The specific cause is a lack of mucous production by the eye, a condition that leaves the eye more vulnerable to surface dirt and bacterial infections.

Xerostomia: Dry mouth caused by damage to the salivary glands; common after cancer treatments to the head and neck area; many lead to serious dental problems if teeth and gum are not kept moist and clean.

Yo-yo dieting: The practice of losing weight and then, only to lose it and regain and again. This practice in animals (and probably human) can make it more difficult to succeed in further attempts to lose weight.

Index